.

Treatment of Depression

Bridging the 21st Century

Contributors

David A. Brent, M.D.

David L. Dunner, M.D.

Ellen Frank, Ph.D.

David Healy, M.D.

Robert M. A. Hirschfeld, M.D.

Steven E. Hyman, M.D.

Donald F. Klein, M.D.

David J. Kupfer, M.D.

Sarah H. Lisanby, M.D.

John C. Markowitz, M.D.

Lata K. McGinn, Ph.D.

Robert Michels, M.D.

Steven O. Moldin, Ph.D.

Charles B. Nemeroff, M.D., Ph.D.

Michael J. Owens, Ph.D.

Eugene S. Paykel, M.D., F.R.C.P., F.R.C.Psych.

A. John Rush, M.D.

Harold A. Sackeim, Ph.D.

William C. Sanderson, Ph.D.

Ezra Susser, M.D., Dr.P.H.

Ming T. Tsuang, M.D., Ph.D., D.Sc.

T. Bedirhan Üstün, M.D.

Treatment of Depression

Bridging the 21st Century

EDITED BY

Myrna M. Weissman, Ph.D.

American Psychopathological Association

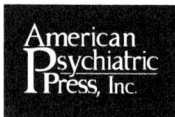

American Psychiatric Press, Inc.

Washington, DC
London, England

Copyright © 2001 American Psychiatric Press, Inc.
ALL RIGHTS RESERVED
Manufactured in the United States of America on acid-free paper

04   03   02   01   4   3   2   1
First Edition

American Psychiatric Press, Inc.
1400 K Street, N.W.
Washington, DC 20005
www.appi.org

Library of Congress Cataloging-in-Publication Data
The treatment of depression : bridging the 21st century / edited by Myrna M. Weissman.– 1st ed.
     p. ; cm.
     Papers from the 89th Annual Meeting of the American Psychopathological Association, held Mar. 1999 in New York, N.Y.
     Includes bibliographical references and index.
     ISBN 0-88048-397-0 (alk. paper)
     1. Depression, Mental–Treatment–Congresses. I. Weissman, Myrna M. II. American Psychopathological Association. Meeting (89th : 1999 : New York, N.Y.)
     [DNLM: 1. Depressive Disorder--therapy–Congresses. WM 171 T78378 2001]
RC537.T738 2001
6616.85'2706–dc21   00-055838

British Library Cataloguing in Publication Data
A CIP record is available from the British Library.

Contents

Section III **Treatment**

Contributors

David A. Brent, M.D.
Academic Chief, Child and Adolescent Psychiatry, and Professor,
    Child Psychiatry, Pediatrics, and Epidemiology, Western Psychiatric
    Institute, Pittsburgh, Pennsylvania

David L. Dunner, M.D.
Professor, Department of Psychiatry and Behavioral Sciences, and Director,
    Center for Anxiety and Depression, University of Washington, Seattle,
    Washington

Ellen Frank, Ph.D.
Professor of Psychiatry and Psychology and Director, Depression and Manic
    Depression Prevention Program, University of Pittsburgh School of
    Medicine, Western Psychiatric Institute and Clinic, Pittsburgh,
    Pennsylvania

David Healy, M.D.
Director, North Wales Department of Psychological Medicine, University of
    Wales College of Medicine, Bangor, Wales

Robert M. A. Hirschfeld, M.D.
Titus H. Harris Distinguished Professor and Chair, Department of Psychiatry
    and Behavioral Sciences, University of Texas Medical Branch, Galveston,
    Texas

Steven E. Hyman, M.D.
Director, National Institute of Mental Health, Bethesda, Maryland

Donald F. Klein, M.D.
Professor of Psychiatry, College of Physicians and Surgeons of Columbia
    University; Director of Research, New York State Psychiatric Institute,
    Department of Therapeutics, New York, New York

David J. Kupfer, M.D.
Professor and Chairman, Department of Psychiatry, and Chair, MacArthur
    Research Network in Psychopathology and Development, University of
    Pittsburgh School of Medicine, Western Psychiatric Institute and Clinic,
    Pittsburgh, Pennsylvania

Sarah H. Lisanby, M.D.
Assistant Professor of Clinical Psychiatry; Director, Transcranial Magnetic
    Stimulation Laboratory; and Co-Director, Brain-Behavior Clinic,
    Columbia College of Physicians and Surgeons, Departments of Psychiatry
    and Biological Psychiatry, New York State Psychiatric Institute, New York,
    New York

John C. Markowitz, M.D.
Associate Professor of Psychiatry, Weill Medical College of Cornell University;
    Director, Psychotherapy Clinic, The Payne Whitney Clinic, New York
    Presbyterian Hospital, New York, New York

Lata K. McGinn, Ph.D.
Associate Professor of Psychology, Ferkauf Graduate School, Yeshiva University,
    Bronx, New York

Robert Michels, M.D.
Walsh McDermott University Professor of Medicine, University Professor of
    Psychiatry, Weill Medical College of Cornell University, New York, New
    York

Steven O. Moldin, Ph.D.
Chief, Genetics Research Branch, National Institute of Mental Health,
    Bethesda, Maryland

Charles B. Nemeroff, M.D., Ph.D.
Reunette W. Harris Professor and Chairman, Department of Psychiatry and
  Behavioral Sciences, Emory University School of Medicine, Atlanta,
  Georgia

Michael J. Owens, Ph.D.
Associate Professor of Psychiatry and Behavioral Sciences, Laboratory of
  Neuropsychopharmacology, Department of Psychiatry and Behavioral
  Sciences, Emory University School of Medicine, Atlanta, Georgia

Eugene S. Paykel, M.D., F.R.C.P., F.R.C.Psych.
Professor of Psychiatry, University of Cambridge, Addenbrooke's
  Hospital, Cambridge, United Kingdom

A. John Rush, M.D.
Betty Jo Hay Distinguished Chair in Mental Health; Rosewood Corporation
  Chair in Biomedical Science; Professor, Department of Psychiatry,
  University of Texas Southwestern Medical Center, Dallas, Texas

Harold A. Sackeim, Ph.D.
Professor of Clinical Psychology in Psychiatry and Radiology and Chief,
  Department of Biological Psychiatry, College of Physicians and Surgeons
  of Columbia University, New York State Psychiatric Institute, New York,
  New York

William C. Sanderson, Ph.D.
Associate Professor of Psychology and Director, Cognitive Behavioral
  Treatment Program for Anxiety and Depression, Department of Clinical
  Psychology, Rutgers University, Piscataway, New Jersey

Ezra Susser, M.D., Dr.P.H.
Professor of Clinical Psychiatry and Clinical Public Health, Joseph L. Mailman
  School of Public Health, Columbia University, New York, New York

Ming T. Tsuang, M.D., Ph.D., D.Sc.
Stanley Cobb Professor of Psychiatry and Director, Harvard Institute of
  Psychiatric Epidemiology and Genetics; Superintendent and Head,
  Harvard Department of Psychiatry, Massachusetts Mental Health Center,
  Boston, Massachusetts

T. Bedirhan Üstün, M.D.
Group Leader, Assessment Classification and Epidemiology Group, World
   Health Organization, Geneva, Switzerland

Myrna M. Weissman, Ph.D.
Professor of Epidemiology in Psychiatry and Chief, Division of Clinical and
   Genetic Epidemiology, College of Physicians and Surgeons of Columbia
   University, New York State Psychiatric Institute, New York, New York

Preface

About the Book

This book compiles the papers from the 89th annual meeting of the American Psychopathological Association (APPA) held in March 1999 in New York city. As president of the APPA, I chose the topic and the speakers, who became the contributors to this volume.

How did I come to choose "Treatment of Depression" as the topic? My experience as an assistant at Yale University to my late husband, Gerald L. Klerman, M.D., and to Eugene Paykel, M.D., on the first study to test drugs and psychotherapy as maintenance treatment for depression led me to graduate school in epidemiology in the 1970s and a career in research. The presidency of the APPA gave me the opportunity to examine where we are now, 25 years later, in the treatment of depression and also what promises the next millennium holds.

The past 25 years have brought new understanding of major depression. The epidemiology and morbidity of depression have been mapped in many parts of the world. Many new treatments—pharmacotherapy and psychotherapy (particularly specified time-limited therapies)—have been introduced and tested for acute and maintenance treatment of depression in adults and to a lesser extent in children and adolescents. Diagnostic methods have been standardized with structured clinical interviews, and their use has improved reliability. New findings and tools in neuroscience and genetics promise to further our understanding of etiology and treatment. Efforts have been made to improve public awareness of the diagnosis and available treatments for depression and to reduce the barriers to treatment produced by stigma and ignorance. The changing health care system has also challenged efforts to bring effective treatment to appropriate patients. This volume is not meant simply to offer congratulations for past accomplishments. The 89th annual meeting of the APPA covered the current status and gaps as well as opportunities in the treatment of depression as we bridge the 21st century.

Part I, introduced by Ezra Susser, M.D., Dr.P.H., gives both an historical and a future perspective. David Healy, M.D., provides an historical and political review of the development and testing of the antidepressants, based on his controversial new book, *The Antidepressant Era*. T. Bedirhan Üstün, M.D., presents a description of the worldwide burden of depression in the 21st century based on World Health Organization and World Bank studies in both developing and developed countries. Robert Michels, M.D., discusses the problems in treating depression in the new health care scene.

Part II, introduced by Ming T. Tsuang, M.D., Ph.D., D.Sc., describes the promise of basic and clinical biologic sciences for developing new treatments. Charles B. Nemeroff, M.D., Ph.D., and Michael J. Owens, Ph.D., review the contribution of the neurosciences in developing new drugs. Steve Hyman, M.D., and Steven O. Moldin, Ph.D., review the promise of genetics. Drawing from their long-term maintenance studies, David J. Kupfer, M.D., and Ellen Frank, Ph.D., Zubin awardees at the meeting, discuss the contribution of psychobiology, particularly sleep and neuroendocrine studies, toward understanding relapse in maintenance treatment.

Part III, introduced by David L. Dunner, M.D., describes the broad range of currently available treatments. Robert M. A. Hirschfeld, M.D., reviews the current status of antidepressants in the United States, what is on the horizon, and future needs. Eugene S. Paykel, M.D., F.R.C.P., F.R.C.Psych., presents a parallel review for the United Kingdom and highlights the numerous promising drugs and psychotherapies available outside the United States. Harold A. Sackeim, Ph.D., and Sarah H. Lisanby, M.D., describe advances in the physical treatment of depression, including electroconvulsive therapy and the newer approaches of transcranial magnetic stimulation and vagus nerve stimulation. David A. Brent, M.D., describes the status of drugs and psychotherapies for the treatment of depression in children and the potential for achieving better outcomes. His topic would not have appeared 25 years ago, when the conventional and mistaken wisdom was that children did not get depressed. Donald F. Klein, M.D., describes the problems in testing new drugs and his ideas on how these problems might be alleviated with new institutional structures. A. John Rush, M.D., the Hoch awardee at the meeting, describes the progress made in practice guidelines and algorithms for the treatment of depression and how it affects managed care.

Part IV, introduced by William C. Sanderson, Ph.D., focuses on the changes that have occurred in psychotherapy as a result of the evolving health care system and the challenges that must be met if psychotherapy is to survive as a reimbursable treatment. William C. Sanderson, Ph.D., and Lata K. McGinn, Ph.D., describe the status of cognitive-behavioral therapy, a well-established and efficacious time-limited treatment for depression. Using interpersonal psychotherapy, another efficacious time-limited treatment for depression, as an example, John C. Markowitz, M.D., describes issues involved in the efficient and effective training of therapists to use these time-limited psychotherapies. Finally, I describe the paradox of both the under- and overuse of psychotherapy for depression, noting that few of the more than 200 identified psychotherapies have been tested.

About the American Psychopathological Association

Because this volume comes from the 89th annual meeting of the APPA, a word about the organization and how this topic fits in is appropriate. The APPA was founded in response to changes in psychiatry in the first decade of the 20th century. Interest was broadening from psychotic hospitalized patients to those who experienced various emotionally distressing conditions, such as headaches, paralysis without demonstrable organic cause, and neurasthenia. With the introduction of psychoanalysis, a therapeutic optimism developed.

The APPA was founded for the promotion of "the study of the scientific problems of abnormal psychology," which included the "abnormal mental processes, their relationship to the organic state of the body as well as social or cultural problems and various means of treatment." The organization was to be small, interdisciplinary, and devoted to the scientific study of psychopathology.

There is a dispute about who founded the organization, and several people have taken credit (Taylor, undated). In *The Life Work of Sigmund Freud*, Ernest Jones (1955) said it was his idea:

> The time not yet being ripe for a purely psychoanalytical society, I proposed that a wider association be formed where psychoanalytical ideas could be discussed. Since psychiatrists were at that time even less interested in psychology than neurologists, we decided to hold our meetings immediately after the annual meeting of the American Neurological Association. So on May 12, 1910, at the Willard Hotel in Washington, D.C., the APPA came into being. (p 76–77)

William James's papers, written in 1899 at Harvard, also claimed credit:

> Recent research into functional disturbances had thrown unexpected light on the constitution of our nature . . . . So far, the laborers in this field have been isolated psychologists, medical men, anthropologists, or psychical researchers. The time seems now to demand more concerted organization. To this end we propose to found an *American Psychopathological Society* for the encouragement of research into the minor mental anomalies, and for the publication of results. (James, undated letter)

Many of the members at that time were heavily involved in psychoanalysis, and the American Psychoanalytic Association was founded at the second APPA meeting. For more than a decade, the two associations were intimately intertwined. In 1919, William A. White, who had been president of the American Psychoanalytic Association, moved that it be dissolved and combined with the APPA. Adolf Meyer, who had been president of the APPA three times in its first decade, objected. Subsequently the APPA emerged as an independent interdisciplinary research organization ready to explore all valid avenues for studying psychopathology. Meetings were held in conjunction with the American Neurological Association for the first 16 years, then with the American Psychiatric Association for 4 years.

The organization was less active during the depression years of the 1930s, but gradually the younger members, Paul Hoch and Joseph Zubin (awards are made each year in their names), took leading roles in planning for the annual meeting and for many years coedited the volumes that constituted the proceedings of the meetings. The publication of such volumes, including this one, continues today.

This current volume on the treatment of depression reflects the historical tradition of the APPA; however, the current content could not have been anticipated when the organization began:

- Psychopathology is now well specified, and efforts to test validity are ongoing.
- Psychopathology is not divorced from neuropathology, at least as a scientific strategy.
- Diagnosis is clearly related to treatment.
- Treatment is multifaceted (i.e., including drugs, psychotherapies, and alternative treatments) with high marks given to evidence for efficacy from controlled clinical trials.
- Development of evidence-based treatments for depressed children and adolescents is a priority.
- Concern exists about how to bring effective treatments to patients who might benefit from them in an era of cost containment.

It is hoped that the 189th APPA president, in preparing the volume in 2099, will find this collection as charming and antiquated as the early writings seem to us now. However, lest we be too smug, it was the vision of Adolf Meyer to hold the APPA meetings in conjunction with the American Neurological Association, which he did for 16 years. In 2099, these disciplines may be seamless, but the understanding of the plasticity of human emotions in a social context will be more deeply understood.

Acknowledgment

Edited books are reflections of the editor's skill in assembling brilliant authors and his or her persistence in getting them to contribute in a timely fashion. The value of the product, however, is in the accomplishments of the contributors, not the editor. Along with my thanks to the contributors, I thank Marlene Carlson, who organized the APPA meeting and worked with all the authors from the beginning. This book was completed at the joyous birth of Rachael, who joined Katherine, Erin, Sarah, and Daniel, who will make their mark in the 21st century.

Myrna M. Weissman, Ph.D.

References

James W: Proposal for an American Psychopathological Society. James Papers. Boston, MA, Houghton Library, Harvard University, undated

Jones E: The Life and Work of Sigmund Freud. New York, Basic Books, 1955, pp 76–77

Taylor E: Who Founded the American Psychopathological Association? Boston, MA, Countway Library of Medicine, undated

Presidents of the American Psychopathological Association, 1911–2000

1911 Morton Prince	1942 Roscoe W. Hall
1912 Adolf Meyer	1943 Frederick L. Wells
1913 James T. Putnam	1944 Frederick L. Wells
1914 Alfred R. Allen	1945 Bernard Glueck
1915 Alfred R. Allen	1946 Robert P. Knight
1916 Adolf Meyer	1947 Frederick L. Wells
1917 Adolf Meyer	1948 Donald J. MacPherson
1918 Smith Ely Jelliffe	1949 Paul Hoch
1921 William A. White	1950 William B. Terhune
1922 John T. MacCurdy	1951 Lauren H. Smith
1923 L. Pierce Clark	1952 Joseph Zubin
1924 L. Pierce Clark	1953 Clarence R. Oberndorf
1925 Albert M. Barrett	1954 David McK. Rioch
1927 Sanger Brown II	1955 David McK. Rioch
1928 Ross McC. Chapman	1956 Oskar Diethelm
1929 Ross McC. Chapman	1957 Howard S. Liddell
1930 William Healy	1958 Leslie B. Hohman
1931 William Healy	1959 Harry C. Solomon
1932 J. Ramsey Hunt	1960 David Wechsler
1933 Edward J. Kempf	1961 William Horsely Gantt
1934 Edward J. Kempf	1962 Lauretta Bender
1935 Nolan D.C. Lewis	1963 D. Ewen Cameron
1936 Nolan D.C. Lewis	1964 Jerome D. Frank
1937 Nolan D.C. Lewis	1965 Franz J. Kallmann
1938 Samuel W. Hamilton	1966 Seymour S. Kety
1939 Abraham Myerson	1967 Bernard C. Glueck, Jr.
1940 Douglas A. Thorn	1968 Benjamin Pasamanick
1941 Roscoe W. Hall	1969 Joel Elkes

1970 Fritz A. Freyhan
1971 Milton Greenblatt
1972 Alfred Freedman
1973 Henry Brill
1974 Max Fink
1975 Charles Shagass
1976 Arnold J. Friedhoff
1977 George Winokur
1978 Gerald L. Klerman
1979 Jonathan O. Cole
1980 Donald F. Klein
1981 Paula J. Clayton
1982 Samuel B. Guze
1983 Robert L. Spitzer
1984 Murray Alpert
1985 James E. Barrett

1986 Robert M. Rose
1987 David L. Dunner
1988 Lee N. Robins
1989 Bernard J. Carroll
1990 Nancy C. Andreasen
1991 Katherine A. Halmi
1992 Elliot S. Gershon
1993 C. Robert Cloninger
1994 Bruce Dohrenwend
1995 Leonard Heston
1996 David Janowsky
1997 Ellen Frank
1998 Judith Rapoport
1999 Myrna M. Weissman
2000 John Helzer
2001 Nina Schooler
2002 Jack Gorman

The Past and the Future

Introduction

Ezra Susser, M.D., Dr.P.H.

The Past

The recognition and treatment of depression changed so profoundly in the second half of the 20th century that it is difficult today to appreciate how scant our knowledge was in the 1950s. As a benchmark, consider the alarm generated by the Midtown Manhattan study (Srole et al. 1962; Susser 1968). In a community prevalence survey in the heart of Manhattan in 1953, about one in five adults was rated as having a mental disorder that caused marked to severe impairment in functioning.

At the time it was first reported, this prevalence was too high to be compatible with common sense. Many researchers inferred that the ratings of disorder and impairment must have been so broad as to have little meaning. Indeed, the criticism was not groundless; there were real weaknesses in the study's assessment of mental disorder and impairment. Others attributed the high prevalence to the modern lifestyle of New York city residents. In lay commentary, the "one in five" became the butt of endless jokes.

In retrospect, however, the Midtown study results do not seem at all unreasonable. The study can now be seen as one of the first in a long line of studies that have documented the high frequency of serious mental disorder in the community. High rates of mental disorder have since been shown to pertain to both urban and rural settings and to both developed and developing countries.

The Midtown results were not diagnostically specific. Subsequent studies have shown that although mental disorder is common almost everywhere, the prevalence of specific diagnoses varies widely across regions and time. Nonetheless, depression and closely related disorders seem to be present in large numbers in virtually every setting and historical period. There is even evidence that the rates of depressive disorders are increasing over time, owing to cohort effects and the changing age structure of populations (Hagnell et al. 1982; Klerman 1976).

Two of the chapters in this section portray, from different perspectives, the dramatic shift that has taken place. In Chapter 1, David Healy describes the process by which the diagnosis and treatment of depression evolved and the array of forces that contributed to the emerging zeitgeist or paradigm. The story includes the role of pharmaceutical companies in legitimizing the notion of depression as a medical illness, which they undertook as a step toward creating markets for their products. His chapter is reminiscent of the brilliant work of Fleck (1935), the predecessor of Kuhn (1962) and the originator of the notion of scientific paradigms. Fleck was the first to capture the haphazard process by which a scientific fact tends to emerge and by which the participants later rewrite the history of that fact.

In Chapter 2, Robert Michels points to what we have learned about the treatment of depression over time. The signal societal event is that the legitimacy of common mental ailments has been widely if not universally accepted, allowing patients with these conditions to receive treatment in the same way that patients with physical ailments receive treatment. Clinicians have come to understand that depression is common, diagnosable, and treatable and that the treatment selected should be evidence based. However, they are still a long way from being able to effectively identify and treat depression in most primary care settings. In the United States, the changes now taking place in the delivery of medical care actually militate against evidence-based treatment of depression. The imperatives of managed care drive the health care system toward decreased use of medical care, both in terms of frequency and duration of care. Yet depression is a common, disabling disorder that is underrecognized and that tends to recur over the life course: Available data indicate that an *increased* frequency and duration of treatment is needed.

The Future

Looking toward the future, the one thing that seems certain is that depressive disorders will increase in prominence. As T. Bedirhan Üstün demonstrates in Chapter 3, health care planners are increasingly interested in the contribution of disorders to disability and loss of productive work time. When disorders are viewed from this perspective, the importance of depression in the community is brought into sharp relief. Because depression is recurrent and often interferes with work and other aspects of daily life, it causes considerable disability over the life course, more than most common physical illnesses.

Perhaps the most profound change we can anticipate is in the recognition and treatment of depression in the nations of the developing world, where the majority of the world's population live. The age structure and health patterns in these nations are being transformed. As perinatal and childhood mortality are brought under control, chronic diseases of midlife and late life are coming to the fore.

At present, depression is unrecognized and untreated throughout the developing countries (Collins and Susser 1999; Weissman et al. 1999). Yet as the work of Üstün and others has shown, depression is already among the primary causes of ill health and disability in these countries. Providing care and hope for the countless millions in the developing world who have this disorder will be one of the most important, and most difficult, challenges of health care in the 21st century.

References

Collins PY, Susser E (eds): Mental health services in the developing world: perspectives on evolution, assessment, and adaptation, 1. Int J Ment Health 28:1–14, 1999

Fleck L: Genesis and Development of a Scientific Fact. Chicago, University Chicago Press, 1935

Hagnell O, Lanke J, Rorsman B, et al: Are we entering an age of melanchology? Depressive illnesses in a prospective epidemiological study over 25 years: Lundby Study, Sweden. Psychol Med 12:122–129, 1982

Klerman GL: Age and clinical depression: today's south in the twenty-first century. J Gerontol 31:318–323, 1976

Kuhn TS: The Structure of Scientific Revolutions. Chicago, University Chicago Press, 1962

Srole L, Langer T, Michael S, et al: Mental Health in the Metropolis: the Midtown Manhattan Study. New York, McGraw-Hill, 1962

Susser M: Community Psychiatry Epidemiology and Social Themes. New York, Random House, 1968

Weissman M, Üstün TB, Eisenberg L, et al: Epidemiologic strategies to address world mental health problems in underserved populations. Int J Ment Health 28:15–37, 1999

CHAPTER 1

The Antidepressant Drama

David Healy, M.D.

The First Act

Imipramine

The orthodox history of the antidepressants begins with the following entry by Roland Kuhn in the clinical notes of Paula JF:

> On 12th January 1956, the treatment is begun with 100 mgs of Tofranil. On 14th January there was an acute symptom of delusion. On 21st January 1956: for three days the patient is a totally changed person. So since the 18th of January, six days from the beginning of treatment, all her manic behavior and restlessness has disappeared. The day before yesterday, she remarked herself that she'd been terribly confused and as stupid as she had ever been before and she didn't know where it had come from but she was only glad that she was better now. (Kuhn 1996, pp. 436)

Several weeks after recording the above impressions, Roland Kuhn wrote to Geigy Pharmaceuticals suggesting that imipramine was an antidepressant.

The conventional story of the antidepressants is that their discovery was second only to the discovery of chlorpromazine as a major breakthrough in the management of mental illness. Furthermore, the use of these two groups of drugs dramatically changed the face of psychiatry.

These impressions are misleading, however. Far from being interested in the possibility that imipramine might be an antidepressant, Geigy, which had been looking for an antipsychotic, was slow to seize the opportunity that an antidepressant offered. At a time when compounds could pass through a clinical testing phase into clinical use within 3 months, imipramine did not reach the market until almost 2 years after Kuhn's first report, and even then it was marketed with what in retrospect looks like reluctance (Healy 1997).

Behind this reluctance is a set of perspectives on the antidepressant story. Imipramine was one of a series of iminodibenzyl compounds that were developed in the late 1940s as possible antihistamines. The first of these compounds, G22150, had been tested in various clinical populations and did not appear to be of particular use. Following the success of chlorpromazine, Geigy revisited G22150 to look at possible psychotropic actions but found nothing clinically useful. The company then examined G22355, also known as imipramine, which was an iminodibenzyl with the same side chain as chlorpromazine. In a study of the drug in a large group of schizophrenic patients at Munsterlingen Hospital in 1955, a number of patients appeared to become more disorganized. Their clinical state worsened, and the company withdrew from the study. Analyzing the protocols from the study, however, Paul Schmidlin noted a mood-elevating effect in some patients (Battegay 2000). Schmidlin's analysis was made essentially on the basis of reported nursing observations. Schmidlin's assessment led representatives of Geigy to ask Kuhn to study the drug in depressed patients. He was initially reluctant but subsequently agreed. The clinical notes at the beginning of this chapter relate to the case of Paula JF, the first patient to receive imipramine as an antidepressant.

With this background in mind, it is difficult to sustain an absolute claim for Kuhn as the discoverer of imipramine's antidepressant effects. However, he has been reluctant to acknowledge the role of any others in the discovery. His basis for claiming priority lies essentially in the contention that what he discovered was not the antidepressant effects of imipramine so much as the contours of a depressive syndrome that would respond to an agent like imipramine. Kuhn argued that the clinical effects of imipramine validated the existence of a form of depression called *vital depression* (endogenous depression), which was to be distinguished from reactive or neurotic depressions. This distinction was at the heart of the views of the Heidelberg school of psychopathology. Because neither Geigy personnel nor the nursing staff had a background in psychopathology, none could have been expected, from Kuhn's point of view, to have appreciated what was being discovered.

Geigy executives were far from persuaded by the reports emerging from Munsterlingen, even reports as dramatic as the case of Paula JF. They had some difficulty understanding the significance of the concept of vital depression. They knew that a treatment—electroconvulsive therapy (ECT)—was available for this condition, and even Kuhn conceded that ECT was probably more effective than G22355 was likely to be. They were also faced with strong indicators that vital depression was not a common disorder. Estimates at the time can have been no greater than 100 cases per 1 million people. These estimates contrast markedly with the current estimates of 100,000 cases per million.

Geigy also was faced with the fact that majority opinion in Europe held that the idea of an antidepressant was almost inconceivable. Depressive disorders were considered reactive in nature or related to some form of object loss, in which case a biologic treatment could not be expected to remedy the problem. In addition, other highly regarded European clinicians, including Hanns Hippius, had given patients imipramine in doses up to 1,500 mg/day, and none reported any effects comparable with those claimed by Kuhn.

It took an accident to further the cause of imipramine. Robert Boehringer, a shareholder in Geigy, became aware of the existence of imipramine and the claims for it. He asked for a supply of the drug to give to a relative who had become severely depressed. His relative responded to the drug. Boehringer then advocated the drug's further development. At the same time, Robert Domenjoz, Geigy's chief pharmacologist, was persuaded of the merits of imipramine and persuaded Paul Kielholz and Roger Coirault to study it. Pierre Deniker had been approached but was reluctant to test the compound because of the risk of suicide associated with inadequate antidepressant treatments. Coirault and Kielholz both reported in 1957 that imipramine had antidepressant effects. Their reports, along with the emergence in 1957 of iproniazid (Marsilid) as an antidepressant, finally led Geigy to market the drug in late 1957 in Switzerland and in 1958 in the rest of the world

(Coirault et al. 1958; Kielholz and Battegay 1958). The imipramine story seems remarkable now, given the acknowledgment of the widespread nature of depressive disorders and the need for their treatment, along with an acceptance of the place of pharmacotherapeutic approaches in the management of these conditions. However, this story was the norm for the time rather than something surprising.

Isoniazid

In 1951 a series of hydrazide derivatives was introduced for the treatment of tuberculosis by the Roche, Squibb, and Eli Lilly pharmaceutical companies. The best known of these derivatives were isoniazid and iproniazid. The impact of these two drugs was remarkable. Terminally ill patients unresponsive to streptomycin were "saved." The most dramatic stories came from New York's Sea View Hospital, from which Irving Selikoff and Edward Robitzek provided the first reports (Robitzek et al. 1952). These electrifying reports captured the attention of the media, and *Life* magazine ran a feature article ("TB Milestone: Two New Drugs Give Real Hope of Defeating the Dread Disease," 1952) that showed previously moribund patients dancing in the wards. These articles caught the attention of many psychiatrists. Psychiatrists throughout the United States were tempted to prescribe these compounds for mental health purposes, given the effects of these drugs to boost appetite, cause weight gain, increase vitality, and improve sleep (J.A. Smith 1953). The conventional wisdom is that no indications emerged from any of these efforts.

Stimulated by the reports of improved sleep and appetite by Robitzek et al. (1952) and probably the feature in *Life*, Max Lurie and Harry Salzer made the first discovery in the antidepressant field in 1952. Following the suggestions that isoniazid appeared to treat tuberculosis and enhance the sense of well-being of the patients receiving the drug, Lurie, like Jackson Smith, thought isoniazid might be a useful agent to help depressed patients (Lurie 1998). Lurie and Salzer began giving it to outpatient and hospitalized depressed patients. They reported a first series of 41 patients in 1953 and a second series of 45 patients in 1955. Of these 86 subjects, 42 had had a previous depressive episode, 32 had had prior treatment with ECT, and 22 had bipolar depression (Salzer and Lurie 1953, 1955). Two of every three patients responded to iso-niazid, and those who responded did so in 2–3 weeks.

Lurie was probably the person who coined the term *antidepressant* in 1952 (Lurie 1998). Kuhn did not describe imipramine as an antide-pressant in the first instance. Under the influence of Jean Delay, re-searchers began to call the first tricyclic antidepressants (TCAs) *thymoanaleptics* or *thymoleptics*. Nathan Kline later discovered the monoamine oxidase inhibitor (MAOI) iproniazid, but he called it a *psy-chic energizer* rather than an antidepressant. The word *antidepressant* cannot be found in *Webster's Third International Dictionary of the En-glish Language* (1966). The *Random House II International Dictionary* (1987) suggests that the term first appeared in the mid-1960s.

Lurie and Salzer's work sank without a trace for several reasons. First, isoniazid, although produced by Roche in 1951 from a parent hy-drazide molecule, had originally been synthesized in 1912. Therefore, it could not be patented. Eli Lilly, Squibb, and Roche all had versions of it. Second, by the time Lurie and Salzer completed their second study, chlorpromazine (Thorazine/Largactil) had hit the market and it appeared as though it would be used as an antipsychotic in large doses and as an anxiolytic or antidepressant in moderate doses. Indeed, sub-sequent trials have shown that chlorpromazine can be used in the treat-ment of depressive disorders (Klein and Fink 1962). Equivalent results are available for many of the other antipsychotics (Robertson and Trim-ble 1982). Against this backdrop, the notion of a specific antidepressant did not register, even though Lurie was providing treatment to outpa-tients, a potentially much larger market than Kuhn saw.

Third, Lurie and Salzer lacked institutional support. They were es-sentially in private practice; therefore, no university supported their work. They were working in Cincinnati, a bedrock of psychoanalytic thinking and practice in the mid-1950s. Being in private practice, they could not take time off to publicize their own work. Finally, they clearly made a mistake publishing the second of their studies in the *Ohio State Medical Journal* (Salzer and Lurie 1955). Even so, their work with iso-niazid was replicated elsewhere. Delay and Buisson in Paris found es-sentially the same outcomes (Delay et al. 1952). Furthermore, other non–MAOI hydrazide tuberculostats, such as cynarizide, were also test-ed in the early 1950s and appeared to have antidepressant properties.

Reserpine

A similar fate befell reserpine, the next antidepressant to be identified. Against a backdrop of reports that this drug made people feel better, then well, and that it was good psychotherapy in pill form, Michael Shepherd and David Davies at the Institute of Psychiatry conducted the first prospective, placebo-controlled, parallel-group randomized control trial in psychiatry using reserpine in outpatients with anxious depression (Davies and Shepherd 1955). They demonstrated clearly that the drug had antidepressant efficacy. This result is of little surprise in one sense because reserpine is a neuroleptic. A large number of traditional neuroleptics, including sulpiride, perphenazine, pimozide, thioridazine, chlorpromazine, and flupenthixol, had been shown to be potentially useful in treating depression, particularly in patients with symptoms of comorbid anxiety (Robertson and Trimble 1982). More recently discovered antipsychotics also appear to be efficacious in treating affective disorders.

The evidence of reserpine's antidepressant efficacy vanished for several reasons. First, as of 1955 the concept of an antidepressant was still lacking. Reserpine was seen as a major tranquilizer. Ciba Pharmaceuticals was not interested in marketing it as an antidepressant. The treatment of psychoses at the time was in the process of becoming respectable medicine, but the treatment of the less severe or minor nervous conditions remained much more contentious. Second, by the late 1950s, 26 different versions of reserpine were on the market; hence, no one company had an incentive to promote it for indications such as mood disorders or to defend the drug when it ran into difficulties.

Third, reserpine ran into some difficulties. The drug was associated with suicide in a number of patients receiving treatment for hypertension. Suicide was liable to occur acutely—within days after the patient began receiving the drug. Physicians reported that the drug appeared to trigger a depressive or psychotic disorder in some patients (Healy and Savage 1998). However, similar reports were being filed for chlorpromazine and other antipsychotics. Psychiatrists who reviewed the problem concluded that reserpine was not doing anything that other antipsychotics were not also doing (Healy and Savage 1998).

A contemporary review of these problems suggests that reserpine was causing akathisia. Symptoms of what would later be termed akathisia were noted as far back as 1955 to be more common in patients receiving reserpine than in those receiving chlorpromazine (Healy and Savage 1998). The term *akathisia*, however, had not entered the psychiatric vocabulary at that time, and general physicians faced with the phenomenon were unlikely to recognize what was happening. The sedative effects of reserpine in animals subsequently became a screening test for new antidepressants. Many of the original TCAs and MAOIs either blocked or reversed reserpine's effects, but the selective serotonin reuptake inhibitors (SSRIs) do not pass the reserpine test; thus, they are antidepressants—but antidepressants that cause akathisia. In addition to these clinical implications, reserpine has startling implications for hypotheses such as the monoamine hypothesis of affective disorders.

Iproniazid

Although Kline's discovery of the antidepressant effects of iproniazid was a more successful development than the discoveries outlined earlier in this chapter, Kline met with the same reluctance that Shepherd, Lurie, and Kuhn had met earlier. In late 1956, Jack Saunders, who had formerly worked for Ciba but who had joined Kline in the research department at Rockland State Hospital in New York, and Harry Loomer, who was a practicing psychiatrist at the hospital, embarked on a study of the psychotropic effects of iproniazid. The patient group included 17 largely retarded and regressed schizophrenic patients along with 7 depressed patients seen in Kline's private practice (Loomer et al. 1957). By early 1957, Kline thought that the drug was promising and approached David Barney, managing director of Roche in the United States, to alert him that iproniazid had promising psychotropic effects. Barney was not interested, however; iproniazid had become a problem for Roche at the time because its use in the treatment of tuberculosis was associated with several adverse mental effects, leading the company to consider removing it from the market.

Despite this early resistance, Kline was in a different position than Lurie, Shepherd, or Kuhn had been. Iproniazid was on the market and selling well. Kline also had access to the professional audiences necessary to disseminate information about the new discovery, and as the discoverer of the psychotropic effects of reserpine and a Lasker Prize winner, he had a track record. On the basis of iproniazid's effects in the 24 patients in the study group, Kline reported to an April 1957 research symposium at an American Psychiatric Association regional meeting in Syracuse, New York, that the drug had psychic energizing properties. He briefed *The New York Times* about the discovery the weekend before the meeting ("Science Notes: Mental Drug Shows Promise" 1957). Within months iproniazid was being widely used for its antinervousness properties (Healy 1997).

In due course, Kline was awarded a second Lasker Prize for this discovery. As part of the award, he was invited in 1964 to write an article on iproniazid and its discovery for the *Journal of the American Medical Association* (Kline 1965). Saunders took exception to Kline's portrayal of the discovery and sued. The issue at stake was who had discovered iproniazid's antidepressant effects. Kline argued that he had discovered the effects when he gave the drug to his depressed outpatients, whereas most of the patients given iproniazid by Loomer and Saunders had been schizophrenic. Saunders's claim was that he had understood that the drug was an MAOI and that on this basis he had expected it to have useful psychotropic effects. Several hearings and contested settlements resulted, and the case was settled only after Kline's death in 1981.

Lurie's work arguably trumped both sets of claims, however, in that isoniazid had antidepressant effects but was not an MAOI. In addition, Lurie's demonstration was more convincing than Kline's, and Kline probably knew about Lurie's work through a number of New York psychiatrists who had given isoniazid to their patients and also found it to have antidepressant effects.

The Second Act

The climate surrounding the antidepressants began to change in 1960 when a number of companies produced amitriptyline. Because process rather than substance patents were the norm of the time, Merck, Lundbeck, Roche, and a Czech group all produced this compound at much the same time. Merck tested the drug for antischizophrenic properties. One of the company's clinical investigators, Frank Ayd, had been present when Kuhn described the antidepressant effects of imipramine in 1957 and had been on the lookout for possible antidepressants because he had a family history of affective disorders. To Ayd, amitriptyline seemed to be producing effects comparable with those of imipramine, and he suggested to Merck that the company investigate its possible antidepressant effects (Ayd 1996). Unlike Roche, Geigy, and other companies, Merck decided to develop amitriptyline as an antidepressant. In addition, Merck bought 50,000 copies of Ayd's 1961 book, *Recognizing the Depressed Patient*, and distributed it along with videos of Ayd interviewing patients. The company recognized that physicians would need to be educated about the existence and management of depressive disorders.

Despite these events, the antidepressants remained the poor cousins in the psychotropic field, and their use remained minimal during the 1960s. Physicians were more likely to interpret community nervousness as anxiety based and were more likely to prescribe a minor tranquilizer than an antidepressant. Only after benzodiazepine dependence was recognized were antidepressants brought out of the shadows.

The emergence of the antidepressants as they are now understood parallels the development of the SSRIs. SSRIs originated in Kielholz's observation in the mid-1960s that some antidepressants appeared to enhance the drive of depressed patients whereas others did something else, which at the time Kielholz expressed as a possible mood enhancement. Reviewing Kielholz's proposals regarding drive and mood enhancement, Arvid Carlsson suggested that the agents that were more drive enhancing were active on the catecholamine system, whereas those that were more mood enhancing had preferential actions on the serotonin system (Kielholz 1971). Carlsson's suggestion led to the proposal that creating a selective serotonin reuptake inhibitor might be worthwhile. Carlsson developed and patented the first SSRI, zimelidine, in 1971 with Hans Corrodi (Carlsson 1996; Carlsson and Wong 1997). The first SSRI to hit the market was indalpine, which was released clinically in France in 1978. Zimelidine and indalpine had to be withdrawn from the market later because of toxicity problems. This left the door open for the subsequent generation of SSRIs, including fluvoxamine, fluoxetine (Prozac), paroxetine, sertraline, citalopram, and others.

Although the SSRIs originated through the observation that not all antidepressants were the same, their marketing has tended to blur these distinctions and to suggest that the SSRIs are essentially the same as the older TCAs except for a relative freedom from side effects and safety in overdose. Evidence does not support this suggestion. SSRIs have benefits in treating a wide range of nervous conditions including posttraumatic stress disorder, social phobia, obsessive-compulsive disorder (OCD), panic disorder, generalized anxiety disorder, body dysmorphic disorder, and mood disorders. They also have significant benefits in treating premature ejaculation. The effects of SSRIs on mood disorders are mixed; patients with melancholic depression and those hospitalized for depression do not respond well to at least some of the SSRIs. Accordingly, the clinical trials submissions to the U.S. Food and Drug Administration for some of these agents did not include any trials of hospitalized depressed patients. This observation is not to suggest that SSRIs are weaker than the TCAs. They clearly are not. Drugs that produce effects in OCD, body dysmorphic disorder, and other similarly severe conditions cannot be described as weak. They are, however, different from the TCAs. Their range of actions begs the question of whether these drugs are not broadly antinervousness agents rather than specifically antidepressants (Healy 1999).

The designation of SSRIs as antidepressants owed a great deal to the problems of benzodiazepine dependence (Healy 1991, 1999). When this dependence was discovered, the word *anxiolytic* became compromised, and clinicians were inclined to suspect that any anxiolytic agent would inevitably cause dependence problems. The door was open for the development of the antidepressant market from the mid-1980s onward. An interesting observation is that benzodiazepine dependence was never as significant a problem in Japan as it was elsewhere. In that country the anxiolytic market remains robust, and as of 1999 no SSRIs had been released for a mood disorder indication. In the West, the management of community nervousness created an antidepressant marketplace, and Peter D. Kramer's 1993 book *Listening to Prozac* marked the community's discovery of the antidepressants, which at that point had already been available for almost 40 years.

The New Industrial State

The thalidomide tragedy in 1962 led to a set of amendments to the 1938 Food, Drugs and Cosmetics Act. The amendments intended, among other things, to constrain drug development to a disease model whereby patients received a tangible benefit that countered the risks of the drug taken. At least initially, the amendments had the outcomes intended. As time goes by, however, it becomes clear that the medicopharmaceutical complex has found ways around the restrictions imposed on the marketing of pharmacologic agents.

Although psychopharmacologic practice has remained something of a cottage industry since the discovery of imipramine in the sense that the quality of outcomes produced clinically has had only limited predictability, neither drug nor market development has remained so primitive. In the intervening period, the pharmaceutical industry has developed a capacity to make markets: If drug availability was to be restricted to diseases, it was perhaps predictable that a mass creation of diseases would result. When the antidepressants were introduced, the general perception was that affective disorders were relatively rare. In the West, until just after World War II, registered rates of affective disorder were on the order of 50–100 per 1 million people. According to current estimates, between 50,000 and 100,000 per million are affected. In order to sell its compounds, the pharmaceutical industry has educated prescribers and the public at large to recognize depression as a widespread disorder affecting more than 350 million people worldwide that leads to considerable disability and economic disadvantage as well as suicide (Murray and Lopez 1996). Thus, depression is accepted as being treatable with antidepressant drugs, even though only minimal evidence indicates that these drugs are helpful for even a significant proportion of these disorders and despite concerns that, in some cases, antidepressants may increase rather than reduce suicide rates (Healy et al. 1999).

Current widespread acceptance of such ideas in the West, however, conceals some extraordinary worldwide variations. For instance, a significant disjunction exists between the East and the West in the antidepressant field. In the West, the 1980s crisis over physical dependence on benzodiazepines led to the eclipse of the minor tranquilizers and, indeed, of the whole notion of anxiolysis. Thus, the antidepressant era was born. Something of a palpable moral relief was felt in some quarters when the benzodiazepines were found to produce dependence. Valium, it seemed to many, had been pitched too clearly at problems of living (M.C. Smith 1991). The Japanese market, as mentioned earlier, provides a striking contrast to what has happened in the West. World-wide, the pattern of psychotropic drug use appears to follow the Japanese model rather than the Western one: benzodiazepines are often prescribed for affective disorders and antidepressants for anxiety states (Üstün and Sartorius 1995). Western practices, for the most part, cannot be assumed to be correct. A more parsimonious interpretation is that such practices are the result of pharmaceutical company market development strategies (Healy 1991).

Similar market developments have occurred in the treatment of OCD, panic disorder, and social phobia, conditions also responsive to antidepressants. OCD was infrequently recognized before 1970 but now is thought to affect 2%–3% of the population. Neither panic disorder nor social phobia were recognized at all before the mid-1960s. Now the conditions are widely recognized even by the public at large. This recognition has followed demonstrations that some of the original antidepressant agents can produce benefits in these conditions. Initially the antidepressants were presumed to help in these conditions by correcting an underlying depressive disturbance. Their benefits are now generally accepted to arise independently of any effects on mood. This widespread selling of nervous diseases, as opposed to nervousness, has made the publication of successive editions of the *Diagnostic and Statistical Manual of Mental Disorders* (DSM) into a cultural event. Not only is reimbursement tied to the treatment of diseases rather than the alleviation of distress, but the problems of living are increasingly expressed in these terms. The psychobabble of yesteryear is being rapidly replaced by a new biobabble.

The critical issue is how the nervousness found in community settings, generally estimated at 15%, is best perceived. Some view it as psychologically based, either the result of poor impulse control, in the case of psychoanalytic theory, or the result of widespread physical, emotional, or sexual abuse. According to sociopolitical views, misery and nervousness are the inevitable results of social or political oppression. Finally, there are biologic views. I have written this chapter based on the premise that although the biologic inputs have a certain primacy, they do not have to be constrained by disease. An alternative is a temperamental or dimensional view of nervous problems, according to which it would be reasonable to expect up to 15% of individuals to be disposed to general or specific nervous disorders by virtue of their genetic inheritance or early epigenetic developments in their biologic functioning. The question is whether neuroscientific and regulatory frameworks to date have favored categorical disease-based models for reasons of convenience rather than accuracy. If the answer to this question is that convenience factors have been important, how long would it take to dismantle current models? In contrast to other areas of business, do pharmaceutical corporations follow what the markets dictate, or like other corporations can they shape the marketplace into which they sell their products?

The Third Act

Background:
Engines of War and Luxury Commodities

The introduction of the antidepressants and the obstacles encountered in their early use stand in marked contrast to the introduction of the antipsychotics, which was a serendipitous breakthrough in the management of severe mental disorders. Within a few years, the use of antipsychotic agents, like that of antibiotics before them, had crossed frontiers and continents regardless of ideologic divides, vividly demonstrating how effective techniques propagate themselves in a way that acclaimed ideas, even in this information age, do not.

The antidepressants, in contrast to the antipsychotics, made it possible to make a difference to a large number of people who might have to be persuaded that they needed this difference in their lives. As early as 1958, Kuhn had noted that some patients with sexual perversion responded to imipramine and that many patients, when they recovered, felt "better than well" while receiving this agent. This observation led Kuhn to state that an agent such as imipramine potentially created significant philosophical and ethical issues (Kuhn 1958). This language is now strongly suggestive of agendas opened up in the mid-1990s by the book *Listening to Prozac* (Kramer 1993), best caught in the term *cosmetic psychopharmacology*, which Kramer introduced. Whereas Kramer's book became a runaway bestseller that seemed in some way to capture the mood of the moment or to articulate possibilities that many thought might be within grasp, Kuhn's speculations had minimal impact. Where philosophers and others had been excited by the advent of LSD and other psychotomimetic compounds, no one was interested in imipramine in 1958.

The argument in this third act is that this developmental course was inevitable and that analyzing the forces that have shaped developments thus far allows a measure of prediction about the future of psychopharmacology and possibly also about psychiatry. For the purposes of this analysis, I divide the field into two areas: The first area is the therapy of severe mental disorders, such as schizophrenia and the dementias, for which the needs are so pressing that any development will be pressed rapidly into use. With these "engines of war," developments are more likely to follow an uncontroversial course because there is a pressing need for effective agents.

The second area involves the "luxury goods"—that is, the other possibilities in psychopharmacology that the antidepressant story creates. Unlike the antipsychotics, which were immediately effective, and the minor tranquilizers, which were immediately appreciated (both because of their sedative effects and because of their pleasurable qualities), the antidepressants represented a technique that had no clear niche. The developmental trajectory of engines of war is determined largely by factors internal to the field. In contrast, the trajectory of luxury goods can be affected critically by external events and factors.

External Factors:
Technical Developments and Accidents

Although in this chapter I focus mainly on the forces that propel development, a series of historical accidents have intervened to channel the developments. The critical external event was the thalidomide disaster, which led in 1962 to the amendments to the Food, Drugs and Cosmetics Act mentioned earlier. To offset the risks of then-available therapies, the thrust of these amendments was to channel drug development and drug availability toward disease indications for which the risks of treatment might be offset by prospective benefits. Pharmaceutical companies were encouraged to develop drugs for disease indications. Drug availability was restricted to prescription-only status and placed in the hands of a set of individuals, who by training would be inclined to make them available for diseases rather than problems. The amendments also endorsed randomized clinical trials (RCTs), an expensive assessment technology that did a great deal to standardize the field through the use of rating scales and operational criteria in a way that the alternative, large, simple trials would not have done. RCTs, however, also forced corporate development by dramatically pushing up development costs.

The premium put on categorical models of disease rather than dimensional models radically changed the face of psychiatry. The exemplar of a categorical disease state was the bacterial infection. In contrast, within psychiatry, dimensional models of pathology were emphasized heavily until the psychopharmacologic era. The Freudian school of thought was dimensional in the extreme. The emerging behaviorism focused on disabilities rather than on disease categories. Dimensional thinking held sway within biology as well, and psychiatric textbooks contained photographs exemplifying different constitutional types—the mesomorphs, endomorphs, and ectomorphs of the American literature or the schizothymes and cyclothymes of the European literature. Hans Eysenck had introduced a personality framework that incorporated notions of inhibition and arousal into introversion–extraversion and neuroticism–stability dimensions onto which the initial sedatives and stimulants appeared to map quite readily. Given their rather minimal treatment effect sizes on the various categories of depressive disorders and their equal effect sizes on a range of other nervous disorders, it is far from clear that the antidepressants would not be better conceived as acting on a dimensional factor.

When psychotropic drugs came on the scene, a number of development routes were possible. The die may have been cast by virtue of the fact that the antipsychotics emerged first and almost immediately became associated with disease management. Had the antidepressants emerged first, they might have been developed as tonics. The era before the 1962 amendments was one in which tonics flourished along with treatments for halitosis and a range of other problems of living. Cyproheptadine, a tricyclic agent that has since been shown to have antidepressant efficacy and to improve sleep and appetite, was promoted first as an appetite stimulant and used widely as a tonic. The idea of a tonic, a usage hallowed by centuries of practice, might have had much greater acceptability among the public at large than the notion of an antidepressant. The antidepressant neologism quickly became associated in the public mind with risks of addiction and other problems, and it has some moral rather than exclusively medical connotations.

Technical Developments

Although antidepressants are not engines of war like penicillin, their development echoes the penicillin story in one important sense. Penicillin was discovered in 1928, but its discovery was of no practical or therapeutic consequence until a cooperative effort between the U.S. government and the pharmaceutical industry during World War II, which involved solving a number of difficult technical problems related to the yield of the agent, brought the discovery online. As this story indicates, creating a technology involves more than the creation of a single technique.

Neuroimaging

In the case of antidepressant psychopharmacology, a number of elements can be specified that the broader technologic base will have to include. Among these elements are neuroimaging and genetic capabilities. Current neuroimaging capabilities have, from the point of view of psychiatry, been rudimentary and do not contribute in any significant way to clinical practice other than in restricted areas of neuropsychiatry. Even so, the early computed tomography (CT) scan reports, which began to appear in the early 1970s, generated considerable anticipatory excitement. This excitement owed little to the results obtained, which have not been replicable or of consequence. Retrospectively, it is difficult to see how anyone could have expected to see more structural features in the brain by crude imaging methods than by close inspection of the brain at postmortem. These techniques, however, signaled a possibility for future convergent developments that have almost certainly underpinned the enthusiasm for these approaches.

Since the 1970s, technical developments driven by factors outside the field of psychiatry have rapidly transformed capabilities. Positron emission tomography (PET) and nuclear magnetic resonance (NMR) machines have hitherto been able to offer only millimeter resolutions that take at least 12 seconds of processing time to achieve. Even so, a series of recent studies has demonstrated variations in receptor densities in healthy volunteer populations and correlations between these variations and personality features (Breier et al. 1998; Farde et al. 1997). The next generation of synchrotron machines will be able to achieve micromolar volumetric resolutions within a second, bringing within reach the realm of in vivo histology and, more important, functional imaging. Issues central to the nature of psychosyndromes will become open to reconceptualization based on clear answers to the questions of whether brain processing is distributed and dynamic (dimensional) or whether it operates on the basis of an if–then motor logic that is subject to discrete lesions (categorical).

Genetics and Pharmacogenetics

Another critical external factor for psychopharmacology hinges on possibilities of enhanced genetic capabilities. This factor is important for a variety of reasons. For example, more precise pharmacogenetic responses to various psychotropic agents need to be established. The incentive to develop specific pharmacogenetic capabilities comes from mainstream medical practice. Once the technology to profile people pharmacogenetically becomes possible, product liability issues will lead to the rapid development of these techniques. These pharmacogenetic developments are likely to become available in the early years of this decade and are liable to have a huge impact in psychiatry quite apart from any effect on litigation issues. Companies have been able to target the whole depression or schizophrenia markets, but in the future they will be able to count on usage only by depressed individuals who have particular pharmacogenetic profiles because of the risk of adverse effects. Treatments will have to become more tailored and individualized than they have been in the past. The problem for companies is that this change may lead to a fracturing of the depressive and schizophrenic monoliths. The benefits for companies are that drug development costs should be reduced and the development process speeded up. The ability to predict which patients are liable to experience adverse reactions will enable drugs to remain on the market that otherwise would have had to be removed. Genetic variants will also yield indicators as to which patients are most likely to respond to a particular drug.

Genetic markers for temperament types are likely to lead to the conclusion that particular antidepressant classes are especially effective along certain personality dimensions rather than for the entire category of depression. Even with the use of older, nonselective agents, up to 50% of the variance in responsiveness to antidepressants stems from constitutional factors (Joyce et al. 1994). The emergence of more selective agents in recent years is likely to lead to a reconsideration of the constitutional backgrounds in which depressive (or nervous) disorders occur, enabling reconceptualization of therapeutic effects. One possibility, for instance, is that selective antidepressants may modulate temperamental inputs to psychosyndromes rather than correct any lesion underpinning these syndromes.

As with the development of neuroimaging, developments relevant to the interface between psychopharmacology and genetics are underpinned by technical developments that are happening outside the field of mental illness. In this case, the underpinning comes from the Human Genome Project, one of the largest developments in a technical infrastructure ever undertaken in terms of investments of either scientific or financial capital, both public and private.

Genomics and Combinatorial Chemistry

Developments in the field of genomics and combinatorial chemistry make it possible to systematically produce compounds that will target the biologic bases of a range of psychologic functions far more selectively than has been possible in the past. The developing capacities are well illustrated by recent findings related to D4 receptor activity in patients with schizophrenia. Following a suggestion of increased D4 receptor density in patients with schizophrenia, Merck, Sharp, and Dohme was able to synthesize a D4 receptor antagonist and complete a clinical trial of this agent in patients with schizophrenia within 2 years (Iversen 1998). The new methods of drug synthesis allow scientific leads to be transformed into market advantages within months.

Quality Standards and the Disease Model

The conjunction of neuroimaging, novel drug development possibilities, and genetic techniques is likely to crystallize new developments in the near future. From this perspective, it seems clear that Kuhn's discovery, in contrast to the development of fluoxetine, could not have gone anywhere: The fact that no one knew how the agent worked made little practical difference to therapeutics, but it cut off significant avenues for development. Part of the promise of fluoxetine, at least the public perception of it as shaped by *Listening to Prozac*, was that this drug had been developed by a process of rational engineering. The notion of rational engineering implies that the effects being produced could be produced as a matter of routine. The implication is that developments have passed a certain quality threshold, whereby *quality* refers to aspects of the reproducibility of the process.

As with psychotherapy, psychopharmacologic practice (as opposed to psychopharmaceutical development) has previously had somewhat of a cottage industry quality to it. It has not been possible to guarantee the quality of the outcomes. In a sense, this uncertainty has not mattered in the therapeutics of severe disorders, in which the patient is in danger and thus doing *something*, even if risky, has been by general consensus preferable to doing nothing. When managing less severe mental (or other) conditions, however, companies and clinicians have run into considerable opposition, in part because of the lack of consistency in outcomes. A disease model offers companies and clinicians an escape from the quality standards that apply to other industries. In a famine, no one sues a food provider if the quality of the goods falls short of accepted standards.

A disease model has also functioned as a means of managing equity in the access to health resources. Since World War II there have been popular difficulties with the notion of inequities in the access to health care resources than, for instance, with access to high-fidelity stereos or computers. Disease models have functioned as a means of managing equity in access to health care. Increasingly, however, as a growing number of agents are developed that potentially modulate lifestyles rather than cure diseases, the public purse will be under strain to maintain open access. Another libertarian element emerges with a disease portrayal, in that the individual experiences something of a moral onus to seek treatment for any diseases that he or she has. This onus does not exist to quite the same extent for the treatment of a risk factor or when it comes to making use of an enhancement technology.

Finally, the dilemmas framed by Kramer (1993) involving the use of fluoxetine for cosmetic psychopharmacology help crystallize other difficulties that stem from the current disease framework. A number of these dilemmas result from fluoxetine's prescription-only status rather than from its effectiveness. As these issues have played in the media, they have been moral problems for physicians who are called on to decide whether it would be a good thing for society to reduce the extent of melancholic temperaments in the community, with the possible loss of spirituality or creativity that might result. These dilemmas are transformed to a great extent if the power to make these decisions is returned to the consumer. Imagine car salespeople being left to decide whether to make a particular brand of car with a new feature available to the public.

Given the preceding analysis, it should be clear why the antidepressant story could not start out in any other way than it did. It should also be apparent, considering these developments, that the technical base is developing rapidly and in a manner likely to produce a range of other possibilities in the near future. The possibility that the quality of outcomes could approach those in other areas of industry raises the question as to whether the new developments will necessarily be restricted to the therapeutic arena. Of critical importance in this area is not the notion that new agents will be more effective than older ones—that antidepressant efficacy will approach that of antipsychotic efficacy—but that the predictability of responses will approach quality standards found elsewhere. The recent emergence of lifestyle agents such as sildenafil (Viagra) owes a great deal to the reliability with which certain responses can be elicited.

Lifestyles and Limits to the Disease Model

When we are told that 10%–15% of the population has a depressive disease and that up to half of the population will have one at some point in their lifetimes, the notion of a disease begins to lose meaning; the implication is that these conditions are defined solely in terms of biologic disruptions of the kind that bacterial infections produce. These figures cannot be understood in terms of the grand melancholias or vital depressions that Kuhn thought he was treating, but they can be understood if the issues are reframed in terms of a general nervousness intimately linked to neuroticism or other dimensional factors and, conversely, if what is aimed at is not so much a cure as the attainment or maintenance of a state of well-being.

Other anomalies in the field of clinical therapeutics suggest that the field comprises a series of diverse domains, many of which may be far removed from the management of bacterial infections. The development and provision of oral contraceptives on a prescription-only basis is underpinned by the same model that underpins the treatment of infections—that is, an understanding that these agents are being used to treat a disease. This notion is faintly ludicrous. Similarly, hormone replacement therapy is dubiously regarded as the treatment of a disease. This therapy is much better seen as an enhancing technology or a cosmetic intervention, and although it seems a good idea to have medical practitioners available to patients as a source of advice, the idea of making these agents available on a prescription-only basis is difficult to defend.

The development of a range of new agents, of which sildenafil is a notable example, further sharpens the issues. Estimates have been made that the use of this agent alone could have substantial cost implications for third-party payers. This development has also drawn attention to the effects on sexual functioning of already available agents such as the SSRIs, which can delay or advance orgasm or otherwise engineer sexual performance but have not been marketed for these indications because of uncertainties about the acceptability of establishing a lifestyle market (Healy 1997). The promotion of sildenafil, therefore, marks an important staging point.

Waiting in the wings are treatments for baldness, agents to reverse age-induced skin changes, and a range of other cosmetic or lifestyle agents. The variety of agents with effects on sexual functioning all allow that function to be manipulated relatively immediately, for defined periods of time, and at an acceptable cost in terms of adverse consequences. The existence of these agents raises in an acute form the question of what a disease is. In recent history a disease has been thought of as an entity established by an underlying biologic lesion. Before that, illnesses were anything that made the individual feel less well, or *dis*-ease, a definition that potentially included halitosis. The emergence of agents that can modify natural variations in hair loss or ejaculatory latency cloud the picture further and potentially push us closer to making explicit one of the currently implicit definitions of disease—that in practice a disease is something for which third-party payers will provide reimbursement.

Against this backdrop, the recent media portrayal of obesity is instructive. From once being seen as all but a moral failing, obesity has in recent years been gradually redefined as a disease. Considerable advantages accrue to such a redefinition. As with other interventions delivered within a medical framework, the product liabilities diminish if the trick can be pulled off. Adherence to a medical model is perhaps best achieved at present by portraying obesity as a risk factor that makes the occurrence of other medical problems more likely. This approach is similar to the one taken with mild hypertension, which is debatably defined as a disease in its own right but is statistically associated with a greater incidence of other medical problems. Some of the interesting issues surrounding the management of obesity are likely to hinge on whether the treatments conflict with vested interests. For instance, agents that retard fat absorption are likely to find much greater support from the food industry than would agents that reduce appetite.

Arguably, the impact of novel psychopharmaceutical technologies will be felt most keenly in the social domain. A current example is alcohol, a psychotropic drug with clear effects on lifestyle. For millennia, alcohol has facilitated social intercourse, almost certainly contributing immeasurably to human civilization in the process. The power of pharmacologic agents to transform social consciousness is difficult to deny in view of the transformations that occurred in social and work relations consequent to the development of oral contraceptives and hormone replacement therapy.

The prospect of "smart drugs" also gives a glimpse of the possible social and political impact of drugs to come. In general, when used in animal populations these drugs offer benefits to less bright, less able, or aged animals compared with younger, more able animals. In today's society, discrimination on the basis of gender, age, race, or religion is unlawful, but discrimination on the basis of intelligence remains legitimate. Clever children get to go to college and are often subsidized to some extent to do so. Thus, they will end up with the better paying and more prestigious jobs. The advantages of natural intelligence and ability, however, stand to be eroded by smart drugs unless, for instance, the use of these drugs is contained to diseases such as age-associated memory impairment (Ray 1998).

New Paradigms

Science is about measurement technologies. Industry is about standards. Measurement technologies within the psychopharmacotherapeutic arena have hitherto been restricted to pen-and-paper interviews using instruments such as the Hamilton Rating Scale for Depression. These instruments were associated with a set of standard views of psychopathology such as neo-Kraepelinism and the monoamine hypotheses of affective disorders. The measurement technologies needed to create new therapeuto-engineering possibilities have begun to emerge. Rating scales that tap into dimensional and personality-based aspects of psychopathology, such as the Cloninger Tridimensional Personality Questionnaire (Cloninger 1987), are gaining widespread use. As with Apple and Microsoft computers, or Betamax and VHS video recorder systems, development trajectories become established when a field settles on a standard, even though that standard may be in many respects inferior to its competitors. The increasing use of the Tridimensional Personality Questionnaire suggests that it is an instrument in the process of becoming a standard; combined with pharmacogenetic and neuroimaging technologies, it is likely to lead to an accelerated set of developments. The genetics of personality traits are likely to be worked out a lot faster than the genetics of risk or protective factors for the major psychosyndromes, if only because the latter factors are bedeviled by complex heterogeneity issues. The question then is whether novel, dimensionally oriented psychopathologies will become the new standards within psychiatry or whether the manipulation of temperamental variables will escape the disease domain entirely.

Current practices are heavily health service and disease oriented. They are dominated by the prescriptive power of medical people and by categorical thinking about disease entities. The focus on a disease model downgraded early etho- and sociopharmacologic findings that drugs taken in different settings may have quite different effects. For example, the disease market has not hitherto distinguished between individuals with depression. If it had, there would have been no means to manage either the variability in human subjects or the lack of specificity of the drugs themselves. Eysenck's early work, which showed that introversion and extroversion dimensions could predict responsiveness to stimulants and sedatives and showed the impact of these dimensions on the acquisition of various reflexes and on performance on a range of tests, gives an indicator of future possibilities. The increasing selectivity of available agents along with an ability to map dimensions to temperament or personality offer an opportunity for behavioral pharmacology to flower.

These advances open up the possibility that it might be more relevant in the future to have a breed of psychopharmacologists, independent of psychiatry, who make their living by advising patients on the use of drugs for behavioral or personality modification purposes. Many of these issues were foreshadowed by Julian Offray de La Mettrie, who prophesied in 1750 that physicians would replace philosophers when it became possible to intervene effectively to shape human behaviors. We have a situation at present where, according to Tom Wolfe, philosophers are deserting their debating chambers in droves and enrolling in neuroscience departments to see at first hand what "the will" looks like. The process seems to be moving one step further, however, in that philosophers and scientists are moving beyond the realm of therapeutics to embrace a domain of biopsychoengineering possibilities.

Possibilities for development in this manner may be available for some time, but nothing will happen unless someone can see a way to make a living out of it. Making a living requires a certain amount of predictability regarding outcomes—that is, a certain level of quality. In our perimillennial society, making a living at something needs to register at a corporate level. Individual entrepreneurial activity makes little difference, but technologies, once they develop, support livelihoods. For this reason, the use of drugs in other than medical settings will generate medical hostility unless the new technologic domain is handed over to medicine.

Psychiatrists and other physicians, meanwhile, have come under public scrutiny because of the poor quality of their services. Various audit procedures, instituted in response to perceptions of marked variations in service delivery, have posed an increasing challenge to the medical professions since the early 1980s. In the United Kingdom, this problem has most recently given rise to the concept of clinical governance. In the United States, managed care companies have for some time been providing data on the quality of intervention outcomes and have moved to a position of not contracting with physicians who cannot provide guarantees of quality to their outcomes. One response to this development might be for psychiatrists to incorporate and form a psychiatric corporation in response to the corporate development within the pharmaceutical industry that has arguably outstripped the monitoring capacities of national psychiatric associations.

A great deal hinges on whether the psychotropic drugs remain available on a prescription-only basis. This outcome is not inevitable. Current agents are much safer than the barbiturates and other agents that were available over the counter before the 1960s. More recently, histamine-2 antagonists have been reclassified from prescription-only to over-the-counter status in a number of countries. These drugs pose risks equivalent to those of many current psychotropic agents. Redesignation of agents as over-the-counter would have several consequences. It might save on public expenditures while maintaining industrial incomes. It would also call into being powerful new consumer agencies that would scrutinize pharmaceutical company claims more vigorously than psychiatrists have done and would by inclination be more likely to approach the issues from the point of view of quality standards rather than disease models. Even after the 1962 amendments to the Food, Drugs and Cosmetics Act, consumers are clearly prepared to consume large amounts of agents to regulate their internal balances. There would seem to be little doubt that an enhancement market, particularly one that offered competitive advantages, would flourish.

Coda

The world is divided by ethnicity, gender, class, wealth, and religion. Political debate pits groups within these domains against one another, often to the detriment of a common good. In contrast to these other domains, health is an arena of common interest, although it has become so only recently. Before the latter third of the 20th century, there was a gross unawareness of health as a distinct domain. Governments did not have departments of health. The media did not cover health-related issues. All this is changing rapidly. Health issues are now front-page news. Popular health and science journals, such as *Scientific American* in the United States and *New Scientist* in the United Kingdom, have begun to outsell political magazines. Where once we depended on wars and politicians to make history, developments within the health field have increasingly been the arena where history is made, with drug brands often marking historical episodes more clearly than anything else—the Valium era, the Prozac era, and now the Viagra era. Health is set to become the central political domain of the 21st century, with various social and technical developments being judged by criteria of whether they further sectional or common interests. This situation uniquely offers the possibility of a common language.

Just as the health domain has emerged only relatively recently to its current position of importance, within this domain depressive conditions have only recently assumed importance. Projections indicate that depression may be the greatest source of disability within health in the 21st century. If it is borne in mind that most health complaints come to medical attention through a filter of well-being or its absence—a filter of neuroticism—then it is clear that nervousness in this sense must inevitably be one of the largest drivers within the health domain, one of the greatest sources of *dis*-ease. How depression is handled in the 21st century will be a question of central importance to humanity.

References

Ayd F: Recognizing the Depressed Patient. New York, Grune & Stratton, 1961

Ayd F: The discovery of amitriptyline, in The Psychopharmacologists, Vol 1. Edited by Healy D. London, Chapman & Hall, 1996, pp 81–120

Battegay R: Forty-four years of psychiatry and psychopharmacology, in The Psychopharmacologists, Vol 3. Edited by Healy D. London, England, Arnold, 2000, pp 371–394

Breier A, Kestler L, Adler C, et al: Dopamine D-2 receptor density and personal detachment in healthy subjects. Am J Psychiatry 155:1440–1442, 1998

Carlsson A: The rise of neuropsychopharmacology, in The Psychopharmacologists, Vol 1. Edited by Healy D. London, Chapman & Hall, 1996, pp 51–80

Carlsson A, Wong DT: A note on the discovery of selective serotonin reuptake inhibitors. Life Sci 61:1203, 1997

Cloninger CR: A systematic method for clinical description and classification of personality variants: a proposal. Arch Gen Psychiatry 44:573–588, 1987

Coirault R, Girard V, Jarrets R, et al: Mode d'action du Tofranil en pathologie mentale. Proceedings 1st Meeting C.I.N.P. Edited by Bradley P. Amsterdam, Elsevier, 1958, pp 520–526

Davies DL, Shepherd M: Reserpine in the treatment of anxious and depressed patients. Lancet 1955, pp 117–120

Delay J, Laine R, Buisson J-F: Note concernant l-action de l'isonicotinyl-hydrazide dans le traitment des etats depressifs. Annales Medico-Psychologiques 110:689–692, 1952

Farde L, Gustavsson JP, Jonsson E: D2 dopamine receptors and personality traits. Nature 380:590, 1997

Healy D: The marketing of 5HT. Br J Psychiatry 158:737–742, 1991

Healy D: The Antidepressant Era. Cambridge, MA, Harvard University Press, 1997

Healy D: The three faces of the antidepressants. J Nerv Ment Dis 187:174–180, 1999

Healy D, Savage M: Reserpine exhumed. Br J Psychiatry 172:376–378, 1998

Healy D, Langmaack C, Savage M: Suicide in the course of the treatment of depression. J Psychopharmacol 13:94–99, 1999

Iversen L: Neuroscience and drug development, in The Psychopharmacologists, Vol 2. Edited by Healy D. London, Chapman & Hall, 1998, pp 325–350

Joyce PR, Mulder RT, Cloninger CR. Temperament predicts clomipramine and desipramine response in major depression. J Affect Disord 30:35–46, 1994

Kielholz P: Diagnose und Therapie der Depressionen fur Praktiker. Munich, Lehmanns JR, 1971

Kielholz P, Battegay R: Behandlung depressiver Zustandbilder, unter spezieller Berucksichtung von Tofranil, einem neue Antidepressivum. Schweizerische Medizinische Wochenschrift 88:763–767, 1958

Klein DF, Fink M: Behavioral reaction patterns with phenothiazines. Arch Gen Psychiatry 7:449–459, 1962

Kline NS: The practical management of depression. JAMA 190:732–740, 1965

Kramer P: Listening to Prozac. New York, Viking Press, 1993

Kuhn R: The treatment of depressive states with G22355 (imipramine hydrochloride). Am J Psychiatry 115:459–464, 1958

Kuhn R: The first patient treated with imipramine, in A History of CINP. Edited by Ban T, Ray O. Brentwood, JM Productions, 1996, p 436

Loomer HP, Saunders JC, Kline NS: A clinical and pharmacodynamic evaluation of iproniazid as a psychic energizer. Psychiatr Res Reps 8:129–141, 1957

Lurie M: The enigma of isoniazid, in The Psychopharmacologists, Vol 2. Edited by Healy D. London, Chapman & Hall, 1998, pp 119–134

Murray C, Lopez A: The Global Burden of Disease. Cambridge, MA, Harvard University Press, 1996

Ray O: A psychologist in American neuropsychopharmacology, in The Psychopharmacologists, Vol 2. Edited by Healy D. London, England, Arnold, 1998, pp 435–454

Robertson MN, Trimble MR: Major tranquillizers used as antidepressants. J Affect Disord 4:173–193, 1982

Robitzek EH, Selikoff IJ, Ornstein GG: Chemotherapy of human tuberculosis with hydrazine derivatives of isonicotinic acid (preliminary report of representative cases). Quarterly Bulletin Sea View Hospital 13:27–51, 1952

Salzer HM, Lurie ML: Anxiety and depressive states treated with isonicotinyl hydrazide (isoniazid). Archives of Neurology and Psychiatry 70:317–324, 1953

Salzer HM, Lurie ML: Depressive states treated with isonicotinyl hydrazide (isoniazid). A follow up study. Ohio State Medicine Journal 51:437–441, 1955

Science notes: mental drug shows promise. New York Times, 7 Apr 1957

Smith JA: The use of the isopropyl derivative of isonicotinyl hydrazide (Marsilid) in the treatment of mental disease. American Practitioner 4:519–520, 1953

Smith MC: A Social History of the Minor Tranquillisers: The Quest for Small Comfort in the Age of Anxiety. New York, Haworth, 1991

TB milestone. Two new drugs give real hope of defeating the dread disease. Life, March 3, 1952, pp 20–21

Üstün T, Sartorius N: Mental Illness in General Health Care. New York, Wiley, 1995

CHAPTER 2

The Worldwide Burden of Depression in the 21st Century

T. Bedirhan Üstün, M.D.

It is far better to foresee even without certainty than not to foresee at all.

Henri Poincare in The Foundations of Science, p. 129

Introduction

Depressive disorders, as mood disorders with accompanying biological, behavioral, and cognitive changes, are the most common forms of mental disorders in community and health care settings (Weissman et al. 1996). Depressive disorders are associated with significant disability. They are not only painful experiences for patients and their families but also greatly disabling because they limit patients' activities and productivity. Depressive disorders constitute a great burden to society. Disability associated with depression is greater than that reported for other chronic physical conditions such as hypertension, diabetes, arthritis, and back pain. These results have been found both in the United States in the Medical Outcomes Study (Wells et al. 1989) and internationally in the World Health Organization's Psychological Problems in General

This chapter was produced in the framework of the World Health Organization/National Institutes of Health Joint Project on Assessment and Classification of Disability (UO1-MH 35883).

Health Care Study (Üstün and Sartorius 1995). In this chapter I introduce the Global Burden of Disease (GBD) study (Murray and Lopez 1996a), which has highlighted the relative importance of depression among all diseases. I discuss the future projections of depressive disorders in light of the evidence available today, including possible developments and their implications for the need for care.

Studying the Future of Depressive Disorders

The future has different meanings and values to all of us, including its predictability, rate of change, and desired features. Whether or not we are deterministic, many of us perceive time as a continuum between past, current, and future. If continuity and discontinuity are studied in a scientific discipline, it may be possible to make plausible projections.

Awareness of future projections has increased markedly in the past decades. The turn of the millennium may have fostered this interest. The need to understand and prepare ourselves for better futures, however, has remained a basic striving of human societies. With regard to health care, studies making future projections may be used at political, managerial, and technical levels for various purposes, from providing inspiration to setting practical indicators and targets. In the field of health care, most countries analyze health policy and formulate plans for the future by asking several questions: How should our health care be organized in the forthcoming years? How will the needs for health care change? How can we be best prepared to respond to future needs? How can we set priorities and allocate resources in a long-term time frame? (van de Water et al. 1998). With escalating health care costs and the inevitability of rationing, research making future projections has received considerable attention. These studies are useful aids in policymaking to study the long-term consequences of current policies and strategies, identify policy change necessary to achieve desired outcomes, induce preparedness and responsiveness to health care transitions, and bring a longer-term life-cycle vision for policy setting. Such research may also help identify the types of information that should be collected now.

Futures research uses projection methods to extrapolate what is

happening today to future years. Given the complexity of social structures, more sophisticated methods are available to forecast different future scenarios taking into account multiple parameters and criteria.
These forecasting studies are referred to as futures, future studies, or futures research, as a discipline drawing heavily from political and social
sciences, economics, computer modeling, ecology, systems thinking,
and theories such as game theory, decision theory, and chaos theory. Futures studies are not a substitute for long-term planning, strategic management, and policy making, although they are closely related to these
processes and can support and complement them.

There are two distinct types of futures studies. The first type are exploratory scenarios (called reference scenarios) that extrapolate to the
future from the past and today. The second type are target-setting scenarios that "backcast" from a desired future point and seek the interventions needed to achieve a target. Futures studies may be approached in
various ways, using either a hard approach (i.e., scientific methods and
technical products) or a soft approach (i.e., speculative methods and
free-ranging products). Such predictions have become a common tool,
especially in management and political sciences, and may help us to ac-
quire a critical awareness of the modern world. However, one should
always be aware of the limitations of these predictions. Although it may
be easy to predict *a* future (e.g., weather for the next day or response to
a treatment), it impossible to predict *the* future. Plausible projections of
the future of health conditions are a useful aid in planning, but making
future predictions about single health conditions may be unreliable. A
focus on individual disease conditions may lack internal consistency in
that the sum of all diseases may easily exceed the real numbers of mortality. One should therefore consider all diseases and consequences
together in a comprehensive way, incorporating epidemiologic knowledge such as base population, rates, and patterns of ill health as well as
socioeconomic, environmental, educational, and technologic factors
and their distributions among populations.

Global Burden of Disease Study

The GBD study was conducted by the World Health Organization and
the World Bank to provide a set of summary health measures that pro-

vide information, including nonfatal health outcomes, for international health policy. To provide unbiased epidemiologic assessments that are uncoupled from advocacy, the GBD study developed internally consistent estimates of the incidence, prevalence, duration, and case fatality for 107 conditions and their 483 disabling consequences. These estimates of burden could also be used in cost-effectiveness analysis and to assess the attributable fraction of risk factors (Murray and Lopez 1996a).

The GBD study created a "Cinderella" effect for mental disorders. Traditional public health measures usually focused on mortality and never ranked mental disorders in the top-ten priority lists. However, when the concept of disability was entered into the equation, as is the case with disability-adjusted life years (DALYs[1]), mental disorders ranked as high as cardiovascular and respiratory diseases, surpassing all malignancies and HIV combined. Looking at the years of life lived with disability (YLD) only, depressive disorders as a single diagnostic category were the leading cause of disability worldwide. The GBD study thus revealed the true magnitude of the long underestimated impact of mental health problems.

Global Burden of Disease Study Projections

The GBD study developed three scenarios for the future (baseline, optimistic, and pessimistic) encompassing mortality and disability for different age-sex groups, causes, and regions. The study used the most important disease and injury trends since 1950 in nine cause-of-death clusters. Regression equations for mortality rates for each cluster by region were developed from:

- Gross domestic product per person (in international dollars)
- Average number of years of education

---

[1] DALYs are based on years of life lost (YLL) because of premature death and years of life lived with disability (YLD). So DALYs = YLL + YLD; thus, the burden equals the sum of mortality plus disability. In summary, one DALY equals one lost year of healthy life. The disability component of this summary health measure, YLD, is weighted according to the severity of the disability. For example, disability caused by major depression was found to be equivalent to blindness or paraplegia, whereas the active psychosis occurring in schizophrenia was estimated as somewhere between paraplegia and quadriplegia in severity of disability.

- Time (in years, as a surrogate for technologic change)
- Smoking intensity, which shows the cumulative effects based on data for 47 countries in 1950 to 1990

Baseline, optimistic, and pessimistic projections of the independent variables were made. Mortality from detailed causes was related to mortality from a cause cluster to project more detailed causes. Based on projected numbers of deaths by cause, years of life lived with disability (YLDs) were projected from different relation models of YLDs to years of life lost (YLLs). Population projections were prepared from World Bank projections of fertility and projected mortality rates.

The findings of the GBD study suggest that health trends through 2020 will be determined mainly by the aging of the world's population; the decline in age-specific mortality rates from communicable, maternal, and nutritional disorders; the spread of HIV; and the increase in tobacco-related mortality and disability (Murray and Lopez 1997). Most important, unipolar major depression ranked second after ischemic heart disease in leading causes of DALYs, surpassing road-traffic accidents, cerebrovascular disease, chronic obstructive pulmonary disease, lower respiratory infections, tuberculosis, war injuries, diarrheal diseases, and HIV. Unipolar major depression could become the second greatest cause of GBD, increasing its share by more than 50%. Figure 2–1 shows the trend of increase in depression and bipolar disorder in comparison with tobacco, HIV, and diarrhea.

Projections of Depressive Disorders

In the light of demographic[2] and epidemiologic[3] transitions (Kalache 1997; Manton 1997; Omran 1971) as well as social factors concerning family structures, urbanization, migration and mobility, and alcohol and drug use, the risks for mental disorders will certainly increase. Increased population, longer life expectancy, possible increases in the rate of depression, and a relative decrease in other communicable condi-

---

[2] Changes in population size and distribution characterized by fertility, birth, and death rates.
[3] Changes in the pattern of diseases from the communicable to noncommunicable diseases.

tions will result in depressive disorders becoming the leading cause of disability and overall burden worldwide. The results of the GBD study have shown variations by country and region, but patterns and trends are remarkably similar worldwide. These findings pose new challenges to mental health policymakers, with unmet and growing needs in both developed and developing countries.

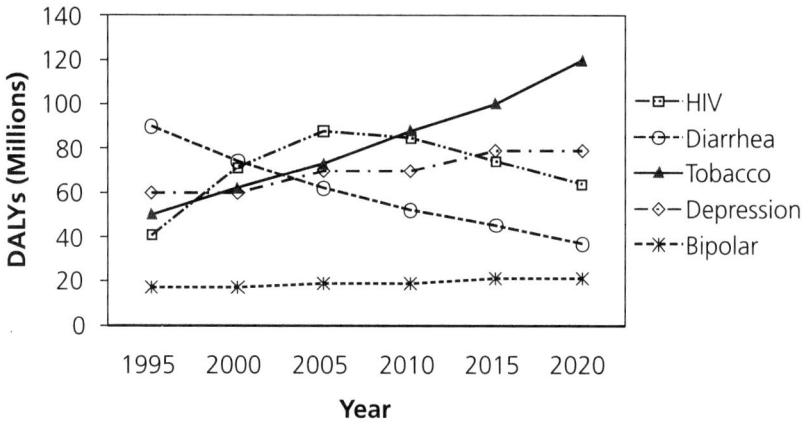

FIGURE 2–1.   Disability-adjusted life years (DALYs) attributable to major causes, 1990–2020 (baseline scenario).
Source.   Data from World Health Organization (1999) and Murray and Lopez (1996b).

The findings also call for debate and for scientific studies to confirm and refine them. Although the results of the GBD study have been extremely useful in mainstreaming mental health, we should be aware of the limitations of these projections as discussed below.

Data and Methods

The GBD study applied basic regression methods statistics to obtain and assess predictions. General disease epidemiology (such as incidence, duration, and change in parameters over time) formed the basic parameters in these predictions. The methodology could be advanced using econometric methods to examine the link between health out-

comes and other determinants of health (such as environmental and behavioral risk factors and socioeconomic determinants) and to consider
applied models of specific disease epidemics in real populations (e.g.,
HIV [Salomon et al. 1999]). These methods aim to generate internally
consistent estimates of total mortality and disability in the world. The
data input to the GBD calculation for depressive disorders, however, remain debatable. Episode incidence was modeled as 2.7% for women
and 1.4% for men; episode average age at onset was 37.1 years, with an
average episode duration of 6 months (Murray and Lopez 1996b, pp.
601–606). Treatment rates for depressive disorders were about 5% in
sub-Saharan Africa and 35% in established market economies (Murray
and Lopez 1996a, Annex Table 4, p. 417). These incidence and prevalence estimates are low compared with the modern psychiatric epidemiologic findings. Annual prevalence of unipolar depression was 12.9%
for women in the National Comorbidity Study (Kessler et al. 1994) as
opposed to the 1.7% prevalence estimate used in the GBD calculations.
Similarly, the GBD age at onset of 37.1 years is much older than the
common finding of between ages 20 and 25 years (Burke et al. 1991).
It may be concluded that GBD results are generally underestimated for
mental and depressive disorders. This discrepancy stems from the uni-
fied approach to creating internally consistent estimates of epidemiologic parameters using the DISMOD computer program, which
assumes a linear relation between incidence, duration, and prevalence.
Future iterations of the GBD study are expected to use more detailed
programming and data from empiric studies.

Conceptualization of Depression

In the GBD study, unipolar depression was modeled as an episodic illness, whereas modern concepts of this disorder suggest a chronic relaps-
ing medical illness model. The requirements and impact of different
modeling are to be studied in future versions of the GBD. Similarly, in
the GBD study depression was considered as an adult disease, and childhood and youth depression were not represented. Life years lost because
of suicide were not included in the depression burden because suicide
is directly studied, independent of depression.

Use of Single Disability Weight for All Types of Depressive Disorders

The disability weight for depressive disorders was taken as 0.6 for untreated cases and 0.3 for treated cases irrespective of severity of depression (mild, moderate, or severe), age, or the part of the world where the cases occurred. It is well known that various severity levels are associated with different degrees of disability. Treatment results may vary by age or social circumstances. Although more detailed models can be made that include these variables, availability of data and the general nature of the GBD exercise did not allow for such detailed estimates.

Comorbidity

The inclusion of comorbidity in the GBD study was limited. With few exceptions (i.e., Down syndrome with mental retardation and mental retardation with cerebral palsy), the GBD study did not explicitly recognize the impact of comorbidity on disability. Given the high rates of comorbidity of depressive disorders with other mental disorders, substance use disorders, and physical disorders, it is important to factor these phenomena in the calculation of GBD. The current model simply takes the comorbidity as additive of two disability weights, which may result in an overestimate.

Dominance of Past Trends

Depression prevalence rates were taken as fixed, although there are indications that they may have increased in recent years (Klerman and Weissman 1989). Given these factors, the GBD estimates were mainly conservative for mental, particularly depressive, disorders.

Considering Future Actions

The GBD study put mental disorders on an equal basis with other disorders. This analysis has indeed mainstreamed mental health. In this context, we should seek applications of the GBD study to policymaking, planning, and programs. By improving input variables of key importance and identifying key actors and their key strategies, we can certainly frame future scenarios by scanning for relevant emerging trends and developing policy options. Envisioning the most likely future and alternative likely futures will allow us to evaluate the feasibility and desirability of an optimal path to a desired future. The GBD study has revealed the importance of mental disorders and has identified depressive disorders as one of the most important targets for the 21st century.

Can we use this information for the management of health policy: How can we cope with the existing burden of depression? How can we decrease the future burden of disease? Most countries have less than $20 (U.S.) per capita available for health care: How can care for depression be incorporated within a comprehensive health care package?

Although the analysis of the current situation is pessimistic, we can still act with hope. Building bridges between burden and effective solutions is necessary. Thinking about the future calls for profound reflection on policies and allocation of resources. Government agencies, care providers, consumers, industry, and researchers should get together to find effective and sustainable ways to combat the increasing burden of depression.

The epidemiologic parameters in projecting depression, such as population dynamics, age at onset, prevalence, and risk factors, may all be debated. However, under the most conservative estimates, the most alarming projection remains that the burden of depressive disorders will increase by at least 50% by 2020.

Given the current gap between treatment efficacy (i.e., success in clinical research trials) and effectiveness (i.e., success in real-world settings), we should develop programs for prevention and find ways of generalizing effective treatment modalities (Üstün 1999). Current trends indicate that the treatment of depressive disorders will move to primary care, that evidence-based guidelines will be used on larger scales to inform care and policy, and that relapses and chronicity of depressive disorders could be prevented. The labor sector has already implemented workplace programs to prevent productivity loss and improve quality of life. Consumer involvement and self-help are growing. We should definitely think about innovative ways to deal with this problem, in particular, strengthening capacities of health systems to identify and manage depression, especially in developing countries.

To combat the burden of depressive disorders we must research the efficacy, effectiveness, cost-effectiveness, and generalizability of mental health interventions. We need to translate the findings of basic science into treatment and prevention interventions. Finally, we must investigate how these interventions might best be implemented in the real world. The changing health care scene, with growing evidence-based medicine and policy, advancing information technology, and developments in neuroscience and genetic research, may help us deal with this burden. Most important, increased public awareness and consumer involvement will enable better dissemination of information and quality assurance for a generalizable and sustainable management strategy.

References

Burke KC, Burke JD Jr, Rae DS, et al: Comparing age at onset of major depression and other psychiatric disorders by birth cohorts in five U.S. community populations. Arch Gen Psychiatry 48:789–795, 1991

Garret MJ: Health Futures: A Handbook for Health Professionals. Geneva, Switzerland, World Health Organization, 1999

Kalache A: Demographic transition poses a challenge to societies worldwide. Trop Med Int Health 2:925–926, 1997

Kessler RC, McGonagle KA, Zhao S, et al: Lifetime and 12-month prevalence of DSM-III-R psychiatric disorders in the United States. Results from the National Comorbidity Survey. Arch Gen Psychiatry 51:8–19, 1994

Klerman GL, Weissman MM: Increasing rates of depression. JAMA 261:2229–2235, 1989

Manton KG: Changes in the age dependence of mortality and disability: cohort and other determinants. Demography 34:135–157, 1997

Murray CJL, Lopez AD: The global burden of disease: a comprehensive assessment of mortality and disability from diseases, injuries, and risk factors in 1990 and projected to 2020. Cambridge, MA, Harvard University Press, 1996a

Murray CJL, Lopez AD: Global health statistics: a compendium of incidence, prevalence and mortality estimates for over 200 conditions. Cambridge, MA, Harvard School of Public Health on behalf of the World Health Organization and the World Bank, 1996b

Murray CJL, Lopez AD: Alternative projections of mortality and disability by cause 1990–2020: Global Burden of Disease Study. Lancet 349:1498–1504, 1997

Salomon JA, Gakidou EE, Murray CJ: Methods for modeling the HIV/AIDS epidemic in sub-Saharan Africa. GPE Discussion Paper No. 3. Geneva, World Health Organization, July 1999

Omran AR: The epidemiologic transition: a theory of the epidemiology of population change. Milbank Memorial Fund Quarterly 49:509–538, 1971

Üstün TB: Global burden of mental disorders. Am J Public Health 89:1315–1318, 1999

Üstün TB, Sartorius N: Mental Illness in General Health Care. Chichester, United Kingdom, Wiley, 1995

van de Water, HPA, Van Herten LM: Health policies on target? Review of the health target and priority setting in 18 European countries, in TNO Prevention and Health. Amsterdam, Elsevier, 1998, 133–135

Weissman MM, Bland RC, Canino GJ, et al: Cross-national epidemiology of major depression and bipolar disorder. JAMA 276:293–299, 1996

Wells K, Stewart A, Hays RD, et al: The functioning and well-being of depressed patients. Results from the Medical Outcomes Study. JAMA 262:914–919, 1989

World Health Organization: The World Health Report 1999: Making a Difference. Geneva, Switzerland, World Health Organization, 1999

CHAPTER 3

Treatment of Depression in the New Health Care Scene

Robert Michels, M.D.

Introduction

Ambiguity exists in the title *Treatment of Depression in the New Health Care Scene*. Surveys of physicians' attitudes toward the managed health care system consistently report dissatisfaction, unhappiness, and even despair. This chapter is, of course, about depressed patients and not depressed physicians, but these two topics are closely intertwined. Physicians complain that the new system limits their professional autonomy, forces them to ration their clinical resources, limits the time available for each patient contact and the possibility of extended or repeated contact, emphasizes cost as the primary determinant in selecting from among alternative treatments, and diminishes their income while offering financial incentives for undertreatment. Physicians believe that these characteristics of the new system interfere with their relationships with patients and reduce the pleasures of medical practice (Michels 1999; Simon et al. 1999). This chapter is about the fate of depressed patients in such a system: How do the system's characteristics—those that depress doctors—affect the experiences of depressed patients?

Changes in the System

The first and most fundamental characteristic of the new system is that it is a system. Formerly, health care was a cottage industry composed of a large number of individuals or small organizations, each doing its own thing, and an even larger number of patients, each negotiating individually for care. Today most patients participate in some kind of organized patient group that does much of their negotiating for them, and most practitioners are linked to an organized provider group. Paradoxically these patient and provider groups may be combined. The largest for-profit behavioral health managed care organization now administers care for more than 60 million people, over 20% of the nation's population.

Second, information systems are widespread. For example, it is possible to track how many patients are given the diagnosis of depression and how many receive adequate treatment (a small minority of the total in the covered population of most behavioral health managed care organizations), how many prescriptions for antidepressants are written (about 0.4 per person per year), and who writes them (one-third by psychiatrists, two-thirds by others) (Hirschfeld 1998).

Third, although the new system has explicitly articulated three goals—improved access, enhanced quality, and controlled cost—only cost control has had a real impact. Although access may have improved for some people, it has grown worse for many more. The proportion of the population that is uninsured or underinsured has grown. Monitoring of quality has begun, but few real quality measures are available, and the goal of enhanced quality has largely been subordinated to the goal of cost control. Quality enhancement efforts have so far focused on the treatment of specific episodes of illness rather than on detection and case finding, management of chronic illness, predisposition or disability, or the effect of the system on the community's overall health. Even cost control has focused almost entirely on short-term direct costs; the structure of the private—and particularly the for-profit—health care system offers little likelihood of longer-term patient–provider relationships and thus little incentive for health care providers to be concerned with future or indirect cost savings.

Fourth, the old system emphasized specialty care, with relative disregard for the care of patients who did not have significant illness. In contrast, the new system emphasizes acute primary care, with problems resulting in the care of patients who have chronic illness, particularly major illnesses with which primary care physicians are not familiar. In general, primary care physicians are not comfortable treating psychiatric illnesses; in particular, they often fail to diagnose and treat depressive disorders.

Fifth, the old system offered incentives to providers for increased intensity of care, whereas the new system offers incentives for decreased care. The result is improved quality in those areas of medicine that had formerly been used in excess, such as hysterectomies or the surgical treatment of back pain, and diminished quality in areas in which use was already low, such as the treatment of depression. An irony exists here in that the so-called medicalization of psychiatry has led to a system that treats psychiatric care as though it had the same problems as general medical care; thus, it uses a single incentive strategy that discourages the use of a broad array of medical and psychiatric treatments, including those that are currently overused and those that are currently woefully underused.

Sixth, in spite of this single incentive strategy, both the old and the new systems handle psychiatric treatment differently than other medical treatment. In the old system the greatest difference was in hospital care, which was often provided in large, isolated public facilities and almost always in separate facilities. In the new system, psychiatric hospital care, at least acute hospital care, has largely been integrated with general health care in community hospitals. However, the widespread practice of so-called behavioral carve-outs has led to separate and unequal outpatient mental health care, with particular problems for the management of conditions that straddle the medical and psychiatric systems, such as those that feature physical symptoms but require psychiatric treatment. Depression is the classic example.

Seventh, the new health care system has almost completely ignored the maintenance and improvement of the health care system itself. Ignored areas include research and development of improved treatments, often made more difficult by the constraints of the managed care system; education, which had been cross-subsidized by the old clinical system but is not in the new system; and human resources issues such as the attractiveness of a career in health care and the satisfaction of health care professionals. I have already commented on the responses of physicians to the new system; dissatisfied doctors are not ideal caretakers.

Finally, the new system is in transition. It is heterogeneous, even chaotic, varying from place to place and from year to year. Its future is also unclear. Many observers believe that the current multiorganizational, largely for-profit managed care system is failing, and that with the next economic downturn the system is likely to be replaced by something more comprehensive and efficient, although possibly even less generous.

We have learned that the fate of depressed patients in any health care system reflects the structure and organizing principles of that system. As the system continues to evolve, if coverage is determined by the attitudes of consumers, employers, or the public, true parity is unlikely and depressed patients will continue to be underserved. If rational cost–benefit analysis determines patterns of care, depressed patients will fare well; the results of treatment are more than worth the cost.

Changes in the
Understanding of Depression

There have been changes not only in the health care system but also in our understanding of depression. The term *understanding* emphasizes not so much what is known about the scientific basis behind depression but rather what has been translated into the useful practical knowledge of psychiatrists, other physicians and professionals, patients, and the general public. This translation is a painfully slow and often irregular process, and the understanding of the average practitioner often lags far behind the cutting edge of new knowledge in the field.

We are increasingly aware that depressive disorders are common; they have both high prevalence and a wide spectrum of clinical presentations. These disorders represent a major cause of morbidity and mortality and are a leading public health problem. There is growing recognition that depression is a disease, not a moral weakness or an inevitable theme of life, and that like other diseases it has symptoms, signs, and a natural course that treatment can influence. Although somewhat less well recognized, depressed patients can present with a medical condition that has physical symptoms or with problems in living and a need for counseling and guidance. Newer treatments are available, both psychologic and pharmacologic, that are safe and effective and that have a high degree of patient acceptability. Perhaps least well known is that depression is frequently a chronic or recurrent condition, and effective management must extend beyond the treatment of the individual episode. Depression is also frequently comorbid with other conditions—medical illnesses, substance abuse, other psychiatric disorders, and social stress and disadvantage. We believe that these comorbid states influence clinical course and treatment response, but we have relatively little scientific knowledge in this area. This means that the clinician's usual problem is not the one that clinical researchers have addressed—how to treat depression—but rather how to treat depression in a specific patient who has been given multiple diagnoses and has comorbid conditions, only one of which is depression. Unfortunately, the current research literature provides relatively little direct assistance in this regard.

A New Notion of Depression: The Changing System

When the new notion of depression is combined with the new health care system, the results can be unfortunate. As in the past, many depressed people do not recognize that they are depressed, or even that they are ill, and fail to seek help. Of those who do seek help, many go outside of the health care system, often seeing well-meaning and humane helpers who do not understand depression, underestimate its prevalence, fail to recognize and diagnose it, and fail to arrange adequate treatment. Such contacts may have a negative impact on the probability of effective treatment by falsely reassuring the patient that he or she is receiving appropriate help when this is not so.

Depressed persons who do enter the health care system may see nonmedical mental health professionals, nonpsychiatrist physicians, or, least likely, psychiatrists. Depression has a low detection rate in the general medical sector, reflecting limitations in the knowledge and skills of primary care physicians and negative attitudes toward psychiatric disorders and patients. The new system has not only failed to address these long-standing problems but has also aggravated them by sharply limiting the time that doctors spend with patients and by adding incentives for doctors to rapidly move patients through the system without inquiring about psychosocial issues, making secondary diagnoses, or providing treatment if patients do not demand it.

Depressed persons who see psychiatrists or other mental health professionals are more likely to receive a diagnosis of depression but not to receive the long-term care required. Here the problem is that the system wants depression to be an acute disease with no need for long-term treatment or follow-up and with treatment selected by cost without regard for patient acceptability or adherence. Unfortunately, the depression that patients have is often not the same as the depression that is acceptable to the world of managed care, and the most appropriate treatment courses are not necessarily the shortest or the least expensive.

Although the new system has an announced goal of improved access, this goal has had little impact on the increasing number of citizens with no insurance coverage. Furthermore, despite the excellent epidemiologic data that would make it easy to estimate the number of insured people who have undiagnosed depression and are not receiving treatment, there has been little interest in identifying them or in providing them with treatment. Essentially, the new health care system provides care for those insured people who recognize that they are sick and seek help. The system has little interest in those who do not recognize that they are sick or have an impaired ability to seek care. One result, perhaps the most disturbing result from the perspective of psychiatric care, has been a steady diminution in the percentage of health care resources directed to mental health services.

The new health care system and our new understanding of depression have also led to positive changes. The leaders of primary care medicine have recognized the need for better training and improved diagnostic tools in the recognition and treatment of depression. The pharmaceutical industry has enthusiastically supported consciousness raising and education of the general public and health professionals. The mental health and psychiatric communities have developed and demonstrated the effectiveness of treatments that can be used by primary care physicians and by specialists and that are acceptable to patients. Modern pharmacologic treatments are safer and have fewer side effects than those of the past, and psychotherapeutic approaches have separated the treatment of depression from the previously dominant undifferentiated treatment of character pathology, with much greater patient acceptability and perhaps greater clinical efficacy as a result.

Solutions

More can and should be done. Competence in general medicine should be defined to include competence in the recognition and diagnosis of depression and should be required for certification and licensure, just as it is with diabetes, hypertension, or glaucoma. Quality in a health care system should be defined as including the identification and provision of treatment for depressed persons for whom the system is responsible and should be measured and incorporated into publicly available measures of quality. System features such as deductibles, copayments, incentives for making or avoiding referrals, capitation, and the like should be evaluated not only for their impact on cost but also for their impact on the care of those whose disorders do not lead them to seek help. Post-episode follow-up and long-term preventive care should be rewarded, not discouraged.

In summary, we know more about depression and have better treatments for it than ever before. Nevertheless, as we enter the 21st century in the United States, the treatment received by the average depressed person is not limited by what is known but rather by characteristics of the health delivery system. This was true long before the new system came into being, but the promises of that new system have not been realized. In fact, the diminution of resources for mental health care, the separation of behavioral from medical care, the lack of interest in those who do not seek care, the disincentives to primary care physicians making secondary diagnoses, the preference for less expensive treatments, and the attempt to limit treatment to specific episodes of illness may have led to an even greater difference between the potential and the actual.

References

Hirschfeld RMA: American health care systems and depression: the past, present and the future. J Clin Psychiatry 59(suppl):5–10, 1998

Michels R: Medical education and managed care (editorial). N Engl J Med 340:959–961, 1999

Simon SR, Pan RJ, Sullivan AM, et al: Views of managed care: a survey of students, residents, faculty and deans at medical schools in the United States. N Engl J Med 340:928–936, 1999

Basic Understanding of Depression

Introduction

Ming T. Tsuang, M.D., Ph.D., D.Sc.

As we enter the 21st century, it is instructive to take stock of our progress thus far in understanding the neurobiology of major depression. To do so, we need to look both forward and backward to get an approximate sense of the road we have worked so hard to traverse. In looking back, one is struck immediately by the distance we have come since the beginning of the 20th century. At that time, the notion that the brain is composed of neurons was still new and still debated by some. Our understanding of emotions in general, let alone disorders of emotion such as depression, was limited to speculation that they had something to do with sensory regions of the brain. It took another 30–50 years before we understood that specific subcortical regions, such as the hypothalamus and other parts of the limbic system, were part of cortical and subcortical neural networks involved in the regulation of affect. It was barely 50 years ago—the middle of the 20th century—that we entered the modern era of pharmacologic treatments for major mental illnesses, and only about 40 years ago was the first antidepressant medication introduced. Moreover, only 35 years ago was an underlying hypothesis put forward to explain why drugs that enhanced catecholamine neurotransmission in the brain might also attenuate symptoms of depression.

What is perhaps most remarkable about these breakthroughs, however, is not that they point out how rudimentary our knowledge has been in the recent past. Rather, they underscore how much we have learned in a relatively short period of time. Monoamine oxidase inhibitors were replaced relatively quickly as treatments of choice for depression by tricyclic antidepressants and then to some extent by selective serotonin reuptake inhibitors (SSRIs). As Nemeroff and Owens point out in Chapter 4 (on the contributions of basic neuroscience to new treatments for psychiatric disorders), the development of fluorescence histochemistry in the 1960s by Falck, Hillarp, and colleagues allowed visualization of norepinephrine-, dopamine-, and serotonin-containing neurons for the first time. Out of this stunning advance evolved the techniques of immunohistochemistry and then in situ hybridization, which allows mRNA to be expressed for neuronal genes. Again these advances took place over a relatively short period of time. Many other such examples illustrate the point that the growth of our knowledge in basic neuroscience is not linear but rather positively accelerated. Most important, as our basic knowledge grows, so does our capacity to generate new, more effective, and more selective treatments for depression. It is this point that has generated much of our current enthusiasm and that allows us some cautious optimism about the future.

Each of the chapters in this section emphasizes aspects of our progress in basic neuroscience and the application of that knowledge to future treatments. Nemeroff and Owens (Chapter 4) identify several likely target systems for therapeutic interventions. For example, they review data that shed light on the nature of serotonergic deficits in depression based on analyses of concentrations of serotonin in synaptic clefts, using single photon emission computed tomography neuroimaging methods. As the deficit becomes more understood at a neuronal level, it may also become possible to predict treatment responses to antidepressant medications sooner. Nemeroff and Owens also review other target systems that are just starting to become amenable to study, such as neurogenesis in the central nervous system. Will it become possible in the near future to treat depression by stimulating the growth of neurons that release neurochemicals with endogenous antidepressant effects? This question could not even be asked a few years ago.

The fields of genetics and molecular biology have witnessed veritable explosions of knowledge in the past 20 years. Nemeroff and Owens (Chapter 4) and Hyman and Moldin (Chapter 5) describe the excitement of these endeavors. Hyman and Moldin emphasize the progress being made by the Human Genome Project, which will identify all of the 80,000 or so genes on the human genome, including the approximately 50,000 or so that are expressed in the brain. Knowledge of these genes will represent a sea change from the 3,000–4,000 genes identified thus far. The potential value of identifying these genes cannot be overstated. The identification of genes that cause diseases such as depression and schizophrenia will be facilitated, and at least two major treatment strategies will result. First, after genes are identified, their products (i.e., the proteins they encode) can also be identified, and the manner in which genes underlie pathophysiologic mechanisms will become amenable for study. At that point, selective drug treatments to intervene in the pathologic cascade of events can be developed. Second, the identification of disease genes will allow the development of targeted strategies for the prevention of disease in high-risk individuals. Kupfer and Frank (Chapter 6) stress methodologic advances in relation to neurobiologic measures. They emphasize their ongoing and productive studies of sleep to develop ways of predicting the long-term course of depression in subjects of different age groups. In addition to emphasizing the need for ongoing longitudinal assessments to enhance the predictive power of their measurements, they stress the importance of obtaining multiple measures to increase predictive power. Their point underscores the growing recognition that multidisciplinary, integrative approaches will be needed to carry us forward into the 21st century.

Thus, as we take stock of our progress, we see that there is still a long way to go before we reach the point at which depression is cured or prevented. At the same time, our review of our progress allows us to hope that such goals will come within our reach in the not-too-distant future.

CHAPTER 4

Contribution of Modern Neuroscience to Developing New Treatments for Psychiatric Disorders

Charles B. Nemeroff, M.D., Ph.D.
Michael J. Owens, Ph.D.

Our hope for the future lies…in organic chemistry or in an approach to [psychosis] through endocrinology. Today this future is still far off, but we should study analytically every case of psychosis because the knowledge thus gained will one day direct the chemical therapy.

Sigmund Freud, in a letter to Marie Bonaparte, 1930

Introduction

In the nearly 70 years that have elapsed since Freud's prophetic statement, remarkable advances have occurred both in our understanding of the pathophysiology of, and in our capacity to treat, many of the major medical disorders that have plagued humankind in the 20th century,

The authors are supported by National Institutes of Health grants MH-42088, MH-39415, MH-40524, MH-51761, MH-58922, DA-09492, DA-08705, and an Established Investigator Award from NARSAD.

including affective disorders and schizophrenia. It is almost a cliché to state that we have learned 90% of our understanding of the central nervous system (CNS) in the past decade. Whether or not this statement is precisely true, little doubt exists that the remarkable advances in the neurosciences will continue to provide the basis for the development of novel strategies for treating the major psychiatric disorders. In this chapter we focus briefly on a few critical advances in the neurosciences that we believe have critically contributed to our understanding of both the pathophysiology and the mechanisms of action of currently available psychopharmacologic agents. The remainder of the chapter consists of several suggested directions for future research and drug development based on recent advances in the neurosciences. Although certainly not gifted with prescience, we hope it serves heuristic purposes to crawl out on a limb with such guesstimates, if for no other reason than to revisit these projections after a decade has passed to determine whether one or more turned out to be correct.

In the field of neuroscience, as in most fields, we stand on the shoulders of giants to glimpse the future. In some ways the CNS is similar to many other organs, and in other ways it is similar to none. Its complexity cannot be overemphasized. For example, the liver was once considered one of the most, if not the most, complex of all organs. Its enzymology, oxidative metabolism, and role in myriad gastrointestinal functions and other vital processes are well established. Yet the cellular structure of the liver, identical in the left and right lobes, is composed of hepatocytes, Kupffer cells, and the portal triad. Consider, in contrast, the mammalian CNS. No single part of the brain is like any other part. Although the cellular composition of the CNS comprises neurons and glial cells, each brain area has its own unique cytoarchitecture, its own unique connections with other neurons, both local and distant, and its own collection of neurons that are chemically defined by the neurotransmitter each uses. How then can we make any sense of this collection of billions of neurons and glial cells and the roles played by a subset of these cells either in health or in disease?

Although the seminal findings in neuroscience that have set the stage for current and future breakthroughs in psychopharmacology are numerous, space constraints preclude their complete discussion. However, a few are worth noting in the context of the present discussion. Luigi Golgi, although incorrect in his monumental war with Santiago Ramón y Cajal about the nature of nerve connections (Golgi believed in the existence of a continuous nerve net, whereas Cajal believed that synapses separate neurons), is notable for developing the Golgi stain. Although this stain allows visualization of only approximately 1% of neurons in a given section, they are seen in their entirety. This method provided remarkable information about the different types of neurons and their dendritic and axonal arborizations.

Falck and Hillarp and their students, Fuxe, Dahlstrom, and Hökfelt, arguably have contributed one of the major breakthroughs in all of neuroscience, namely, the technique of fluorescence histochemistry, which has evolved into both immunohistochemistry and in situ hybridization. This technique, in its original iteration, allowed for the direct visualization of serotonin (5-HT), dopamine, or norepinephrine (NE) in tissue slices after exposure to paraformaldehyde gas, permitting for the first time a comprehensive description of several chemically defined neural circuits. Immunohistochemistry, a more refined method, uses antibodies to neurotransmitters or their synthetic enzymes, providing a simpler, more specific, and more sensitive method to chemically identify neurons. Most recently, in situ hybridization has allowed the demonstration of mRNA expression for particular genes in neurons, including genes that code for neurotransmitter transporters, preprohormones, receptors, and myriad intracellular structural and signaling proteins. Figure 4–1 presents the distribution of arginine-vasopressin mRNA expression in the mouse hypothalamus, an example of the remarkable results that can be obtained using such methodology. Armed with this formidable technology, a generation of chemical neuroanatomists have characterized in detail the distribution of neuropeptide- and monoamine-containing perikarya and nerve terminals in the mammalian CNS as well as the projections of these neurons from the brain stem to various forebrain and spinal cord projection areas.

Monoamine Mechanisms in Depression: Pathophysiology and Treatment

The serotonergic projections from the raphe nuclei in the brain stem have been characterized in considerable detail as part of a topographi-

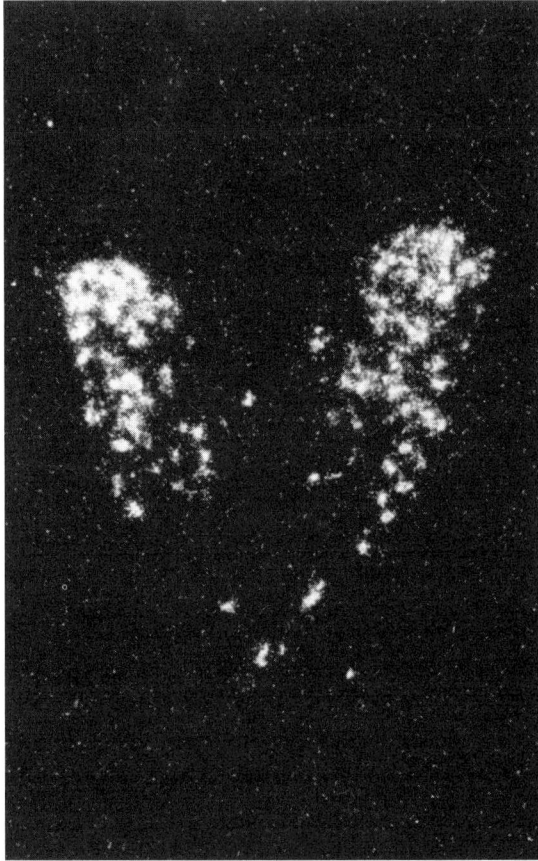

FIGURE 4–1.   Arginine vasopressin mRNA as determined by in situ hybridization using a ^{35}S-labeled antisense riboprobe. Darkfield photomicrograph shows dense hybridization over the hypothalamic paraventricular nucleus in a coronal brain section (30 mm) from a mouse. Magnification ×100.
Source.   Provided by Dr. Larry Young, Department of Psychiatry and Behavioral Sciences, Emory University.

cally widespread projection system, which fits well with their postulated role in the pathophysiology of depression. Because depression as a syndrome includes symptoms in a number of physiologic and behavioral arenas (i.e., disrupted sleep, appetite, libido, mood, autonomic nervous system function, and immune function) as well as mood and endocrine alterations, any single neurotransmitter system posited to be integral to the disease process must innervate myriad brain regions known to sub-serve each of the physiologic functions altered in depression. In addi-tion to the widespread innervation of the CNS by serotonergic neurons is the remarkable density of this innervation (Table 4–1). Each raphe neuron provides 500,000 varicosities in the cerebral cortex, resulting in a density of 5-HT–containing varicosities of 5,800,000 per mm^3 of tissue.

TABLE 4–1. *Quantitative data on serotonin (5-HT) neurons innervating the neostriatum, cerebral cortex, and hippocampus*

Variable	Neostriatum	Cerebral cortex	Hippocampus
Varicosities per mm^3 of tissue	2.6×10^6	5.8×10^6	2.7×10^6
5-HT content per varicosity (concentration)	0.2 fg (1800 μg/g)	0.05 fg (535 μg/g)	0.06 fg (450 μg/g)
Varicosities per target neuron	100–200	145–230	20–130
Varicosities per cell body of origin	60,000	500,000	150,000
Frequency of junctional varicosities	~20%	30%–40%	Very low

Source. Adapted from Descarries L, Audet MA, Doucet G, et al: "Morphology of Central Serotonin Neurons: Brief Review of Quantified Aspects of Their Distribution and Ultrastructural Relationships." *Ann N Y Acad Sci* 600:81–92, 1990. Used with per-mission.

Thus, the serotonergic system meets the criteria for both wide-spread topographic distribution and density of innervation, and as all students of the biology of depression know, a vast database supports the hypothesis that alterations in 5-HT–containing neurons or their recep-tors are intimately involved in the treatment and, perhaps, the patho-genesis of depression (Owens and Nemeroff 1998). These data include the following: 1) decreased concentrations of 5-HT or its major metab-olite 5-hydroxyindoleacetic acid (5-HIAA) in the cerebrospinal fluid (CSF) of medication-free depressed patients; 2) reduced 5-HT uptake and 5-HT transporter binding sites in the brain and platelets of de-pressed patients; 3) increased density of 5-HT$_2$ receptor binding sites in the brain and platelets of depressed patients; 4) reduced plasma concentrations of tryptophan, the 5-HT precursor, in medication-free depressed patients compared with control subjects; 5) blunted neuroendocrine responses to fenfluramine and other serotonergic provocative stimuli in depressed patients compared with control subjects; 6) altered regional CNS glucose use, as revealed by positron emission tomography (PET) in response to fenfluramine, in depressed patients compared with control subjects (Mann et al. 1996); 7) the efficacy of selective serotonin reuptake inhibitors (SSRIs) in the treatment of depression; and 8) the loss of efficacy of SSRIs after tryptophan depletion in depressed patients.

Given this evidence and the efficacy of the SSRIs, why is there such an intensive ongoing search for novel antidepressants? First and foremost, not all depressed patients respond to treatment with these agents. Depending on one's definition of response, approximately 30% of depressed patients do not respond to SSRIs. Such estimates typically use a 50% reduction in one or another depression severity scale as the definition of response. In addition, a sizable group of patients are partial responders—that is, they improve, but certain depressive symptoms such as insomnia, decreased ability to concentrate, or depressed mood persist. In addition, the SSRIs, although clearly a remarkable advance over the older tricyclic antidepressants (TCAs) and monoamine oxidase inhibitors (MAOIs), are not without side effects. Most of these side effects, including nausea and headache, exhibit tachyphylaxis with continued use; other effects, most prominently sexual dysfunction, do not, which is one of the leading reasons that patients discontinue SSRIs during the maintenance phase of antidepressant therapy.

What strategies might be used to circumvent SSRI-induced sexual dysfunction? As discussed in detail by Mansour et al. (1995), the specificity of the 5-HT signal is provided not by differential 5-HT release in different brain areas but by the relative distribution of myriad postsynaptic 5-HT receptors. Table 4–2 summarizes the 5-HT receptors cloned thus far and their CNS mRNA distribution.

The question that has eluded investigators thus far is which 5-HT receptors mediate the SSRI-induced therapeutic effects of increased 5-HT concentrations in the synapse and which mediate the side effects, specifically sexual dysfunction. This knowledge is essential if a new, more selective class of antidepressants that act on serotonergic circuits

TABLE 4–2. *Serotonin (5-HT) receptor protein mRNA distribution*

	Anatomic distribution	Pre- versus postsynaptic
5-HT_{1A}	Limbic brain areas (hippocampus, septum, amygdala) and raphe nuclei (somatodendritic)	Pre- and postsynaptic
5-HT_{1B}	mRNA expression in raphe neurons and hippocampus (CA_1), striatum, and cortex	Pre- and postsynaptic
5-HT_{1D}	mRNA found in hippocampus, striatum, and amygdala	Pre- and postsynaptic
5-HT_{1E}	Binding in human cortex, amygdala, and septum	?
5-HT_{1F}	mRNA found in neocortex, hippocampus, and dorsal raphe	Pre- and postsynaptic
5-HT_{2A}	mRNA localized in neocortex (1.V), claustrum, pontine nuclei, striatum, and hippocampus	Postsynaptic
5-HT_{2B}	mRNA expression in brain (low levels)	?
5-HT_{2C}	High level of mRNA expression in choroid plexus; also expressed in subiculum, hypothalamus, and dorsal raphe	Postsynaptic/ presynaptic?
5-HT_3*	mRNA expression in cortex, hippocampus (CA_1), amygdala, and dorsal raphe	Pre- and postsynaptic
5-HT_4	Binding in hippocampus, striatum, and midbrain	Postsynaptic?
5-HT_6	mRNA found in hippocampus, striatum, nucleus accumbens, and cortex	Postsynaptic
5-HT_7	mRNA expression in hippocampus, hypothalamus, amygdala, and raphe nucleus	Pre- and postsynaptic

*Ligand-gated ion (Ca^{++}) channel.

Source. Reprinted from Mansour A, Chalmers DT, Fox CA, et al.: "Biochemical Anatomy: Insights Into the Cell Biology and Pharmacology of Neurotransmitter Systems in the Brain, in *The American Psychiatric Press Textbook of Psychopharmacology.* Edited by Schatzberg AF, Nemeroff CB. Washington, DC, American Psychiatric Press, 1995, pp 45–63. Used with permission.

is to be developed. Two major strategies have emerged. The first strategy posits development of a novel antidepressant composed of an SSRI and a selective 5-HT receptor antagonist that blocks the action of 5-HT at the receptor that, when activated, causes sexual dysfunction. Unfortunately, that receptor or combination of receptors has not been identified. Nevertheless, this strategy should be successful. For example, although currently cost prohibitive, the $5-HT_3$ receptor antagonists granisetron and ondansetron, which are indicated for the treatment of chemotherapy-induced emesis, block SSRI-induced nausea. There is one case report of granisetron blocking SSRI-induced sexual dysfunction. After the receptor that mediates 5-HT–induced sexual dysfunction is identified definitively, a combination of an antagonist at that receptor coupled with an SSRI should result in the usual SSRI therapeutic effects without this troubling side effect. Such a strategy would be unsuccessful only if the receptor that mediates both the side effect and the therapeutic effect of the SSRI were identical, a possibility considered unlikely by most investigators. Such a combination drug would also confer additional patent life on any given SSRI, with all of the associated financial implications for its manufacturer.

An alternative strategy is the development of a selective 5-HT receptor agonist that acts at the 5-HT receptor believed to mediate the therapeutic effects of the SSRIs. Theoretically, this approach should result in therapeutic efficacy without any of the side effects that have plagued the SSRIs. One likely candidate is the $5-HT_{1A}$ receptor. Several $5-HT_{1A}$ receptor agonists have been developed, including gepirone, ipsapirone, and flesinoxan; however, these three compounds have thus far failed to exhibit sufficient efficacy in the treatment of mood or anxiety disorders to gain approval by regulatory agencies. Virtually all drugs used to treat psychiatric disorders (e.g., antipsychotics and antidepressants) are receptor antagonists or transporter inhibitors. With the exception of benzodiazepines, few psychopharmacologic agents currently in use are receptor agonists, owing partly to the problem of rapid tachyphylaxis to the effects of receptor agonists. This strategy may well be effective if an intermittent dosing schedule to activate, but not downregulate, postsynaptic 5-HT receptors can be developed by the use of, for example, intermittent release from a programmable capsule (as developed by Alza Corporation) during the 18–24 hours of gastrointestinal transport time.

Perhaps if we understood the exact nature of the serotonergic deficit, we could more readily develop novel treatment strategies and better understand why SSRIs and related drugs are effective. Perusal of the data presented in Table 4–1, coupled with the recent report of reduced raphe 5-HT transporter binding (Malison et al. 1997), might shed light on this quest. If one posits a 10% reduction in the number of 5-HT–containing neurons in the raphe nuclei in the brain stem, then a corresponding 10% reduction in the number of 5-HT–containing varicosities in the cerebral cortex would translate into a loss of 5 million of these varicosities in each mm^3 of tissue. Treatment with SSRIs should theoretically increase the concentration of 5-HT in the synaptic cleft, reversing the 5-HT deficiency that is associated with such a reduction in raphe neurons. That is precisely what the single photon emission computed tomography (SPECT) imaging data with β-CIT (2β-carbomethoxy-3β-[4-iodophenyl]tropane) in depressed patients has revealed. If this finding is confirmed with more specific ligands, then we can ask the next logical questions: Do SSRI responders show this deficit preferentially and do SSRI nonresponders not show this finding? And are nonresponders more likely to respond to other antidepressants such as MAOIs, bupropion, or pure norepinephrine uptake inhibitors such as reboxetine? Our group, led by Kilts and Goodman, has recently developed selective and specific ligands for the 5-HT transporter that can be used in SPECT or PET studies. Such experimental approaches may yield the laboratory predictors of response that we have long sought. Such techniques, if successful, would be cost effective because they would result in fewer treatment failures.

Characterization of the 5-HT transporter and the gene that codes for it has allowed for studies of the distribution of both the transporter protein and the mRNA that encodes it (Blakely et al. 1991). Using human endothelial kidney cells that lack any other neurotransmitter transporters or receptors, we have measured the potency of various antidepressants in this system (Owens et al. 1997), largely confirming results obtained previously in brain homogenates (Figure 4–2). Moreover, polymorphisms of the 5-HT transporter have been identified and implicated in certain personality characteristics and in certain psychiatric disorders. Whether these polymorphisms are associated with vulnerability to a mood disorder remains unclear, as does the possibility

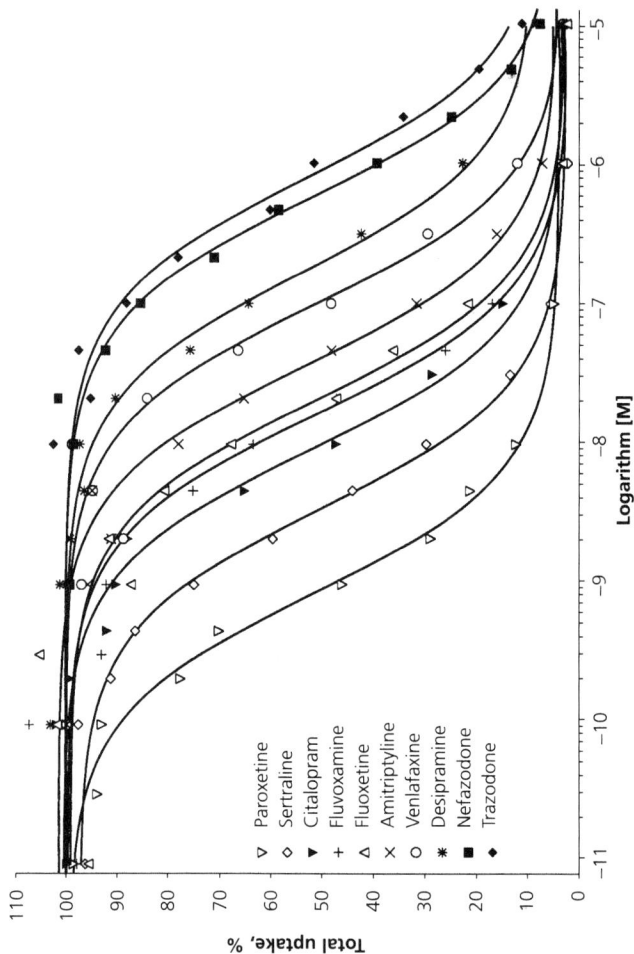

FIGURE 4–2.   Averaged competition curves for 3H-5HT uptake in hSERT cells. The amount of uptake for each individual curve was converted to percentage total uptake, and the mean of three to six separate experiments is plotted as the average curve for each drug.
Source.   Adapted from Owens et al. 1997

that alterations in the transporter gene might confer resistance or susceptibility to affective or anxiety disorders.

As noted earlier in this chapter, overwhelming evidence indicates a preeminent role for alterations in the 5-HT system in the pathophysiology of depression, but it is clearly not the only neurotransmitter system so implicated. For many years the most prominent theory for the pathogenesis of depression was the catecholamine hypothesis originally promulgated by Schildkraut (1965). Similar to the 5-HT system, the norepinephrine projection to the forebrain from the locus coeruleus in the brain stem is topographically diffuse. Considerable evidence supports this norepinephrine hypothesis of mood disorders, including alterations in CSF and urinary metabolites of norepinephrine in depressed patients, as well as altered neuroendocrine (growth hormone) responses to noradrenergic probes such as clonidine. In addition, drugs that block norepinephrine reuptake, such as maprotiline, have long been known as effective antidepressants. With the identification of the norepinephrine transporter and the gene that codes for it, we have been able to use the human endothelial kidney cell cultures described earlier to characterize the effects of various antidepressants (Owens et al. 1997). The results are compatible with previous findings, with a few notable exceptions. One of the results may explain in part why some patients who do not respond to one SSRI may respond to another. Figure 4–3 illustrates our results with the norepinephrine transporter. Note the relatively high potency of paroxetine in inhibiting binding to the norepinephrine transporter (Owens et al. 1997). By our calculations, plasma levels attained in patients given the clinically used dose range of paroxetine will result in measurable norepinephrine reuptake inhibition, and preliminary in vivo studies conducted in our laboratory have confirmed this (Owens et al. 2000).

The same strategy described earlier to diminish the side effects of the SSRIs could also be used to reduce the side effects associated with norepinephrine reuptake inhibitors or 5-HT/norepinephrine reuptake inhibitors. One potential side effect of such agents is hypertension; another is sweating. The combination of a selective norepinephrine uptake inhibitor with a selective antagonist at the adrenergic receptor that mediates these side effects might result in an effective combination with few side effects provided that no new adverse events arise secondary to

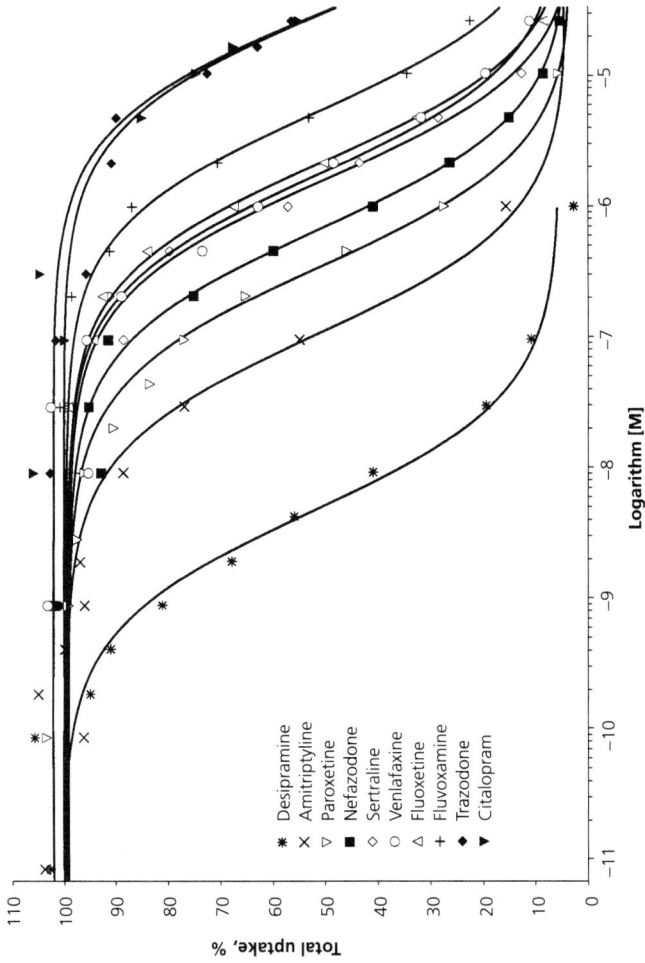

FIGURE 4–3.   Averaged competition curves for 3H-NE uptake in hNET cells. The amount of uptake for each individual curve was converted to percentage total uptake, and the mean of three to six separate experiments is plotted as the average curve for each drug.

Source.   Adapted from Owens et al. 1997

peripheral adrenergic receptor antagonism. Alternatively, an adrenergic receptor agonist acting at the receptor subtype believed to mediate the therapeutic effects of a selective norepinephrine reuptake inhibitor might also represent a successful strategy. Finally, development of a selective PET or SPECT imaging ligand for the norepinephrine transporter might be useful in identifying patients who have norepinephrine neuronal alterations; presumably, these patients would be more likely to respond to norepinephrine uptake inhibitors than to SSRIs. Such a ligand is not yet available.

Neuropeptides in Mood Disorders: Focus on Corticotropin-Releasing Factor

Although evidence of a preeminent role for 5-HT– and norepinephrine-containing circuits in the pathophysiology of depression has increased since the 1960s, an arguably equally impressive literature exists on the contributions of hyperactivity of neurons that use corticotropin-releasing factor (CRF). For reviews of this literature, see Arborelius et al. (1999), Heit et al. (1997), and Nemeroff (1996). In this section we review the evidence that CRF is hypersecreted in depressed patients and discuss the potential therapeutic implications of these findings.

Perhaps the most venerable finding in all of biologic psychiatry is the increase in hypothalamic-pituitary-adrenal (HPA) axis activity in medication-free depressed patients. There is considerable consensus that this endocrinopathy is caused partly, and perhaps largely, by hypersecretion of CRF, the hypothalamic hypophysiotropic hormone that stimulates the secretion of adrenocorticotropic hormone (ACTH) from the anterior pituitary gland. CRF is also found in extrahypothalamic areas, particularly in the areas believed to play a role in the regulation of affect, including the amygdala, cerebral cortex, locus coeruleus, raphe, and other limbic system sites. When injected directly into the CNS of laboratory animals, CRF produces many effects that are similar to the signs and symptoms observed in depressed patients. These signs and symptoms include decreased appetite and weight loss, decreased sexual behavior, decreased sleep, increased neophobia, and psychomotor alterations.

Several investigators have reported that depressed patients exhibit elevated CSF concentrations of CRF (Banki et al. 1987; Nemeroff et al. 1984). Chronic administration of CRF to healthy volunteers results in HPA axis alterations that are virtually indistinguishable from those observed in patients with major depression. Acute administration of CRF to depressed patients results in a blunted ACTH and β-endorphin response (Gold et al. 1986; Holsboer et al. 1984; Krishnan et al. 1993; Young et al. 1990) consistent with the hypothesis of CRF hypersecretion and anterior pituitary CRF receptor downregulation in response to such peptide hypersecretion. Our group has also reported downregulation in CRF receptor number in the frontal cortex of depressed patients compared with control subjects (Nemeroff et al. 1988), and we have recently confirmed this finding. Perhaps the most compelling evidence of CRF hypersecretion in depression has been provided by Raadsheer et al. (1994, 1995). They reported in postmortem brain tissue studies that compared with control subjects, depressed patients exhibit a marked increase in the number of hypothalamic paraventricular neurons that express CRF (1994); in a second study, these authors reported that paraventricular neuron CRF mRNA expression is also markedly elevated in depressed patients compared with control subjects (1995).

What are the therapeutic implications of these findings? First, considerable evidence, provided from studies in our laboratory and studies by our colleague Plotsky, indicates that untoward early life experience is associated with a persistent increase in CRF gene expression and CRF neuronal activity, which may underlie the vulnerability of individuals exposed to child abuse or neglect to develop depression in adulthood (Coplan et al. 1996; Ladd et al. 1996). In preclinical and clinical studies, treatment with antidepressants (paroxetine, fluoxetine, venlafaxine, and mirtazapine) is associated with a reduction in indices of CRF neuronal activity; however, as we noted earlier, the currently available antidepressants are not without side effects. Might a strategy that reduces neurotransmission in CRF-containing circuits represent a novel form of antidepressant treatment? Two CRF receptors (CRF_1 and CRF_2) have been cloned that have distinct distributions in the CNS. Evidence indicates that the recently discovered neuropeptide urocortin is the endogenous ligand for the CRF_2 receptor. Several pharmaceutical companies have developed CRF receptor antagonists as potential novel antidepressants or anxiolytics. The vast majority are CRF_1 receptor antagonists, although at least one selective CRF_2 receptor antagonist has been developed. The first open-label trial of a CRF_1 antagonist for the treatment of major depression has recently been reported, with very promising results (Zobel et al. 2000).

In addition to the CRF receptor antagonist approach, an antisense methodology could theoretically be used to reduce CRF neurotransmission. Antisense technology is increasingly being applied to therapeutics in others areas of medicine (e.g., in the treatment of cystic fibrosis). What is antisense technology, and how can it be applied to the development of novel treatments of depression? Once a gene sequence is known, the complementary mRNA sequence that the gene encodes is also known. An antisense probe, usually of 15–25 bases in length, directed against the mRNA sequence will prevent translation of the protein encoded by the gene. We first demonstrated in vitro a reduction in pituitary CRF binding site density (Owens et al. 1995) after exposure to a CRF antisense probe. Almost simultaneously, Holsboer's group demonstrated anxiolytic effects of a CRF receptor antisense probe after direct intra-amygdaloid injection in rats (Liebsch et al. 1995).

Molecular Neurobiology

The theoretical specificity associated with antisense knockdown techniques is just one aspect of the powerful tools that molecular biology has made available to modern neuroscience. Although not a be-all and end-all, laboratory techniques that target DNA and RNA have led to revolutionary developments in neuroscience. Three techniques that are, or we believe will be, important are broadly termed *transgenic animals*, *gene chips/arrays*, and *viral-vector-mediated gene transfer*.

Through the process of homologous recombination, specific genes can be induced to be overexpressed or, more commonly, switched with nonfunctioning versions of the genes (called knockout genes). These nonfunctioning versions do not produce a functional gene product. Although functional adaptations may sometimes render interpretation difficult, knockout animals represent one means by which the function of any protein in the brain can be assessed. As shown at the level of the hypothalamus in Figure 4–4, a homologous oxytocin knockout mouse completely lacks oxytocin immunoreactivity compared with normal levels in wild-type mice.

It has become quite clear that a single biochemical abnormality does not account for any of the major psychiatric illnesses. Moreover, none of the few hundred proteins in the brain (e.g., receptors, enzymes) that have been studied have unequivocally been linked to the pathophysiology or treatment of psychiatric illnesses. Proteins that have been studied, or rather have been amenable to study, represent a minority of the many proteins produced in the brain. Recently developed techniques, including differential-display reverse transcriptase polymerase chain reaction (RTPCR), RNA fingerprinting, and gene chips/arrays, allow relatively efficient screening for RNA species that are differentially expressed among various experimental groups (see Watson and Akil 1999 for review). These techniques are now allowing investigators to find known and unknown proteins that are differentially expressed in control versus ill groups or in response to pharmacotherapy even in a single cell. It is expected that these techniques will identify novel targets for medications development.

Following identification of appropriate genes for targeting, virally mediated gene transfer can allow for direct modification of gene expression. Although a number of nuances relate to timing and localization of the gene targeting, the technique works via the ability of a virus to insert the genetic information it carries into the host's genome. In the laboratory, several types of viruses are modified to be made nonvirulent, and specific genetic material from laboratory animals or humans is incorporated into the viral vectors. When these viral vectors are injected into specific regions of the brain, for example, the viral particles, through their normal mechanisms, invade cells or neurons near the injection site and incorporate their genetic material into the host's. The artificial gene is then expressed in the host cell for variable amounts of time. Akin to the studies using transgenic animals, genes of interest can then be made to be overexpressed or knocked down. Unlike transgenic animals in which homeostatic changes are thought to sometimes cloud the issue regarding the function of specific gene products, viral-vector-mediated gene transfer can be performed at select locations, times, and lengths of treatment. Thus, in the absence of selective, small-molecule

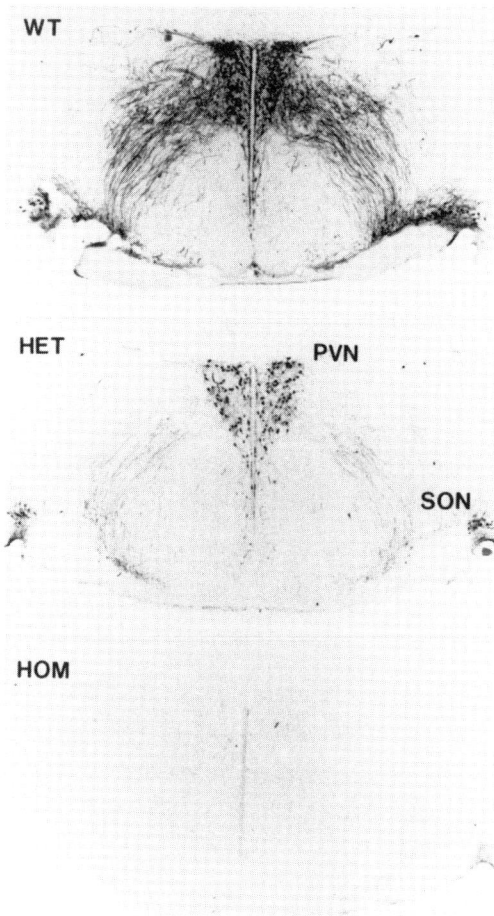

FIGURE 4–4. Immunocytochemistry reveals hypothalamic oxytocin-containing neurons in the mouse. The top panel shows pronounced oxytocin immunoreactivity in paraventricular (PVN) neurons and their efferents in a wild-type (WT), or control, mouse. The middle panel shows significantly reduced oxytocin immunoreactivity in a heterologous (HET) knockout (one of the two alleles is nonfunctional). The bottom panel reveals a complete absence of oxytocin immunoreactivity in a homologous (HOM) knockout. The absence is for the entire body and not just in the hypothalamus. SON = supraoptic nucleus.
Source. Young LJ, Winslow JT, Wang Z, et al.: "Gene Targeting Approaches to Neuroendocrinology: Oxytocin, Maternal Behavior, and Affiliation." *Hormones and Behavior* 31:221–231, 1997. Used with permission.

drugs, this technique or modifications of it may be used in selectively modifying the production of important proteins in the CNS. Even if additional research determines that this approach is not technically feasible as a therapeutic modality in humans, we expect to learn much about the roles of various brain peptides and proteins in the pathophysiology and treatment response of many psychiatric illnesses.

Neurogenesis

Although it is well known that neurons are plastic in nature and can form new connections, it was previously thought that the adult human brain did not produce new neurons. Landmark research has shown that neurogenesis does occur in adult primate brain and that environmental and chemical factors can modify neurogenesis (Eriksson et al. 1998; Gould et al. 1999; Kempermann and Gage 1999). Neurobiologists have known that considerable neural regeneration occurs in the damaged brain of reptiles and other lower vertebrates. More discrete neurogenesis (i.e., in limited regions of the brain) has been demonstrated in songbirds and rodents, but only recently has neurogenesis, so far limited to the hippocampus, been observed in mature primate brain. In the dentate gyrus of the hippocampus, unspecialized neuronal stem cells are found at the boundary of the granule cell layer and hilus. These stem cells continuously replicate and can migrate into the granule cell layer, where they can differentiate into granule cells that send out normal dendrites and axons along paths used by neighboring granule cells. This process is complex in that various factors control the survival of the immature stem cell progeny, their migration into the granule cell layer, and ultimately their differentiation into mature neurons. Recent studies have shown that neurotransmitters, glucocorticoids, and environmental conditions that alter neurotransmission (e.g., novelty, learning) potently regulate these processes.

We foresee that in the near future, therapy aimed at modifying this process either through growth factor augmentation of stem cell proliferation or through conscious efforts at limiting environmental factors that inhibit neurogenesis (e.g., stress) will become increasingly important. Finally, it has recently become possible to harvest and grow human embryonic stem cells, which may lay the foundation for transplantation studies that may be of great benefit for the treatment of various neurodegenerative diseases (Pedersen 1999).

Conclusion

Since the introduction of the first antidepressant in the late 1950s, the field has witnessed remarkable progress. We have developed safer and more selective antidepressants, and we will undoubtedly improve on these successes. Advances in diverse subfields of neurobiology most certainly will contribute to further advances. Whether these future advances are discovered from studies of signal transduction, growth factors, receptor cycling, cytokines, or novel proteins remains unclear. What is quite clear is that the future of this field is indeed bright.

References

Arborelius L, Owens MJ, Plotsky PM, et al: The role of corticotropin-releasing factor in depression and anxiety disorders. J Endocrinol 160:1–12, 1999

Banki CM, Bissette G, Arato M, et al: Cerebrospinal fluid corticotropin-releasing factor–like immunoreactivity in depression and schizophrenia. Am J Psychiatry 144:873–877, 1987

Blakely RD, Berson HE, Fremeau RT, et al: Cloning and expression of a functional serotonin transporter from rat brain. Nature 354:66–70, 1991

Coplan JD, Andrews MW, Rosenblum LA, et al: Persistent elevations of cerebrospinal fluid concentrations of corticotropin-releasing factor in adult non-human primates exposed to early life stressors: implications for the pathophysiology of mood and anxiety disorders. Proc Natl Acad Sci U S A 93:1619–1623, 1996

Descarries L, Audet M, Doucet G, et al: Morphology of central serotonin neurons: brief review of quantified aspects of their distribution and ultrastructural relationships. Ann N Y Acad Sci 600:81–92, 1990

Eriksson PS, Perfilieva E, Bjork-Eriksson T, et al: Neurogenesis in the adult human hippocampus. Nat Med 4:1313–1317, 1998

Gold PW, Loriaux DL, Roy A, et al: Responses to corticotropin-releasing hormones in the hypercortisolism of depression and Cushing's disease: pathophysiologic and diagnostic implications. N Engl J Med 314:1329–1335, 1986

Gould E, Beylin A, Tanapat P, et al: Learning enhances adult neurogenesis in the hippocampal formation. Nature Neuroscience 2:260–265, 1999

Heit S, Owens MJ, Plotsky P, et al: Corticotropin-releasing factor, stress, and depression. The Neuroscientist 3:186–194, 1997

Holsboer F, von Bardelieben V, Gerker A, et al: Blunted corticotropin and normal cortisol response to human corticotropin-releasing factor in depression. N Engl J Med 311:1127, 1984

Kempermann G, Gage FH: New nerve cells for the adult brain. Sci Am 280:48–53, 1999

Krishnan KRR, Rayasam K, Reed D, et al: The corticotropin-releasing factor stimulation test in patients with major depression: relationship to dexamethasone suppression test results. Depression 1:133–136, 1993

Ladd CO, Owens MJ, Nemeroff CB: Persistent changes in corticotropin-releasing factor neuronal systems induced by maternal deprivation. Endocrinology 137:1212–1218, 1996

Liebsch G, Landraf R, Gerstberger R, et al: Chronic infusion of a CRH1 receptor antisense oligodeoxynucleotide into the central nucleus of the amygdala reduced anxiety-related behavior in socially defeated rats. Regul Pept 59:229–239, 1995

Malison RT, Pelton G, Carpenter L, et al: Reduced midbrain serotonin transporter binding in depressed vs healthy subjects as measured by [^{123}I] β-CIT SPECT (abstract). Neuroscience 23:1220, 1997

Mann JJ, Malone KM, Diehl DM, et al: Demonstration in vivo of reduced serotonin responsivity in the brain of untreated depressed patients. Am J Psychiatry 153:174–182, 1996

Mansour A, Chalmers DT, Fox CA, et al: Biochemical anatomy: insights into the cell biology and pharmacology of neurotransmitter systems in the brain, in The American Psychiatric Press Textbook of Psychopharmacology. Edited by Schatzberg AF, Nemeroff CB. Washington, DC, American Psychiatric Press, 1995, pp 45–63

Nemeroff CB: The corticotropin-releasing factor (CRF) hypothesis of depression: new findings and new directions. Molecular Psychiatry 1:336–342, 1996

Nemeroff CB, Widerlov E, Bissette G, et al: Elevated concentrations of CSF corticotropin-releasing factor–like immunoreactivity in depressed patients. Science 226:1342–1344, 1984

Nemeroff CB, Knight DL, Krishnan KRR, et al: Marked reduction in the number of platelet [^{3}H]-imipramine binding sites in geriatric depression. Arch Gen Psychiatry 45:919–923, 1988

Owens MJ, Nemeroff CB: The serotonin transporter and depression. Depression 8 (suppl 1):5–12, 1998

Owens MJ, Mulcahey JJ, Kasckow JW, et al: Exposure to an antisense oligonucleotide decreases CRF receptor binding in rat pituitary cultures. J Neurochem 64:2358–2361, 1995

Owens MJ, Morgan WN, Plott SJ, et al: Neurotransmitter receptor and transporter binding profile of antidepressants and their metabolites. J Pharmacol Exp Ther 283:1305–1322, 1997

Owens MJ, Knight DL, Nemeroff CB: Paroxetine binding to the rat norepinephrine transporter in vivo. Biol Psychiatry 47:842–845, 2000

Pedersen RA: Embryonic stem cells for medicine. Sci Am 280(4):68–73, 1999

Raadsheer FC, Hoogendijk JJ, Stam FC, et al: Increased number of corticotropin-releasing hormone neurons in the hypothalamic paraventricular nucleus of depressed patients. Neuroendocrinology 60:436–444, 1994

Raadsheer FC, van Heerikhuize JJ, Lucassen PJ, et al: Increase corticotropin-releasing hormone (CRH) mRNA in paraventricular nucleus of patients with Alzheimer's disease or depression. Am J Psychiatry 152:1372–1376, 1995

Schildkraut JJ: The catecholamine hypothesis of affective disorders: a review of supportive evidence. Am J Psychiatry 122:509–522, 1965

Watson SJ, Akil H: Gene chips and arrays revealed: a primer on their power and their uses. Biol Psychiatry 45:533–543, 1999

Young EA, Watson SJ, Kotun J, et al: β-lipotropin/β-endorphin response to low dose ovine corticotropin-releasing factor in endogenous depression. Arch Gen Psychiatry 47:449ñ457, 1990

Zobel A, Nickel T, Künzel H, et al: Effects of the high affinity corticotropin-releasing hormone receptor 1 antagonist R121919 in major depression: the first 20 patients treated. J Psychiatr Res 34:171–181, 2000

CHAPTER 5

Genetic Science and Depression

Implications for Research and Treatment

Steven E. Hyman, M.D.

Steven O. Moldin, Ph.D.

Summary

Data from family, twin, and adoption studies demonstrate the involvement of genetic factors in the transmission of major depression. However, the mode of inheritance is complex, and familial transmission is not accounted for by a single major gene. Indeed, the evidence to date suggests that vulnerability is produced by multiple loci of small effect, some of which may have small independent additive effects and others of which may act epistatically. In addition, nongenetic effects appear to play a role both in creating vulnerability and in triggering episodes. As a result, the correlation between genotype and phenotype is obscured; that is, genotype is connected to phenotype more loosely in depression than it is in illnesses such as Huntington disease. Despite these challenges, as the Human Genome Project and other initiatives provide denser genetic maps, faster sequencing methods, state-of-the-art DNA array technologies, and full-length complementary DNA (cDNA) clones containing an entire protein coding sequence, the stage will be set for a new era of gene identification and functional studies in psychiatry. Perhaps of greatest relevance to clinical care is the promise the isolation of vulnerability genes holds for significantly advancing drug discovery and individualized treatment selection. This current genetic revolution will have major public health implications and is expected to revolutionize our understanding of pathophysiology, diagnosis, treatment, and ultimately prevention of major depression.

Genetic factors contribute to virtually every human disease by conferring susceptibility or resistance, affecting the severity or progression of disease, and interacting with environmental factors that modify disease course and expression. Much of current biomedical research is based on the expectation that understanding the genetic basis of disease will revolutionize diagnosis, treatment, and prevention. Human molecular genetics may ultimately prove to be the single most powerful tool we have for understanding how the brain malfunctions in depression and other mental disorders (Hyman 1999). Defining and understanding the role of genetic factors in depression will also facilitate our ability to understand environmental contributions that interact with genes to cause disease.

Tremendous advances have occurred in mapping and cloning genes for rare diseases that are attributable to a single major locus, so-called Mendelian disorders (Bassett et al. 1997). In a historical trend that would have defied credulity not long ago, systematic discovery of these disease genes has generally occurred without any prior biologic knowledge of how they function. In contrast, the discovery of genes that influence vulnerability to major depression, schizophrenia, bipolar disorder, autism, and other mental disorders has proceeded slowly (Risch and Botstein 1996; Risch et al. 1999). The complex etiology of these diseases, in which vulnerability is produced by the interaction of multiple genes of small effect and nongenetic factors, poses major challenges for gene hunters and for the neurobiologists, pharmacologists, and epidemiologists who hope to use those genes.

A common assumption is that the biggest direct clinical payoff from discovering genes for depression will be the development of a genetic test, presumably used to identify at-risk individuals. However, the greater the level of complexity underlying the penetrance of a disease phenotype and the manner in which it is expressed, the lesser the likelihood of a truly useful predictive test. The greatest benefits from genetic research are likely to result from the generation of powerful new tools to understand pathophysiology, development of new therapeutic compounds, and a revitalization of the epidemiologic study of risk. In this chapter, we briefly review our knowledge of the genetics of depression and discuss new genomic tools and technologies (Table 5–1) that will be brought to bear to understand the etiology and pathophysiology of depression. (Burmeister [1999] provides nongeneticists with a useful review of basic terminology and concepts used when studying complex genetic diseases.) Finally, we discuss how such tools and technologies may be used to develop new compounds and enhance the efficiency of drug regimens.

Genetic Basis of Depression

Various research designs are used to investigate genetic and nongenetic factors that produce disease vulnerability. Family studies implicate genes as the source of familial aggregation of a disorder; twin and adoption studies specifically test the hypothesis that familial aggregation is attributable to genetic effects.

Major depression is a familial disorder in which the risk to first-degree relatives of depressed probands ranges from 5% to 25% across several studies (Moldin et al. 1991; Tsuang and Faraone 1990). This risk is significantly greater than the risk to first-degree relatives of control subjects (Gershon et al. 1975, 1982; Weissman et al. 1984; Winokur et al. 1982).

Adoption studies support the role of heredity in disease transmission (Cadoret 1978; Mendlewicz and Rainer 1977; Wender et al. 1986), as do twin studies. The monozygotic twin concordance rate of about 40% for unipolar depression is more than twice the corresponding dizygotic concordance rate (Allen et al. 1974; Bertelsen et al. 1977; Kendler et al. 1992; McGuffin et al. 1996; Torgersen 1986), clearly implicating genetic factors. Twin studies also implicate nongenetic factors, given concordance rates of less than 100% in monozygotic twins (who share 100% of their DNA). Twin studies have shown that vulnerability to major depression is produced by both genetic and nongenetic factors but that the

TABLE 5–1.   *Genomic tools to be applied in the study of major depression*

Tool	Description	Application
Genetic maps	Physical and genetic maps of ESTs and STSs	Discover vulnerability genes
SNPs	Sequence variation at a single nucleotide base	Discover vulnerability genes; identify new drug targets
Genome-wide association analysis	Analytic method to search for differences in the frequencies of specific genetic variants	Discover vulnerability genes
Complete human DNA sequence	Finished sequence of the genome, including the identification and location of all human genes	Discover vulnerability genes; identify new drug targets
Full-length cDNAs	DNA sequence complementary to mRNA, containing the entire protein coding sequence of a gene	Study gene expression patterns in the brain; understand gene and protein function
DNA arrays	An ordered set of DNA molecules used for the automated matching of known and unknown DNA samples, based on base-pairing rules	Study gene expression profiles; screen for disease mutations; discover and score SNPs; simultaneously genotype hundreds of SNPs; identify new drug targets

Note.   ESTs = expressed sequence tags; SNPs = single nucleotide polymorphisms; STSs = sequence tagged sites.

nongenetic factors are not caused by the shared familial environment (McGuffin et al. 1996). Although these nongenetic factors may include specific environmental events (that would ultimately be targets of preventive interventions), we cannot rule out epigenetic effects such as chemical modifications of DNA (e.g., methylation [Surani 1998]) and stochastic (random) factors that act during brain development.

Analyses of patterns of familial aggregation have failed to unambiguously support a single major locus (Cox et al. 1989; Crowe et al. 1981; Goldin et al. 1983; Marazita et al. 1997; Price et al. 1987; Tsuang et al. 1985). The proportion of genetic variance in familial risk to depression, termed *heritability*, is moderate, but estimates vary considerably from 40% to 70% (Kendler et al. 1992; McGuffin et al. 1996; Thapar and McGuffin 1994). Such imprecision is thought to reflect the roles of both etiologic heterogeneity and differences across studies in the definition of depression. The broad diagnostic category of major depression described in DSM-IV (American Psychiatric Association 1994) is useful for current clinical purposes but is not optimal for genetic studies.

Researchers have sought clinical criteria to identify subtypes of depressed patients who have familial unipolar illness. Perhaps the most promising subclassification is based on patients with early onset depression (typically before age 20 or 30 years) who have a history of recurrent episodes. Relatives of probands with early onset recurrent depression show increased risk for depression (Bland et al. 1986; Kupfer et al. 1989), and early onset depression is more heritable in twins than is late onset depression (Lyons et al. 1998). Rates of mood disorder are nearly twice as high in the first-degree relatives of children with prepubertal-onset major depression with recurrence (60%) than in first-degree relatives with no recurrence of major depression (Weissman et al. 1999). Analyses in a large twin sample identified the number of previous episodes as a significant predictor of risk for major depression (Kendler et al. 1999).

Molecular Genetic Studies

The goal of molecular genetic studies is the identification and cloning of vulnerability genes. A first stage in such studies is the identification of chromosomal regions that appear to contain a genetic locus that contributes to vulnerability. The genetic analysis of family data by linkage methods has been successful in establishing the chromosomal localization of a large number of disorders that are caused by a single major locus (Ott 1991). In this approach, investigators look within families for coinheritance of chromosomal regions linked to a disease or other trait of interest. With genes of small effect size, however, or with genes that exert no effect in the absence of other genes, such linkage methods lack the power to define loci involved in genetically complex phenotypes such as mood disorders (Risch and Merikangas 1996).

Another approach is to identify a candidate gene, based on knowledge of pathogenesis, and test the hypothesis that the gene is a vulner- ability gene by conducting association analysis in unrelated affected individuals and control subjects (Burmeister 1999; Spielman et al. 1993). The study of individual candidate genes, such as genes encoding neurotransmitter receptors or transporters, has proved frustrating in psy- chiatric genetics in general and in mood disorders in particular be- cause, given our current knowledge of pathophysiology, convincing candidates are lacking. Most candidates have been based on the action of antidepressant drugs, which is widely acknowledged as a weak source of clues about pathogenesis. For example, the report of an association between unipolar depression and a polymorphism in the human sero- tonin transporter gene on chromosome 17q (Ogilvie et al. 1996) has been followed by two nonreplications (Kunugi et al. 1996; Stober et al. 1996). A weak and nonreplicated association between depression and the dopamine D4 receptor gene has been found in another sample (Manki et al. 1996).

In summary, the mode of inheritance of major depression is complex, and if transmission is caused by a single major locus in any family, we have not yet detected such a locus. At least for most families, multiple genes of small effect in interaction with one another (Frankel and Schork 1996) and with nongenetic events during brain development produce a com- plex vulnerability to the disorder. A subtype of depression, defined by re- current episodes and early age at onset, holds promise as the basis of a phenotype for molecular genetic studies, but the subtype has not been ad- equately delimited. Future gene discovery and the application of knowl- edge gained to the development of new treatments and therapeutic regimens will require the application of state-of-the-art tools and technol- ogies developed in the sciences of *genomics* (the study of genomes) and *genetics* (the study of how genetic variation contributes to phenotypic dif- ferences). Before discussing these exciting developments, we present a brief discussion of key molecular genetics concepts to facilitate under- standing of the neurobiology of gene action in the brain.

Genes and the Genome

DNA contains the human genetic blueprint. It transmits information across generations and is the repository of information needed for both the development of an organism and for the cells within that organism in interaction with environmental signals. DNA is a linear polymer; its information is contained in its sequence of nucleotide bases. This physical arrangement makes it an ideal template for the synthesis of other macromolecules by the sequential reading of its order of DNA nucleotides. Although the DNA double helix is ideal for stable information storage and transfer, its chemical simplicity and relative rigidity mean that the information it contains must be expressed through other molecules—RNA and protein. DNA is transcribed to produce both structural RNA molecules and messenger RNAs (mRNAs) that are the required intermediates in the synthesis of proteins, the key building blocks of cells.

Within cells, DNA is organized into very long molecules called *chromosomes*, in which the DNA is associated with both structural and regulatory proteins. The human genome comprises 23 pairs of chromosomes—one pair that determines gender and 22 remaining pairs of identical chromosomes (*autosomes*). Genes are stretches of DNA that encode a single structural RNA or a single mRNA that can be translated (depending on how it is processed or spliced) into one or more proteins. Genes themselves contain two classes of sequences: 1) regions that are transcribed into RNA molecules and 2) regulatory regions that are not transcribed but that control the time, place, and level at which a gene is transcribed. Mutations in DNA sequence within the regulatory or coding regions of genes may alter the timing, cell type, or spatial location in which a structural RNA or protein is expressed. They may also result in failure to express the protein or in the expression of an altered protein with loss of function or with a new function that might be adaptive, neutral, or toxic to cells. Such mutations may produce significant alterations in phenotype.

The total number of human genes has been estimated at 60,000–100,000 (Fields et al. 1994; Rowen et al. 1997), of which at least 30,000 unique genes have been placed on a publicly available genetic-physical map (Deloukas et al. 1998). In fact, most of the DNA that comprises chromosomes is void of genes. It is estimated that only approximately 4% of the human genome is occupied by genes and that genes are not spread evenly across the genome. There are gene-rich chromosomes and chromosomal regions as well as gene-poor regions. Mutations outside of genes have unknown, if any, biologic consequence. As a result, diminished selection pressure is placed on these regions, and they may have a higher mutation rate than DNA regions within genes.

The DNA contents of specific cell types are virtually identical; what makes the cell types different is the pattern of genes expressed in the cell. Because of the extreme diversity of cell types in the brain, a large percentage of the genome is expressed in the brain. Some genes are common ones that are essential for general cell maintenance (house-keeping genes); the expression of others may be restricted largely to a specific cell type (tissue-specific gene expression). This differential expression results from the earlier-described action of the control regions within DNA.

Gene Mapping

Central to current efforts in human genetics is a reference sequence of the entire human genome, which will be the main product of the Human Genome Project (see next section). A reference mouse sequence will follow soon after. The ability to compare two mammalian genomes will have an enormous impact on our ability to extract information because conservation of sequences across evolutionary time is an important indicator of functional importance. In addition, substantial efforts have been made in the public and private sectors to provide a comprehensive catalog of human DNA sequence variation. After all, the impact of variation on individual phenotypes is at the heart of genetics. Our knowledge of the genomic location and sequence of individual genes ultimately will intersect with our knowledge of sequence variation within the genome, providing genetic tools of enormous power.

Before the 1980s, the idea of constructing comprehensive human genetic maps was only a distant dream. Human genetics is descriptive rather than experimental in the sense that breeding experiments to examine whether two loci are linked is out of the question. In the pre–molecular biology era this left only the possibility of constructing genetic maps based on polymorphic markers that could be detected at the protein level. These maps would be useful if they represented loci at which at least two *alleles* (alternate forms of a gene differing in DNA sequence) were present at significant frequencies in the population and if these alleles were not necessarily related to disease or to gene action. As long as the markers were adequately polymorphic and showed segregation patterns predicted by Mendel's laws, a map could be constructed. The problem was with the limited number of suitable polymorphic markers that could be readily detected at the protein level at the time, notably blood group, human leukocyte antigen type, and serum protein markers.

With the introduction of the tools of molecular biology and the ability to sequence DNA, the scientific community became aware of the existence of a substantial level of variation in DNA sequence that occurs naturally in mammalian populations. Botstein et al. (1980) proposed to treat differences in the DNA sequence (whether or not they occurred in genes; more commonly they did not) like allelic variants of a gene and to use them as genetic markers for mapping. Based on a molecular technique described by Southern (1975), these differences could be visualized using restriction enzymes with different sequence specificities that cut genomic DNA into fragments of various lengths. Polymorphisms obtained in this fashion are called *restriction fragment length polymorphisms* (RFLPs); they generally represent anonymous markers (i.e., sequences of DNA that have no known biologic function).

The next breakthrough came as a result of the identification of markers far more polymorphic and easier to detect than RFLPs. Minisatellite markers of intermediate size and smaller microsatellite markers were identified that are easily detected by polymerase chain reaction methods. When the chromosomal location of a marker, such as a unique microsatellite marker, is known, it is referred to as a sequence tagged site (STS). Readily detected STSs now form the basis of the human physical map.

Markers of various types can be placed on two distinct types of maps—linkage and physical—that can be derived for each chromosome in the genome. Linkage and physical maps are distinguished by the methods by which they are derived and the metrics that are used for measuring distances on them. In theory, these maps should provide consistent and closely related information on chromosomal assignment and the ordering of loci.

Linkage maps can be constructed only for loci that occur in two or more alleles. The linkage map assigns the relative order of loci and the distances that separate them, as measured in centimorgans (cM). Linkage maps have been enormously valuable in assigning genes that cause Mendelian human diseases to relatively small areas on chromosomes. As a genetic distance the centimorgan represents a variable physical distance as measured in base pairs.

All physical maps are based on the direct analysis of DNA. Physical distances between loci are measured in terms of DNA base pairs (bp), 1,000 base pairs (kilobase; Kb), or 1 million base pairs (megabase; Mb). The entire human genome is 3,000 Mb, or 3 billion base pairs. A map consisting of data from over 41,000 STSs, representing about 30,000 human genes, has been assembled (Deloukas et al. 1998). Physical maps are used to examine in more detail the chromosomal regions implicated in genetic studies to determine the precise location of the disease gene.

The Human Genome Project

The Human Genome Project is an international effort with the ultimate aim of determining the complete human DNA sequence. The impact of having a complete sequence will be profound; the genetic capacity of the human organism will become entirely known and researchers will have the opportunity to find and study every genetic element. This multi-billion-dollar multiyear effort began in the 1980s and was planned in the United States by the Department of Energy and the National Institutes of Health (NIH). Initially, major goals included 1) completion of a high-resolution linkage map, which was accomplished in 1994 (Cooperative Human Linkage Center 1994); 2) completion of an ordered map of 30,000 STSs at a resolution of 100 kb; and 3) determination of the complete DNA sequence of the human genome. Work continues to progress on identifying genes in the mouse, the premier model system for studies of mammalian development.

In 1998, a new plan for the Human Genome Project was presented in which human DNA sequencing would be the major emphasis (Collins et al. 1999). The plan also included goals for sequencing technology development; for studying human genome sequence variation; for developing technology for functional genomics; for completing the sequence of two model systems (*Caenorhabditis elegans* and *Drosophila*) and the mouse genome; for studying the ethical, legal, and social implications of genome research; for initiating bioinformatics studies; and for the training of genome scientists. Sequencing goals for the human genome were revised recently to complete a working draft by spring 2000 and an accurate, finished version by 2003 (Marshall 1999a). As announced by President Clinton on June 26, 2000 (http://www.white-house.gov/WH/New/html/20000626.html), a "rough draft" of the human genome has been completed by the international Human Genome Project and a private company (Celera Genomics). Although additional work will be required to produce a "finished," highly accurate sequence, completion of this rough draft is a landmark scientific achievement that will be a critical milestone in deciphering the specific function of individual genes.

Human DNA Sequence Variation

Natural DNA sequence variation is found in all genomes. The most common polymorphisms in the human genome are single base-pair differences, termed *single nucleotide polymorphisms* (SNPs; pronounced "snips") (Chakravarti 1998; Collins et al. 1997; Lander 1996; Risch and Merikangas 1996). Their density in the human genome is estimated to be on average 1 per 1,000 base pairs; hence, several million exist and it is estimated that, on average, four SNPs may be found in each human gene. SNPs that affect biologic functions occur both within control or protein-coding regions of genes and outside such regions. According to recent reports, about half of SNPs found in coding regions are protein altering (Cargill et al. 1999; Halushka et al. 1999). Of greatest interest to researchers studying depression will be the protein-altering SNPs that occur within genes expressed in brain regions of interest.

Because of their abundance and wide distribution across the genome as well as their potential for large-scale automated analysis, SNPs will be critical for genetic studies of complex diseases such as depression. Rather than conducting association analyses by choosing candidate genes, researchers may use a systematic, brute-force approach to association analysis by surveying thousands of SNPs to search for variants in disease genes across the entire genome. (Association studies look for differences in the frequencies of specific genetic variants between unrelated affected individuals and control subjects [Burmeister 1999].)

The greatest value of SNPs for gene discovery will be their use in whole-genome association studies, of which there are two types (Collins et al. 1997). *Direct association analysis* assumes that the SNP variant in question has a causative role in disease; *indirect association analysis* (also called linkage disequilibrium mapping) assumes that the SNP in question is in the neighborhood of an altered gene that has a causative role. Direct association approaches require the identification of all biologically significant variations within human genes. The indirect strategy of linkage disequilibrium mapping requires a dense SNP map, for which thousands of SNPs across the genome are analyzed in a highly parallel and cost-effective manner (e.g., by using DNA arrays; see next section). Such whole-genome association studies have been proposed as a powerful approach for detecting the subtle effects of genes that confer susceptibility to mental disorders and other common, complex diseases (Collins et al. 1997; Lander 1996; Risch and Merikangas 1996). As many as 500,000 SNPs may be required for whole-genome studies (Kruglyak 1999).

As part of the Human Genome Project, new technologies for rapid, large-scale identification and scoring of hundreds of thousands of SNPs are being developed. Exciting collaborations have been developed between academic laboratories and biotechnology companies. The greatest utility of these approaches involves the marriage of large-scale automated analysis with DNA array technologies (see next section). Ten large pharmaceutical companies and the Wellcome Trust in the United Kingdom have established a consortium to discover 300,000 SNPs (Marshall 1999b).

Functional Analysis

The Human Genome Project, along with parallel efforts to identify expressed sequences—both expressed sequence tags (ESTs) and full-length cDNAs—will enable neuroscientists and other biologists to study the expression of genes (and eventually proteins) on a global scale, across the entire genome. *Functional genomics* refers to a broad range of methods that permit the elucidation of patterns of gene expression that result from the interaction of different genomes with their environments. Similar systematic studies of proteins have been termed *proteomics*. Large-scale characterization of gene transcripts expressed in the human brain and their protein products will greatly accelerate our understanding of underlying biologic mechanisms in the normal human brain that may be disturbed in major depression. Functional genomics approaches typically involve isolating mRNA from tissue and then reverse transcribing it into DNA. This approach produces a cDNA that is complementary to the mRNA transcript found in the tissue. cDNAs are organized into libraries, which are representative collection of copies of transcripts from a given tissue.

A new project, the Brain Molecular Anatomy Project, sponsored by the National Institute of Mental Health (NIMH) and the National Institute of Neurobiological Disorders and Stroke (NINDS), is aimed at accelerating the discovery of genes expressed in the mammalian brain and placing these genes on anatomic and genetic maps. cDNA libraries have been created using tissue from the spinal cord and 10 specific brain regions of interest (prefrontal cortex, hippocampus, hypothalamus, amygdala, striatum, basal ganglia, brain stem, cerebellum, olfactory bulb, and pineal gland). To date, more than 20,000 ESTs have been generated from this project; these represent about 11,000 unique mouse genes, of which half are newly discovered.

Full-length cDNAs that contain the entire protein sequence are needed to study and understand the function of the protein encoded by the gene and to make functional genetically altered (transgenic) mice. The NIH has launched an initiative to generate a complete set of such full-length cDNA clones and their sequences for all human, mouse, and other mammalian genes. The goal is to make many valuable resources—sequences, clones, annotation of gene function and structure, and analytical tools—available to the scientific community; it is anticipated that such resources will be widely used and highly valuable to neuroscientists.

A new technology is revolutionizing how neuroscientists study genes. DNA *arrays*, or DNA (gene) chips, are fabricated by high-speed robotics on glass or nylon substrates, for which probes are used to determine complementary binding (Chee et al. 1996; Watson and Akil 1999). This technology provides a systematic way to survey DNA and

RNA variation across the entire genome. An experiment with a single DNA array can dramatically increase throughput and provide researchers with information on thousands of genes simultaneously. These arrays are likely to become a standard tool for both molecular biologic research and clinical diagnostics (Lander 1999). Array technology has expanded rapidly with investments from the public and private sectors and has been applied to quantifying in a highly parallel way gene expression profiles (Lipshutz et al. 1999), screening for disease mutations with pronounced allelic heterogeneity (Hacia et al. 1996), comparing genomes of different organisms (Behr et al. 1999), discovering and scoring SNPs (Cargill et al. 1999; Halushka et al. 1999), simultaneously genotyping hundreds of SNPs (Wang et al. 1998), and identifying appropriate targets for therapeutic interventions (Debouck and Goodfellow 1999). We expect comparable applications of arrays in the study of depression and other mental disorders, making use of both animal models and postmortem human tissues.

Genetically Informed Therapeutics

The greatest benefit from genetic research is likely to come in the development of platforms for drug discovery and for understanding the genetic contributions to drug action. Because genes are the blueprints that code for the protein building blocks of cells, the discovery of alleles that confer vulnerability to depression or other diseases will direct attempts to compensate for the resulting alterations in expression pattern or function of the affected protein. Moreover, because proteins interact with one another within cells, identification of vulnerability genes will direct attention to biochemical pathways that could provide multiple targets for new therapies.

Many pharmaceutical companies are now intensely interested in the search for complex disease genes. Given a conservative estimate of 500–1,000 unique genes that contribute to risk for 100 important multifactorial diseases, and with each gene product interacting with 3–10 other proteins in the signaling pathways, approximately 3,000–10,000 interesting new molecular sites for intervention (drug targets) are expected to emerge over the next few years compared with the roughly 500 targets on which today's drug therapies are based (Drews 1998). If 10 genes influence the risk of depression, there may be 30–100 interesting new drug targets. Many biotechnology companies are mining large genetic EST and SNP databases to gather information on gene coding regions and to look for previously unknown proteins that may be new drug targets. Once promising genes are identified, the protein products are screened in cells and animals.

DNA arrays are now available to simultaneously analyze thousands of genes expressed in the brain. Such profiles will reveal in which cells or tissues these genes are up- or downregulated and under which specific environmental or developmental conditions. Candidate targets can be specified and subsequently expressed. The opportunity to compare the expression of thousands of genes simultaneously between disease and normal tissues or in animal models before and after some manipulation will allow the identification of multiple new drug targets (Debouck and Goodfellow 1999). The proteins thus isolated can be used to develop appropriate screening assays, which can then be followed by combinatorial chemistry techniques and high-throughput screening to develop and test a large number of new compounds.

In addition, genes will be identified that control the activation, distribution, and elimination of many drugs used to treat clinical disease. Mutations in a given gene lead to variations in the amount of the protein synthesized, its properties, and its final destination. Such genetic mutations may produce a variant protein that can cause an altered drug response; hence, proteins are the direct link between genetic constitution and individual-specific drug response. The emerging field of *pharmacogenomics* is concerned with genetic effects on therapeutic drugs themselves and with the genetic variation that contributes to the variable effects of drugs in different individuals.

By focusing on the genes that affect drug action rather than on genes involved in disease pathophysiology, molecular methods can be used to identify common SNPs that alter the structure and function of the expressed protein or its level of expression. From this perspective, all human genes may be available as potential targets. Thus, genomic science may make a tremendous contribution by focusing our attention on genetic effects on metabolism that alter pharmacokinetics and on effects on pathways of drug action that alter pharmacodynamics.

Although a distant hope, it may one day be possible to selectively prescribe drugs to patients and to develop individual pharmacologic response profiles. Side effects and other adverse events may also be correlated with underlying patterns of genetic variation (Houseman and Ledley 1998).

Conclusion

Evidence gathered from previous studies has implicated heredity as playing a role in the transmission of major depression. A single major gene is an unlikely contributor to etiology; rather, multiple genes of small effect contribute with nongenetic factors in producing vulnerability to the illness. Large-scale family genetic and association studies are currently under way in the United States and other countries to provide the materials to map and ultimately identify the specific genes that are involved. Once these genes are identified, many powerful genomic tools and technologies developed in the Human Genome Project and other initiatives may be applied. One way to remain apprised of these developments is to consult World Wide Web sites devoted to advances in genetic research (Table 5–2).

New advances in genomic science bring with them a potential to accelerate our understanding of disease pathophysiology, as we understand what goes wrong in the brains of depressed individuals. Large-scale characterization of gene transcripts expressed in the human brain and their protein products will provide tools for functional studies that may greatly advance our understanding of disturbed underlying neurobiologic mechanisms. Perhaps of greatest direct relevance to clinical care is the promise that genomic science has for significantly advancing drug discovery and differential therapeutics. Efficient treatment regimens that take into account individual side effect and antidepressant treatment response profiles may be tailored to specific genetic profiles. In this way, clinical applications of genetics will allow individual clinicians to consider the profound variability in patient populations. The ultimate benefit will be safer and more efficacious treatments that can reduce or eliminate the marked impairments that so frequently accompany major depression.

TABLE 5–2. *Selected genetics resources on the World Wide Web*

URL	Description
http://genetics.nature.com	*Nature Genetics*
http://www.faseb.org/genetics/ashg/jou-ashg.htm	*American Journal of Human Genetics*
http://www.ornl.gov/TechResources/Human_Genome/home.html	Human Genome Project
http://www.hgmp.mrc.ac.uk/GenomeWeb/	Human genome databases
http://www.ncbi.nlm.nih.gov	National Center for Biotechnology Information
http://www.nhgri.nih.gov	National Human Genome Research Institute
http://www.nih.gov/science/models/mouse/	Trans-NIH Mouse Initiative
http://www.genome.ad.jp/kegg/	Kyoto encyclopedia of genes and genomes (links to many genome databases)
http://www.ornl.gov/TechResources/Human_Genome/publicat/primer/intro.html	Primer on molecular genetics
http://www.affymetrix.com/	Affymetrix, a DNA array biotechnology company
http://www.ncbi.nlm.nih.gov/SNP/	Public SNPs database
http://www.wellcome.ac.uk/en/1/awtprerel0499n123.html	SNPs consortium of pharmaceutical companies and the Wellcome Trust
http://www-grb.nimh.nih.gov	NIMH-funded genetics research

Note. NIH = National Institutes of Health; NIMH = National Institute of Mental Health; SNPs = single nucleotide polymorphisms.

References

Allen MG, Cohen S, Pollin W, et al: Affective illness in veteran twins: a diagnostic review. Am J Psychiatry 131:1234–1239, 1974

American Psychiatric Association: Diagnostic and Statistical Manual of Mental Disorders, 4th Edition. Washington, DC, American Psychiatric Association, 1994

Bassett DE, Boguski MS, Spencer F, et al: Genome cross-referencing and XREFdb: implications for the identification and analysis of genes mutated in human disease. Nat Genet 15:339–344, 1997

Behr MA, Wilson MA, Gill WP, et al: Comparative genomics of BCG vaccines by whole-genome DNA microarray. Science 284:1520–1523, 1999

Bertelsen A, Harvald B, Hauge MA: A Danish twin study of manic-depressive disorders. Br J Psychiatry 130:330–351, 1977

Bland RC, Newman SC, Orn H: Recurrent and nonrecurrent depression. Arch Gen Psychiatry 43:1085–1089, 1986

Botstein D, White RL, Skolnick MH, et al: Construction of a genetic linkage map in man using restriction fragment length polymorphisms. Am J Hum Genet 32:314–331, 1980

Burmeister M: Basic concepts in the study of diseases with complex genetics. Biol Psychiatry 45:522–532, 1999

Cadoret R: Evidence for genetic inheritance of primary affective disorder in adoptees. Am J Psychiatry 133:463–466, 1978

Cargill M, Altshuler D, Ireland J, et al: Characterization of single-nucleotide polymorphisms in coding regions of human genes. Nat Genet 22:231–238, 1999

Chakravarti A: It's raining SNPs, hallelujah? Nat Genet 19:216–217, 1998

Chee M, Yang R, Hubbell E, et al: Accessing genetic information with high-density DNA arrays. Science 274:610–614, 1996

Collins FS, Guyer MS, Chakravarti A: Variations on a theme: cataloging human DNA sequence variation. Science 278:1580–1581, 1997

Collins FS, Patrinos A, Jordan E, et al: New goals for the U.S. Human Genome Project: 1998–2003. Science 282:682–689, 1999

Cooperative Human Linkage Center: A comprehensive human linkage map with centimorgan density. Science 265:2049–2054, 1994

Cox NJ, Reich T, Rice JP, et al: Segregation and linkage analyses of bipolar and major depressive illness in multigenerational pedigrees. J Psychiatr Res 23:109–123, 1989

Crowe RR, Namboodiri KK, Ashby HB, et al: Segregation analysis and linkage analysis of a large kindred of unipolar depression. Neuropsychobiology 7:20–25, 1981

Debouck C, Goodfellow PN: DNA microarrays in drug discovery and development. Nat Genet 21:48–50, 1999

Deloukas P, Schuler GD, Gyapay G, et al: A physical map of 30,000 human genes. Science 282:744–746, 1998

Drews J: Biotechnology's metamorphosis into a drug discovery industry. Nat Biotechnol 16:22–24, 1998

Fields C, Adams MD, White O, et al: How many genes in the human genome? Nat Genet 7:345–346, 1994

Frankel WN, Schork NL: Who's afraid of epistasis? Nat Genet 14:371–373, 1996

Gershon ES, Mark A, Cohen N, et al: Transmitted factors in the morbid risk of affective disorders: a controlled study. J Psychiatr Res 12:283–299, 1975

Gershon ES, Hamovit JH, Guroff JJ, et al: A family study of schizoaffective, bipolar I, bipolar II, unipolar, and normal control probands. Arch Gen Psychiatry 39:1157–1167, 1982

Goldin LR, Gershon ES, Targum SD, et al: Segregation and linkage analyses in families of patients with bipolar, unipolar, and schizoaffective mood disorders. Am J Hum Genet 35:274–287, 1983

Hacia JG, Brody LC, Chee MS, et al: Detection of heterozygous mutations in *BRCA1* using high density oligonucleotide arrays and two-color fluorescence analysis. Nat Genet 14:441–447, 1996

Halushka MK, Fan J-B, Bentley K, et al: Patterns of single-nucleotide polymorphisms in candidate genes for blood pressure homeostasis. Nat Genet 22:239–247, 1999

Houseman D, Ledley FD: Why pharmacogenomics? Why now? Nat Biotechnol 16:2–3, 1998

Hyman S: Introduction to the complex genetics of mental disorders. Biol Psychiatry 45:518–521, 1999

Kendler KS, Neale MC, Kessler RC, et al: A population-based twin study of major depression in women: the impact of varying definitions of illness. Arch Gen Psychiatry 49:257–266, 1992

Kendler KS, Gardner CO, Prescott CA: Clinical characteristics of major depression that predict risk of depression in relatives. Arch Gen Psychiatry 56:322–327, 1999

Kruglyak L: Prospects for whole-genome linkage disequilibrium mapping of common disease genes. Nat Genet 22:139–144, 1999

Kunugi H, Tatsumi M, Sakai T, et al: Serotonin transporter gene polymorphism and affective disorder. Lancet 347:1340–1341, 1996

Kupfer DJ, Frank E, Carpenter LL, et al: Family history in recurrent depression. J Affect Disord 17:113–119, 1989

Lander ES: The new genomics: global views of biology. Science 274:536–539, 1996

Lander ES: Array of hope. Nat Genet 21:3–4, 1999

Lipshutz RJ, Fodor SPA, Gingeras TR, et al: High density synthetic oligonucleotide arrays. Nat Genet 21:20–24, 1999

Lyons MJ, Eisen SA, Goldberg JTW, et al: A registry-based twin study of depression in men. Arch Gen Psychiatry 55:468–472, 1998

Manki H, Kanba S, Muramatsu T, et al: Dopamine D2, D3 and D4 receptor and transporter gene polymorphisms and mood disorders. J Affect Disord 40:7–13, 1996

Marazita ML, Neiswanger K, Cooper M, et al: Genetic segregation analysis of early-onset recurrent unipolar depression. Am J Hum Genet 61:1370–1378, 1997

Marshall E: Human Genome Project: sequencers endorse plan for a draft in 1 year. Science 284:1439–1441, 1999a

Marshall E: Drug firms to create public database of genetic mutations. Science 284:406–407, 1999b

McGuffin P, Katz R, Watkins S, et al: A hospital-based twin register of the heritability of DSM-IV unipolar depression. Arch Gen Psychiatry 53:129–136, 1996

Mendlewicz J, Rainer JD: Adoption study supporting genetic transmission in manic-depressive illness. Nature 268:326–329, 1977

Moldin SO, Reich T, Rice JP: Current perspectives on the genetics of unipolar depression. Behav Genet 21:211–242, 1991

Ogilvie AD, Battersby S, Bubb VJ, et al: Polymorphism in serotonin transporter gene associated with susceptibility to major depression. Lancet 347:731–733, 1996

Ott J: Analysis of Human Genetic Linkage, Revised Edition. Baltimore, John Hopkins University Press, 1991

Price RA, Kidd KK, Weissman MM: Early onset (under age 30 years) and panic disorder as markers for etiologic homogeneity in major depression. Arch Gen Psychiatry 44:434–440, 1987

Risch N, Botstein D: A manic depressive history. Nat Genet 12:351–353, 1996

Risch NJ, Merikangas K: The future of genetic studies of complex human diseases. Science 273:1516–1517, 1996

Risch NJ, Spiker D, Lotspeich L, et al: A genomic screen of autism: evidence for a multilocus etiology. Am J Hum Genet 65:493–507, 1999

Rowen L, Mahairas G, Hood L: Sequencing the human genome. Science 278:605–607, 1997

Southern EM: Detection of specific sequences among DNA fragments separated by gel electrophoresis. J Mol Biol 98:503–517, 1975

Spielman RS, McGinnis RE, Ewens WJ: Transmission test for linkage disequilibrium: the insulin gene region and insulin-dependent diabetes mellitus (IDDM). Am J Hum Genet 52:506–516, 1993

Stober G, Heils A, Lesch KP: Serotonin transporter gene polymorphism and affective disorder. Lancet 347:1340–1341, 1996

Surani WA: Imprinting and the initiation of gene silencing in the germ line. Cell 93:309–312, 1998

Thapar A, McGuffin P: A twin study of depressive symptoms in childhood. Br J Psychiatry 165:259–265, 1994

Torgersen S: Genetic factors in moderately severe and mild affective disorders. Arch Gen Psychiatry 43:222–226, 1986

Tsuang MT, Faraone SV: The Genetics of Mood Disorders. Baltimore, MD, John Hopkins University Press, 1990

Tsuang MT, Bucher KD, Fleming JA, et al: Transmission of affective disorders: an application of segregation analysis to blind family study data. J Psychiatr Res 19:23–29, 1985

Wang DG, Fan J-B, Siao C-J, et al: Large-scale identification, mapping, and genotyping of single-nucleotide polymorphisms in the human genome. Science 280:1077–1082, 1998

Watson SJ, Akil H: Gene chips and arrays revealed: a primer on their power and uses. Biol Psychiatry 45:533–543, 1999

Weissman MM, Gershon ES, Kidd KK, et al: Psychiatric disorders in the relatives of probands with affective disorders. Arch Gen Psychiatry 41:13–21, 1984

Weissman MM, Wolk S, Wickramaratne P, et al: Children with prepubertal-onset major depressive disorder and anxiety grown up. Arch Gen Psychiatry 56:794–801, 1999

Wender PH, Kety SS, Rosenthal D, et al: Psychiatric disorders in the biological and adoptive families of adopted individuals with affective disorders. Arch Gen Psychiatry 43:923–929, 1986

Winokur G, Tsuang MT, Crowe RR: The Iowa 500: affective disorder in relatives of manic and depressive patients. Am J Psychiatry 139:209–212, 1982

Can Psychobiology Contribute to Understanding Maintenance Treatment of Depression?

David J. Kupfer, M.D.
Ellen Frank, Ph.D.

Overview

The earliest approach to the psychobiology of depression concentrated almost exclusively on single parameters: electroencephalographic (EEG) sleep; hypothalamic-pituitary-adrenal axis abnormalities, especially those represented in the dexamethasone suppression model; and biogenic amine metabolites. These parameters were typically examined as individual correlates of acute clinical states, usually comparing depressed patients with control subjects (Kupfer 1978) or examining the relationship of the variable to severity of depression (Brown et al. 1994; Frank et al. 1994). Ultimately this proved not to be a particularly fruitful approach in helping us understand the biology of either short- or long-term treatment of depression.

As we matured somewhat in our view of depression and the relationship of psychobiologic parameters to the disorder, we began to

This research was supported in part by grants from the National Institute of Mental Health to Ellen Frank (MH29618; MH49115), David J. Kupfer (MH30915, MH24652), and to Neal Ryan (MH41712–13).

think about a state–trait approach to the problem (Kraemer et al. 1994). We began to see that there were abnormalities (i.e., differences from values observed in nondepressed control subjects) that were present only when the patient was in the state of depression. Other abnormalities remained even after depression had remitted (Kupfer et al. 1994). Because we could identify potential research subjects only after they had had a first episode of depression (thus making them a part of the population of interest), we were initially unable to determine whether these abnormalities represented preexisting traits, scars, or residua of previous depressive illness. This led to important studies of high-risk subjects. Looking for these same kinds of abnormalities in individuals who had never experienced an episode of depression but were, on the basis of their family histories at high risk for the disorder, proved to be a relatively useful strategy with respect to EEG sleep (Giles et al. 1998) but failed to unlock the broader mystery of vulnerability to depressive illness or depressive episodes.

Now, after nearly three decades of this work, why are the psychobiologic parameters that reliably predict treatment outcome or course still not identified? Perhaps the wrong parameters have been examined. Or perhaps the correct parameters have been examined, but the measures used were not sufficiently sensitive or the wrong analyses were used to examine the data.

We would argue that the problem lay elsewhere. We would posit that we have been held back in these efforts because we have been looking only at single biologic systems, when simultaneous exploration of multiple systems is required. We would argue further that those multiple, interacting biologic systems probably need to be understood in the context of the psychosocial aspects of the individual's life. Finally, we would argue that we have been hampered by what may well be a misguided view of disorder itself, misguided at least if one is trying to understand the relationship of psychobiology to course and outcome. Although the *Research Diagnostic Criteria* and the *Diagnostic and Statistical Manual of Mental Disorders* were extremely important in moving us forward in the reliability of our epidemiology and in the early studies of treatments for major depression, an approach that looks at softer forms of disorder may be much more helpful in sorting out the psychobiology of these conditions.

As we enter the 21st century, we have come to have a somewhat different view of depressive illness than that which held sway when we first began to conduct studies of the psychobiology of depression. In the mid-1970s, we viewed depression as an acute illness. Among the many benefits we have received from the high-quality psychiatric epidemiology that has been done in the decades since the 1970s is a very different understanding of depressive illness. We have come to see that unipolar depression is probably as much a lifelong condition as is bipolar disorder. We now recognize that unipolar depression recurs frequently and often requires lifelong treatment. This knowledge should provide some important clues about how we ought to be studying the psychobiology of depression.

We will be in our best position to understand the relationship of psychobiology to course and outcome when we embed studies of psychobiology either in long-term treatment studies or in long-term follow-up studies. To date, however, there has been a paucity of longitudinal studies that examine the psychobiology of major depressive disorder. As we proceed, we will argue that longitudinal studies of psychopathology, especially treatment trials, provide a unique opportunity to begin to approach a true understanding of the psychobiology of depression.

Studies of EEG Sleep and Long-Term Outcome

The particular question that we now try to address with data we have collected at the University of Pittsburgh is whether the major biologic correlates of treatment outcomes studied to date, primarily sleep physiologic measures, include common features across the age span or are age dependent. We begin to address these issues with data from two long-term treatment trials, one in midlife depressive illness and a second in late-life depressive illness. Finally, we describe data from longitudinal follow-up studies of depressed children.

Maintenance Treatment of Depression

Several reports from our laboratory have pointed to preliminary relationships between sleep physiologic measures and the recurrence of depression during prophylactic treatment. In 1990 we demonstrated that reduced delta sleep ratio (total delta counts in the first non–rapid eye movement [NREM] sleep stage to total delta counts in the second NREM stage) represented a marker of vulnerability to recurrence. In short, patients with the lowest sleep delta ratios were most likely to experience a recurrence of depression (Kupfer et al. 1990). Second, when repeated sleep EEG studies were conducted throughout a 3-year maintenance treatment period, we found that patients who continued to receive active imipramine treatment continued to demonstrate consistent REM sleep alterations and high sleep continuity (Kupfer et al. 1994). Third, in elderly depressed patients we noted that the recurrence of major depression during the first year of maintenance nortriptyline treatment is associated with lower phasic rapid eye movement (REM) activity and lower subjective sleep quality but not with abnormalities in delta activity (Buysse et al. 1996).

In summary, the available data and analyses did not provide a satisfactorily clear and consistent picture of the relationship of EEG sleep to long-term maintenance and the likelihood of recurrence of depression. To provide a maximal-size sample of patients receiving treatment in a maintenance protocol, we sought to combine the data from the original Pittsburgh Study of Maintenance Therapies in Recurrent Depression (Frank et al. 1990) and the newly completed study of Maintenance Treatment in Late-Life Depression (Reynolds et al. 1999). In the original Pittsburgh study, we randomly assigned 128 patients with recurrent unipolar depression who had responded to acute and continuation treatment with imipramine and interpersonal psychotherapy (IPT [Klerman et al. 1984]) to one of five maintenance treatment conditions: 1) active imipramine and maintenance interpersonal psychotherapy (IPT-M), 2) active imipramine and medication clinic visits, 3) placebo and medication clinic visits, 4) placebo and IPT-M, and 5) IPT-M alone (Frank et al. 1990). The treatment outcome in this study demonstrated the usefulness of maintenance drug treatment in these patients as well as the significant role of IPT-M in prolonging the period before recurrence as compared with placebo. We have now reported results from our IPT-M in Late-Life Study, which is a comparable study of 108 elderly patients (average age, 67 years) who entered a four-cell protocol and were assigned to the following four maintenance conditions: 1) nortriptyline and monthly IPT-M, 2) nortriptyline and monthly medication clinic visits, 3) placebo and monthly IPT-M, and 4) placebo and monthly medication clinic visits (Reynolds et al. 1999). Similar to the midlife study of major depression, the length of time before recurrence of a major episode was significantly greater for all active treatments than for placebo. In addition, combined treatment with nortriptyline and IPT was superior to IPT plus placebo.

Because systematic EEG sleep studies were conducted in both long-term maintenance trials, we were able to examine sleep variables at three time points: 1) baseline sleep measures taken prior to active treatment when all subjects were medication free; 2) during continuation treatment when all patients were receiving both active medication (imipramine or nortriptyline) and IPT; and 3) during maintenance treatment, which in all cases represented 1–3 months after maintenance treatment assignment. Thirteen variables were selected to provide measures of sleep continuity, sleep architecture, and specific REM sleep variables. On the basis of previous investigations, sleep variables included the following: total recording period, time spent asleep, sleep efficiency, percent REM, REM latency, REM time, REM activity, REM counts (whole night), REM counts (first REM period), and delta sleep ratio (0.5–3.0 Hz) (Kupfer et al. 1993). Given the randomization scheme for the maintenance treatment assignments in the midlife study, 55% of the total group of patients were not receiving active medication in maintenance. To examine the relationship of sleep to the length of time before recurrence, we eliminated from the group of 234 patients the 27 who had experienced a recurrence or who were terminated from the protocol within the first 8 weeks of maintenance treatment. Log rank statistics were computed on the sleep variables in a Kaplan–Meier survival analyses with treatment group as the stratification variable. This nonparametric test is computed by pooling over the defined strata (treatment group). A significant result indicates that the sleep variable is associated with survival time (Collett 1994).

As noted in Table 6–1, the 207 patients had a median duration of illness of 16.8 weeks prior to their entry into acute treatment. The median age at onset of disorder for the entire group was 33 years, and patients had experienced a median of four previous episodes of depression. Their median baseline depression severity as measured by the Hamilton

Rating Scale for Depression at the time of entrance to the study was 21. The median Global Assessment of Functioning score was 54. The median age of the sample, almost 75% of whom were female, was 57 years.

TABLE 6–1.   *Clinical characteristics of patients in maintenance treatment**

Clinical characteristic	Mean ± SD	Median
Duration of current episode, *wk*	27.0 ± 28.2	16.8
Age at onset, *y*	37.2 ± 17.6	33
Previous episodes, *n*	5.9 ± 6.3	4
Baseline Hamilton Rating Scale for Depression	21.7 ± 4.5	21
Baseline Global Assessment of Functioning	52.8 ± 7.8	54
Age, *y*	52.5 ± 16.4 (Range, 21–79)	57
Gender	75% female	

*(N = 207).

When we examined the relationship of sleep variables to survival time in maintenance, we found no significant relationships between baseline sleep variables and survival time in maintenance. The same was true for EEG sleep assessed at entry to the continuation treatment period. Indeed, the only significant findings were noted for several sleep variables studied during maintenance. There was only a trend ($P = 0.06$) for REM percent, but REM sleep time ($P < 0.02$), manually scored REM activity ($P < 0.05$), and automated REM counts for the entire period of sleep ($P < 0.03$) were all significantly related to survival time. A negative correlation appeared to exist between REM sleep and survival time—that is, increased REM predicted early recurrence of depression (Table 6–2).

Because there were, in essence, four different treatment conditions in these studies during the maintenance treatment protocol, we decided to examine whether any of these conditions was primarily responsible for the overall significant findings relating maintenance sleep to maintenance treatment outcome. On the basis of previous studies, we decid-

TABLE 6–2. *Relationship of sleep variables to survival time in maintenance*

Variable	Baseline, *P*	Continuation, *P*	Maintenance, *P*
Total recording period	0.81	0.55	0.41
Time spent asleep	0.45	0.81	0.14
Sleep efficiency	0.38	0.90	0.45
Percent REM	0.89	0.66	0.06
REM latency	0.91	0.16	0.28
REM time	0.86	0.87	0.02
REM activity	0.87	0.56	0.05
REM counts (whole night)	0.15	0.73	0.03
REM counts (first REM period)	0.16	0.99	0.13
Delta sleep ratio (0.5–3.0 Hz)	0.37	0.41	0.13

ed to investigate the two conditions in which active medication was discontinued and patients continued to receive either IPT-M or medication clinic visits with placebo. As noted in Table 6–3, a significant difference existed between the relationship of sleep variables to survival time in the two conditions. In the group of 58 patients who continued to receive psychotherapy, no significant relationships existed. However, in the 34 patients in whom both active medication and psychotherapy had been discontinued, a number of sleep variables showed highly significant relationships to survival time. Time spent asleep ($P < 0.003$) and total recording period ($P < 0.03$) were related to the length of remission, as were several REM sleep variables, particularly REM sleep time ($P < 0.006$) and manual ($P < 0.03$) and automated REM activity ($P < 0.03$). These findings suggested that in patients in whom both medication and psychotherapy had been withdrawn, a highly significant relationship existed between sleep parameters and risk of recurrence. In contrast, withdrawal of medication alone, with continuation of psychotherapy, did not yield significant relationships. In our concluding note we comment on the significance of these findings.

TABLE 6–3. *Relationship of sleep variables to survival time in maintenance (subgroups)*

Variable	Psychotherapy plus placebo (*n* = 58)	Medication clinic plus placebo (*n* = 34)
Total recording period	0.18	0.03
Time spent asleep	0.68	0.003
Sleep efficiency	0.38	0.78
Percent REM	0.16	0.09
REM latency	0.50	0.47
REM time	0.35	0.006
REM activity	0.45	0.03
REM counts (whole night)	0.16	0.03
REM counts (first REM period)	0.19	0.07
Delta sleep ratio (0.5–3.0 Hz)	0.61	0.89

Long-Term Follow-Up Studies of Depressed Children and Control Subjects

Although no studies have examined maintenance treatment in childhood and adolescent depression, we examined the current longitudinal data sets to determine what could be concluded at the present time. One major study of childhood depression included both baseline biologic measures and the follow-up of clinical course (Dahl et al. 1989; Rao et al. 1995). In these studies, children were age 8–12 years at the time of initial assessment during an episode of major depressive disorder (N = 46). Initial biologic measures (time 1) were obtained for all subjects (28 depressed, 35 nondepressed controls). Clinical assessment 7 years later showed a retention of 94% of the sample (Rao et al. 1996). The clinical follow-up yielded four groups for reanalysis of time 1 biology, which consisted of 1) subjects who had a major depression but no further episodes during follow-up (*n*=6), 2) subjects who had major depressive disorder with a recurrent unipolar course (*n*=13), 3) a small group of control subjects who subsequently developed major depressive disorder (*n*=5), and 4) the control subjects who remained free of psychopathology ($n=23$). When several key sleep variables and sleep-onset cortisol were examined, a number of findings emerged. No significant differences were found in the overall group for REM latency, even though the REM latency tended to be longest in the control group (Table 6–4). With respect to REM density, a highly significant difference existed between the subjects who had at least one episode of major depressive disorder and the control group that had no episodes of depression on follow-up ($F = 4.6$, $P = 0.008$). There was also a significant elevation in sleep-onset cortisol in the group of patients with a recurrent major depressive disorder course. ($F = 2.9$, $P = 0.05$). Although these findings are consistent with our earlier notions of biologic relationships between episodes of depression and long-term course, in the absence of longitudinal studies, the findings need to be viewed with some caution. The findings in childhood and adolescence strongly support the sleep physiology findings in midlife and late life that REM sleep parameters are strongly related to recurrence of depression.

Conclusion

At this point we would have to conclude that we have not learned a great deal that is helpful in predicting the long-term course of depressive disorders in the majority of children, adults, and the elderly who have these conditions. When we consider the findings that represent practical tools for the clinician, we have little to offer. EEG sleep, although a wonderful window into the brain, is not a practical tool in the hands of the frontline clinician. Thus, it is incumbent on us to work on the development of efficient and inexpensive proxies for the all-night-sleep EEG. Research aimed at the development of such proxy measures is being initiated at the Western Psychiatric Institute and Clinic.

What other kinds of studies will help us to predict the long-term course of depressive illness? As we have implied, we need to be thinking about longitudinal assessment; however, we also need to be thinking about assessment of multiple parameters over time. By that we mean both multiple biologic parameters (i.e., looking at multiple biologic systems at the same time) and psychosocial variables (Kupfer and Frank 1997). The key is not likely to be in any single relationship but in rela-

TABLE 6–4.   *Adolescent electroencephalographic sleep and plasma cortisol measures and clinical outcome at follow-up[a]*

Variables	Patients with MDD with no further episodes at follow-up (n = 6)	Patients with MDD with unipolar course (n = 13)	Control subjects who developed depression (n = 5)	Control subjects with no psychopathology at follow-up (n = 23)[b]	F	P
Sleep latency[c]	17.9 ± 19.9	25.0 ± 13.5	21.6 ± 14.5	18.2	1.1	0.38
REM latency[c]	81.0 ± 45.4	76.8 ± 31.2	67.3 ± 20.2	104.1 ± 48.2	1.8	0.15
REM density	1.3 ± 0.2	1.4 ± 0.2	1.5 ± 0.3	1.1 ± 0.3	4.6	0.008
Percentage of 24-hour cortisol near sleep onset	7.3 ± 5.3	10.8 ± 4.7	8.7 ± 5.2	6.7 ± 2.7	2.9	0.05

Note.   EEC = electroencephalogram; MDD = major depressive disorder; REM = rapid eye movement.
[a]Values are means (± SD).
[b]Sample size (n = 20) for sleep variables.
[c]Analyses were performed on the logarithm.
Source.   Reprinted by permission of Elsevier Science from "The Relationship Between Longitudinal Clinical Course and Sleep and Cortisol Changes in Adolescent Depression" by Rao U, Dahl RE, Ryan ND, et al. *Biological Psychiatry* 40:474–484, Copyright 1996 by the Society of Biological Psychiatry.

tively complex interaction effects. Some such work is just beginning to take place. For example, we are now examining the relationship among very carefully measured life stress using George Brown's Life Events and Difficulties Schedule (LEDS) methodology (Brown et al. 1994), EEG parameters, and treatment outcome. The kinds of relationships that are beginning to emerge from this three-way interaction paradigm appear to be much stronger than the kinds of relationships presented earlier in this chapter.

Embedding such longitudinal assessments in treatment studies in which there are ill subjects at the beginning of the trial, mostly well subjects somewhere in the middle of the trial, and then some who remain well and others who do not, should enable us to parse the variance in a more efficient way. With this sort of design we can examine whether ill-state (i.e., baseline) parameters or well-state, traitlike (i.e., remission) parameters are most associated with the course of maintenance treatment or with long-term follow-up.

A comparable advantage can probably be achieved by embedding such studies in longitudinal assessment of high-risk individuals. Perhaps, however, we should be thinking about high risk in broader terms than as high risk for single entity disorders. If we focus on individuals at high risk for more complex combinations of depression and anxiety, some of which may be fully syndromal and some of which may be subsyndromal, we are likely to begin to truly understand the contribution of psychobiology to the course of mood disorders and mood disorder treatment. In addition, it will probably prove useful to focus on prodromes or early signs of impending onset. Clearly, the challenges for the 21st century will be the hypothesis-driven use of more refined and sophisticated combinations of previously studied parameters, such as EEG sleep and neuroendocrine functioning coupled with the powerful new brain imaging techniques, in the context of treatment or follow-up studies as well as the hypothesis-driven use of molecular biology and genetics and genomics.

More practical challenges for the future will be to find the funding for, and the subjects willing to sustain participation in, such highly expensive and personally demanding studies. However, we remain optimistic that this is possible. We believe that this is precisely the kind of optimism that Joe Zubin would have had. On the eve of his 90th birthday, Joe submitted a letter of intent for a prospective study of relapse in schizophrenia. He died before he was able to carry out the study; however, if we maintain his tenacity about the possibilities of empiric research, we will surely get to the right answers eventually.

Acknowledgment

The lecture on which this chapter is based was dedicated to the memory of Joe Zubin, who was an inspiration to us in many respects. Perhaps most important, when few in the area of psychopathology were focused on carefully designed empiric studies, that is precisely where Joe focused his energy. It was the foundation of his work. We were also inspired by Joe's endless curiosity and optimism about the possibilities of learning more in our field. For the psychologists among us, he was a particular inspiration. He arrived at the University of Pittsburgh just as Ellen Frank was beginning her doctoral studies in psychology. To have a psychologist who studied patients with serious mental disorders, rather than an unhappy college sophomore, appear in the classroom was an important moment in her training. What it told her was that the study of real patients who had severe illnesses was a possibility for clinical psychologists as well.

Finally, Joe's insistence on a stress-diathesis model of psychopathology enabled us to think that it would be possible to combine the streams of influence that were important to both of us in our intellectual development as psychopathology researchers: a strong belief in psychosocial influences on the etiology of mental illnesses and an equally strong belief in the neural basis of mental disorders. Joe enabled us to see how those two streams of influence could be melded in order to have a truly complete understanding of mental disorders.

References

Brown GW, Harris TO, Hepworth C: Life events and endogenous depression: a puzzle reexamined. Arch Gen Psychiatry 51:525–534, 1994

Buysse DJ, Reynolds CF, Hoch CC, et al: Longitudinal effects of nortriptyline on EEG sleep and the likelihood of recurrence in elderly depressed patients. Neuropsychopharmacology 14:243–252, 1996

Collett D: Modelling Survival Data in Medical Research. London, Chapman & Hall, 1994

Dahl R, Puig-Antich J, Ryan N: Cortisol secretion in adolescents with major depressive disorder. Acta Psychiatr Scan 80:18–26, 1989

Frank E, Kupfer DJ, Perel JM, et al: Three year outcomes for maintenance therapies in recurrent depression Arch Gen Psychiatry 47:1093–1099, 1990

Frank E, Anderson B, Reynolds CF, et al: Life events and the research diagnostic criteria endogenous subtype: a confirmation of the distinction using the Bedford College methods. Arch Gen Psychiatry 51:519–524, 1994

Giles De, Kupfer DJ, Rush AJ, et al: Controlled comparison of electrophysiological sleep in families of probands with unipolar depression. Am J Psychiatry 155:192–199, 1998

Klerman GL, Weissman MM, Rounsaville BJ, et al: Interpersonal Psychotherapy of Depression. New York, Basic Books, 1984

Kraemer HC, Gullion CM, Rush AJ, et al: Can state and trait variables be disentangled? A methodological framework for psychiatric disorders. Psychiatry Res 52:55–69, 1994

Kupfer DJ: Application of EEG sleep for the differential diagnosis and treatment of affective disorder. Pharmakopsychiatric-NeuroPsychopharmacologie 11:17–26, 1978

Kupfer DJ, Frank E: The role of psychosocial factors in the onset of major depression, in The Integrative Neurobiology of Affiliation. (This volume is a result of a conference entitled "The Integrative Neurobiology of Affiliation" sponsored by the New York Academy of Sciences and held March 14–17, 1996, in Washington, DC). Edited by Carter CA, Lederhendler IL, Kilpatrick B. New York, New York Academy of Sciences, 87:429–439, 1997

Kupfer DJ, Frank E, Grochocinski VJ, et al: Delta sleep ratio: a biological correlate of early recurrence in unipolar affective disorder. Arch Gen Psychiatry 47:1100–1105, 1990

Kupfer DJ, Frank E, McEachran AB, et al: EEG sleep correlates of recurrence of depression on active medication. Depression 1:300–308, 1993

Kupfer DJ, Ehlers CL, Frank E, et al: Persistent effects of antidepressants: EEG sleep studies in depressed patients during maintenance treatment. Biol Psychiatry 35:781–793, 1994

Rao U, Ryan ND, Birmaher B, et al: Unipolar depression in adolescents: clinical outcome in adulthood. J Am Acad Child Adolesc Psychiatry 34:566–578, 1995

Rao U, Dahl RE, Ryan ND, et al: The relationship between longitudinal clinical course and sleep and cortisol changes in adolescent depression. Biol Psychiatry 40:474–484, 1996

Reynolds CF, Frank E, Perel JM, et al: Nortriptyline and interpersonal psychotherapy as maintenance therapies for recurrent major depression: a randomized controlled trial in patients older than 59 years. JAMA 281:39–45, 1999

Treatment

Introduction

David L. Dunner, M.D.

Lithium carbonate was introduced as a treatment for acute mania and as a maintenance treatment for bipolar disorder in the United States in the early 1970s. This compound had been studied in Europe for two decades prior to its approval for clinical use in psychiatry in the United States. This timeline is likely related to the difficulty of American psychiatrists in diagnosing mania and the lack of commercial sponsorship for lithium, a common salt that would have provided the impetus for lithium studies in acute mania and for maintenance therapy of bipolar disorder.

The changes in diagnostic classification from DSM-II to DSM-III likely reflected the need of American psychiatry to adopt a system that allowed for and indeed encouraged the diagnosis of bipolar disorders. This change in nomenclature also helped to focus attention on major depression at a time when the treatments for major depression largely consisted of tricyclic antidepressants, monoamine oxidase inhibitors, electroconvulsive therapy (ECT), and analytically oriented psychotherapy.

The last three decades of the 20th century are notable for the development of changes in classification of depression to include subtypes in DSM-IV that are treatment related (e.g., melancholic, atypical, seasonal, psychotic, and catatonic) and the introduction of newer antidepressant entities that have greater tolerability than the tricyclic antidepressants. These advances have made it easier for depression to be diagnosed and treated in the primary care setting. Interestingly, there has also been a parallel development of specific brief psychotherapies found to be effective for the treatment of depression, notably interpersonal psychotherapy and cognitive-behavioral therapy. However, the development of new treatments has increased the acute treatment costs of depression, resulting in new economic considerations.

What new treatments can we anticipate in the 21st century? The investment in new treatments is of considerable importance because of increased recognition that available treatments are not completely effective. Some patients have disorders that are resistant to treatment. Thus, the development of treatments that work by novel mechanisms may be beneficial. However, the development of such treatments is linked to their economic success. The restriction of treatments for depression by third-party insurers seems shortsighted and, in the long run, not cost effective when the impact of depression on total medical care costs is considered. Psychiatrists and their patients must be forceful in their economic arguments to ensure that new treatments for depression continue to be developed.

This section of the book focuses on treatments for depression. Included are chapters on the history, current status, and future needs of antidepressants in the United States (Chapter 7) and on practices in the United Kingdom (Chapter 8). Advances in techniques for the administration of ECT—one of the first effective treatments for depression—and the development of newer treatments such as rapid transcranial magnetic stimulation and vagus nerve stimulation are described in Chapter 9. Chapter 10 examines the increased recognition of mood disorders in children and the development of effective and safe treatments for this population. Clinical trials of depressed patients over time have shown increasing placebo response rates. In Chapter 11, better strategies for demonstrating efficacy and for administration as well as scientific and new structures for efficient testing are described for newer treatments. As a range of new treatments emerge, guidelines for treatment become necessary; these are provided in Chapter 12.

Finally, clinical trials of depressed patients over time have shown increasing placebo response rates. Are there better strategies than placebo for demonstrating efficacy of newer treatments? These seven chapters review the past, discuss the present, and propose an optimistic future for the treatment of depression.

CHAPTER 7

Antidepressants in the United States

Current Status and Future Needs

Robert M. A. Hirschfeld, M.D.

Background

Antidepressant medications in the United States are big business. In 1998, retail domestic sales for fluoxetine (marketed under the trade name Prozac) were reported at nearly $2 billion (Cardinale 1998). Three of the top ten best-selling pharmaceuticals in the United States in 1998 were antidepressants: fluoxetine (number 2), sertraline (Zoloft) (number 5), and paroxetine (Paxil) (number 7).

The popularity of antidepressants is a relatively recent phenomenon. The number of prescriptions written for antidepressants was low prior to the mid-1980s, and none of the antidepressants were among the top 20 prescribed pharmaceuticals. In 1988 only 2.5 million prescriptions were written for antidepressants in the United States each month. In 1998 more than 10 million prescriptions were written each month (Walsh America PMSI, Phoenix, AZ).

This increased use of antidepressant medications in the United States resulted largely from the introduction of new classes of antidepressants. Compared with older antidepressants, these newer medications have greatly reduced side effects and are much safer in overdose. Before 1988 the antidepressant market consisted of tricyclic antidepressants (TCAs) and the monoamine oxidase inhibitors (MAOIs), which were associated with many unpleasant side effects that made them undesirable to patients and limited their marketability.

Tricyclic and Heterocyclic Antidepressants

Tricyclic and heterocyclic antidepressants are characterized by a molecular structure consisting of three or more rings. In general, these drugs inhibit the reuptake of both norepinephrine and serotonin (5-HT). Many of the side effects of the TCAs are caused by histaminergic, cholinergic, and adrenergic receptor activity. Antihistaminic effects are weight gain and drowsiness. Anticholinergic side effects include blurred vision, constipation, drowsiness, and dry mouth. Adrenergic side effects include postural hypotension, dizziness, and drowsiness (Stahl 1996). The narrow therapeutic index of the TCAs increases the risk of blood toxicity, central nervous system toxicity, and overdose (Potter et al. 1995).

Monoamine Oxidase Inhibitors

Monoamine oxidase (MAO) is an enzyme found throughout the body that metabolizes various neurotransmitters. Two forms of MAO exist: MAO-A and MAO-B. MAO-A preferentially metabolizes 5-HT, whereas MAO-B preferentially oxidizes dopamine. Both forms also oxidize other neurotransmitters.

The MAOIs prevent or inhibit the metabolism of the monoamines by MAO. The original MAOIs (e.g., tranylcypromine and phenelzine) were irreversible inhibitors of MAO. More recently, a group of reversible inhibitors of MAO-A (RIMAs) have been developed (e.g., moclobemide).

Selective Serotonin Reuptake Inhibitors

Fluoxetine was the first of a new class of medications, the selective serotonin reuptake inhibitors (SSRIs). These medications were as effective as the then-existing antidepressants but had a much more benign side effect profile, which made them more palatable to patients. In January 1988, fluoxetine was approved by the U.S. Food and Drug Administration (FDA) for the treatment of depression. Fluoxetine received enormous media attention. It was featured on the cover of *Newsweek* magazine and other national publications and became the subject of best-selling books. In February 1992 the FDA approved the second SSRI for the treatment of depression, sertraline, which was followed in February 1993 by paroxetine.

In early 1994 the sales of the three SSRIs exceeded the sales of all the older antidepressants combined; this pattern has continued ever since. Although the number of prescriptions for the older medications has remained constant for the past decade, the number of prescriptions for the newer antidepressants has continued to grow.

More New Antidepressants

The FDA has approved four additional antidepressants for the treatment of depression, bringing to 20 the total number of antidepressants approved for use in the United States (Table 7–1). These medications include nefazodone (Serzone), venlafaxine (Effexor), mirtazapine (Remeron), and citalopram (Celexa). In addition, bupropion (Wellbutrin) is an antidepressant with a chemical structure unlike the others. Its mechanism of action is largely unknown, although it does possess noradrenergic and dopaminergic reuptake blocking properties (Golden et al. 1998). These newer antidepressants spawned a host of new class names based on their putative mechanisms of action, such as selective norepinephrine reuptake inhibitors (SNRIs), norepinephrine and dopamine reuptake inhibitors (NDRIs), noradrenergic and specific serotonergic antidepressants (NaSSAs), and serotonin-2 antagonist reuptake inhibitors (SARIs). The efficacy of these medications is roughly equal to that of the older antidepressants, but the newer medications have much more benign side effect profiles and better safety due to their specificity of action on receptor activity.

Are We Overprescribing Antidepressants?

The national publicity and burgeoning sales of antidepressants has caused much controversy. Some people believe that antidepressants are

TABLE 7–1.   *Antidepressants available in the United States in 1999*

Class	Agents
Tricyclic antidepressants and heterocyclics	Imipramine
	Amitriptyline
	Nortriptyline
	Protriptyline
	Amoxapine
	Doxepin
	Desipramine
	Trimipramine
	Maprotiline
Monoamine oxidase inhibitors	Phenelzine
	Tranylcypromine
Norepinephrine and dopamine reuptake inhibitors	Bupropion
Selective serotonin reuptake inhibitors	Fluoxetine
	Sertraline
	Paroxetine
	Fluvoxamine
	Citalopram
Serotonin-2 antagonist/reuptake inhibitors	Trazodone
	Nefazodone
Serotonin-norepinephrine reuptake inhibitors	Venlafaxine
Noradrenergic and specific serotonergic antidepressants	Mirtazapine

overprescribed and overused (Ruthven 1998). Reports such as the story of Wenatchee, Washington, where a substantial proportion of the town had been prescribed Prozac (Egan 1994), have fueled this controversy.

A review of the evidence does not support this assertion, however. In fact, the vast majority of patients with major depression receive little or no treatment at all. For example, a study conducted across various medical and mental health settings reported that only 11% of patients with depression of low severity received an antidepressant and only 29% of patients with depression of high severity received an antidepressant (Hirschfeld et al. 1997). Furthermore, of those who received an antidepressant, less than half received an adequate dose for a minimum period of time.

In 1998 a door-to-door survey conducted by Yale researchers identified 312 people with major depression (Druss et al. 1998). Of these people, only 7.4% were taking an antidepressant medication. Thus, approximately 92% of those with major depression received no antidepressant medication (Druss et al. 1998). Despite the tremendous attention given to antidepressants and the substantial increase in their usage, depression continues to be substantially underrecognized and undertreated.

Problems With Existing Antidepressants

Clinical response to antidepressants usually becomes apparent after 2 weeks or more, and full efficacy may take several months. In patients who have chronic depression, the response may take even longer. For example, in the Chronic Depression Maintenance Study involving 635 patients, 22% demonstrated only a partial response after aggressive treatment with either imipramine or sertraline for 12 weeks. When these patients continued taking the same medication for an additional 16 weeks, 33% achieved full response (Keller et al. 1998).

Nonetheless, some improvement may be noted within the first 1–2 weeks of treatment. Montgomery (1995) has reported drug–placebo differences as early as 1–2 weeks (Dunbar et al. 1991; Tollefson and Holman 1994) that are sustained throughout treatment. According to Montgomery (1995), the "appearance of some clinical effect" is usually too subtle to be considered a response and therefore often goes unnoticed.

Adverse Events

The newer generation of antidepressants represents great progress in terms of safety and tolerability. Lethality from overdose is extremely rare (Barbey and Roose 1998). In contrast, TCAs and MAOIs can be lethal in overdose (Carvey 1998; Janicak et al. 1997).

The side effects of dry mouth, blood pressure problems, constipation, sedation, weight gain, and nausea had an adverse effect on compliance for patients receiving the older agents. Substantial dietary restrictions make the MAOIs particularly difficult to manage. The side effect profiles of the newer drugs are considerably better, but side effects remain. This is an important issue, particularly for long-term treatment. Compliance is much less of a problem when patients are acutely symptomatic. Following recovery, the presence of side effects greatly influences compliance. For example, the sexual side effects of the SSRIs are a relatively minor issue in acute treatment but may become a major impediment to long-term compliance.

Differences Among the Antidepressants

In general, all of the antidepressants are equally efficacious. Overall, approximately two-thirds of patients respond to an antidepressant in comparison with the approximately one-third who respond to placebo (Janicak et al. 1997). Considerable controversy exists over whether the so-called dual-action antidepressants (e.g., most of the TCAs, venlafaxine, and mirtazapine) have increased efficacy compared with so-called single-action drugs (e.g., the SSRIs) (Hirschfeld 1999). Some evidence supports this possibility. In a French study of hospitalized patients with severe melancholic depression, venlafaxine was compared with fluoxetine. Baseline scores for both groups on the Hamilton Rating Scale for Depression (Ham-D) were approximately 30. The mean doses of the drugs were 200 mg for venlafaxine and 40 mg for fluoxetine. After 3 weeks, the patients taking venlafaxine showed a statistically significantly greater decrease in Ham-D scores than did those taking fluoxetine. This disparity increased to approximately seven Ham-D points by the end of the study at 6 weeks (Clerc et al. 1994).

Another study compared venlafaxine, fluoxetine, and placebo in depressed outpatients. Venlafaxine dosing ranged from 75 to 150 mg, and fluoxetine dosing ranged from 20 to 40 mg. Although venlafaxine and fluoxetine were both better than placebo in reducing mean scores on the Ham-D, Montgomery-Åsberg Depression Rating Scale, and Clinical Global Impressions Scale after 8 weeks of treatment, no significant differences were observed between the two drug groups. The relatively low dosing of venlafaxine precludes definitive conclusions regarding relative efficacy (Costa e Silva 1998).

In a study of mirtazapine versus fluoxetine, differences were reported at 3 weeks in favor of mirtazapine; the differences persisted throughout the 6-week study ($P = 0.054$) (Wheatley et al. 1998). In a study of mirtazapine versus paroxetine, a statistically significant comparative improvement occurred in the patients receiving mirtazapine versus those receiving paroxetine at week 1 but did not persist throughout the study (Benkert et al. 1998).

How Well Do the Antidepressants Work and What Do They Do?

The efficacy of antidepressant medications has been well studied. Clinical trial methodology involving double-blind conditions, random assignment, and standardized objective measures has been used in a large number of studies. Studies usually include 6–8 weeks of active treatment, although some studies are as short as 4 weeks and others last 12 weeks or longer.

In his meta-analysis of the literature, Janicak et al. (1997) analyzed 79 studies of TCAs involving 5,159 patients. They reported that the response rate in patients taking the active drug was 63%, whereas the rate for patients taking the placebo was 36% — a difference of 27%. Response rate in general is defined as at least a 50% drop in baseline Ham-D scores. Similarly, for the MAOIs these authors reported a response rate of 66% for active drug compared with 32% for placebo, a difference of 34%. These differences are highly statistically significant; the probability of the results occurring by chance were 1 in 10^{-40} for the TCAs and 10^{-12} for the MAOIs.

What does a 50% drop in the Ham-D total score signify? The Ham-D includes 17 items that assess depressed mood, vegetative features (e.g., appetite, sleep, and sexual drive), motivation, and cognitive items (Hamilton 1960). The scale focuses on clinical symptoms of depression to the exclusion of other qualities that may be affected by depression such as the psychosocial variables of marital and family relationships, occupational functioning, and social and leisure activities.

Problems With Assessment of Response

A 50% drop in the Ham-D scale does not necessarily mean that a patient is no longer depressed. For example, a patient with moderate major depression might enter a study with a Ham-D score of 22, which is generally indicative of substantial clinical impairment. A 50% drop would bring the patient to a score of 11. Although a drop of this magnitude represents marked improvement overall, it still falls shy of the "7 or less" standard, according to which the patient would generally be considered as not depressed (Endicott et al. 1981). Moreover, a severely ill depressed patient might enter a study with a Ham-D score of 30. In this situation, a 50% drop would bring the score to 15, which would still qualify the patient for most clinical trial treatments of dysthymia. Furthermore, an 8-week study by Nierenberg et al. (1999) found that even with so-called full responders (i.e., patients whose posttreatment Ham-D scores were 7 or less), symptoms of major depression still persisted in most patients despite their improvement. In this study, 56.5% of the full responders still had two or more symptoms, and less than 20% of the full responders were free of all symptoms. Thus, a response may signify substantial clinical improvement, but the patient is far from well.

In addition, none of the existing antidepressants cures the depression. They provide symptomatic relief, and premature discontinuation of the medications often results in relapse. Several studies of continuation therapy have demonstrated a significantly lower relapse rate in patients receiving drug therapy (11%–16%) compared with a placebo (31%–46%) (Doogan and Caillard 1992; Montgomery and Dunbar 1993; Montgomery et al. 1993). In addition, Reimherr (1998) suggested that continuation therapy must continue for 6–9 months following symptomatic improvement to prevent relapse.

For patients who are at risk for recurrence, long-term antidepressant therapy is indicated. Patients who have had prior recurrent depression, more severe depression, or poor control during the continuation period (Hirschfeld 1998) should be considered at risk for recurrence. In such patients, the rate of recurrence is lowered substantially by maintenance treatment with the antidepressant. For example, in the Kupfer et al. (1992) studies, patients were followed-up for as long as 5 years in maintenance therapy. They were placed in one of five treatment groups that involved various combinations of imipramine, interpersonal psychotherapy, and placebo. The active medication group had a mean survival time (i.e., time until recurrence) of 99 weeks, whereas the placebo group had a mean survival time of 54 weeks. In a recent study of chronic

depression, Keller et al. (1998) demonstrated that sertraline maintenance treatment is effective in preventing recurrence or reemergence
of symptoms.

Treatment of Specific Symptom Clusters

Traditional clinical lore has held that medications address and improve
the biologic somatic symptoms of drive disturbances (e.g., sleep, appetite, sexual disturbances, energy) and that psychotherapy addresses and
improves cognitive and other thinking disturbances associated with depression, including pessimism, hopelessness, difficulty concentrating,
and suicidal ideation.

The Ham-D scale has been used to measure the overall severity of
depression. However, the Ham-D also has been divided into subscales.
Evaluation of the improvements in the subscales can address the question of differential efficacy among symptom clusters. For example, in a
study of mirtazapine versus placebo, Claghorn and Lesem (1995) found
that anxiety/somatization disturbances and retardation improved over
the course of the study. Improvements in cognitive disturbance subfac-
tors were also observed. These results and results from other studies
(e.g., Mendels et al. 1999) support the notion that antidepressants are
not specific in their salutary effects. Rather, when they work, they appear to work across the board. This observation is at odds with the traditional clinical lore.

Similarly, studies of psychotherapy report that clinical improvement tends to occur across all symptom clusters when it happens and
not in specific cognitive symptoms (Rush 1999). Some evidence suggests that the susceptibility to relapse may be lower with psychotherapy
than with pharmacotherapy for patients whose depression was treated
successfully (Segal et al. 1999). In addition, prophylactic continuation-
phase cognitive therapy for depressed outpatients may reduce relapse
of depression (Jarrett et al. 1998). Thus successful treatments for depression tend to address all symptoms of depression, both somatic and psychologic. Evidence for targeted improvement by one mode of therapy
or by a particular medication is lacking.

The Future

The number of prescriptions written for antidepressants has grown markedly since the introduction of fluoxetine. Various pharmacologic treatment options are available for the treatment of depression. These treatments are effective, they have benign side effect profiles, and they are safe in overdose; however, substantial numbers of people who could benefit from treatment do not receive it.

The antidepressant medications are moderately effective, but a significant number of people either do not respond or respond only partially. Although benign, side effects (e.g., sexual dysfunction and weight gain) continue to create problems for patients. None of the currently available treatments cures depression. We look forward to the future for treatments with a faster onset of action, improved side effect profiles, and better long-term efficacy.

References

Barbey JT, Roose SP: SSRI safety in overdose. J Clin Psychiatry 59(suppl 15):42–48, 1998

Benkert O, Szegedi A, Kohnen R: Rapid onset of therapeutic action in major depression: a comparative trial of mirtazapine and paroxetine. Poster presented at the 37th annual meeting of the American College of Neuropsychopharmacology, Las Croabas, Puerto Rico, December 14–18, 1998

Cardinale V: Drug Topics Red Book. Montvale, NJ, Medical Economics, 1998

Carvey PM: Drug Action in the Central Nervous System. New York, Oxford University Press, 1998

Claghorn JL, Lesem MD: A double-blind placebo-controlled study of Org 3770 in depressed outpatients. J Affect Disord 34:165–171, 1995

Clerc GE, Ruimy P, Verdeau-Palles J: A double-blind comparison of venlafaxine and fluoxetine in patients hospitalized for major depression and melancholia. The Venlafaxine French Inpatient Study Group. Int Clin Psychopharmacol 9:139–143, 1994

Costa e Silva J: Randomized, double-blind comparison of venlafaxine and fluoxetine in outpatients with major depression. J Clin Psychiatry 59:352–357, 1998

Doogan DP, Caillard V: Sertraline in the prevention of depression. Br J Psychiatry 160:217–222, 1992

Druss BG, Rohrbaugh R, Kosten T, et al: Use of alternative medicine in major depression. Psychiatr Serv 49:1397, 1998

Dunbar GC, Cohn JB, Fabre LF, et al: A comparison of paroxetine, imipramine and placebo in depressed outpatients. Br J Psychiatry 159:394–398, 1991

Egan T: A Washington town full of Prozac. The New York Times, January 30, 1994.

Endicott J, Cohen J, Nee J, et al: Hamilton Depression Rating Scale. Extracted from regular and change versions of the Schedule for Affective Disorders and Schizophrenia. Arch Gen Psychiatry 38:98–103, 1981

Golden RN, Dawkins K, Nicholas L, et al: Trazodone, nefazodone, bupropion, and mirtazapine, in Textbook of Psychopharmacology, 2nd Edition. Edited by Schatzberg AF, Nemeroff CB. Washington, DC, American Psychiatric Press, 1998, pp 251–269

Hamilton M: A rating scale for depression. J Neurol Neurosurg Psychiatry 23:56–62, 1960

Hirschfeld RM: Long-term nature of depression. Depression and Anxiety 7(suppl 1):1–4, 1998

Hirschfeld RM: Efficacy of SSRIs and newer antidepressants in severe depression: comparison with TCAs. J Clin Psychiatry 60:326–335, 1999

Hirschfeld RMA, Keller MB, Panico S, et al: The National Depressive and Manic-Depressive Association consensus statement on the undertreatment of depression. JAMA 277:333–340, 1997

Janicak PG, Davis JM, Preskorn SH, et al: Principles and Practice of Psychopharmacology, 2nd Edition. Baltimore, MD, Williams and Wilkins, 1997

Jarrett RB, Basco MR, Risser R, et al: Is there a role for continuation phase cognitive therapy for depressed outpatients? J Consult Clin Psychol 66:1036–1040, 1998

Keller MB, Kocsis JH, Thase ME, et al: Maintenance phase efficacy of sertraline for chronic depression: a randomized controlled trial. JAMA 280:1665–1672, 1998

Kupfer DJ, Frank E, Perel JM, et al: Five-year outcome for maintenance therapies in recurrent depression. Arch Gen Psychiatry 49:769–773, 1992

Mendels J, Kiev A, Fabre LF: Double-blind comparison of citalopram and placebo in depressed outpatients with melancholia. Depression and Anxiety 9:54–60, 1999

Montgomery SA: Are 2-week trials sufficient to indicate efficacy? Psychopharmacol Bull 31:41–44, 1995

Montgomery SA, Dunbar G: Paroxetine is better than placebo in relapse prevention and the prophylaxis of recurrent depression. Int Clin Psychopharmacol 8:189–195, 1993

Montgomery SA, Rasmussen JGC, Tanghoj P: A 24-week study of 20 mg citalopram, 40 mg citalopram, and placebo in the prevention of relapse of major depression. Int Clin Psychopharmacol 8:181–188, 1993

Nierenberg AA, Keefe BR, Leslie VC, et al: Residual symptoms in depressed patients who respond acutely to fluoxetine. J Clin Psychiatry 60:221–225, 1999

Potter WZ, Manji HK, Rudorfer MV: Tricyclics and tetracyclics, in Textbook of Psychopharmacology, 2nd Edition. Edited by Schatzberg AF, Nemeroff CB. Washington, DC, American Psychiatric Press, 1995, pp 141–160

Reimherr FW, Amsterdam JD, Quitkin FM, et al: Optimal length of continuation therapy in depression: a prospective assessment during long-term fluoxetine treatment. Am J Psychiatry 155:1247–1253, 1998

Rudorfer MV, Potter WZ: Pharmacokinetics of antidepressants, in Psychopharmacology: The Third Generation of Progress. Edited by Meltzer HY. New York, Raven, 1987, pp 1353–1364

Rush AJ: Psychotherapies for Major Mood Disorders: From Efficacy to Effectiveness, in Cost-Effectiveness of Psychotherapy: A Guide for Practitioners, Researchers, and Policy Makers. Edited by Miller ME, Magruder KM. New York, Oxford University Press, 1999, pp 211–223

Ruthven L: It's time to stop over-prescribing antidepressants. Employee Benefit News 12:1–2, 1998

Segal ZV, Gemar M, Williams S: Differential cognitive response to a mood challenge following successful cognitive therapy or pharmacotherapy for unipolar depression. J Abnorm Psychol 108:3–10, 1999

Stahl SM: Essential Psychopharmacology: Neuroscientific Basics and Practical Applications. New York, Cambridge University Press, 1996

Tollefson GD, Holman SL: How long to onset of antidepressant action: a metanalysis of patients treated with fluoxetine or placebo. Int Clin Psychopharmacol 9:245–250, 1994

Wheatley DP, van Moffaert M, Timmerman L, et al: Mirtazapine: efficacy and tolerability in comparison with fluoxetine in patients with moderate to severe major depressive disorder. Mirtazapine-Fluoxetine Study Group. J Clin Psychiatry 59:306–312, 1998

CHAPTER 8

Treatment of Depression in the United Kingdom

Eugene S. Paykel, M.D., F.R.C.P., F.R.C.Psych.

Introduction

In this chapter I provide an overview of historical and current trends in the treatment of depression in the United Kingdom. The United States and the United Kingdom have been described as two countries divided by a common language, but the language really is one, and the two variants, having diverged, are now increasingly convergent because of television and films. Similarly, in a time when the Atlantic Ocean has shrunk to an unexciting air journey taking only part of a day, treatment approaches have converged and the countries do not differ very much. Therefore, after my overview of treatment approaches in the United Kingdom I focus on one aspect of my own research: the problem of high relapse rates in depression, in particular, a large controlled trial of cognitive therapy in residual depression.

Antidepressants

Modern treatment starts with the antidepressants, and the watershed event occurred with their general introduction at the end of the 1950s. Historically, British psychiatry was Kraepelinian and somatic in its approach, and the antidepressants came into widespread use rapidly. An early milestone was the first placebo-controlled trial of imipramine (Ball and Kiloh 1959). Sargent and colleagues' vigorous enthusiasm for monoamine oxidase inhibitors (MAOIs) resulted in the greater use of these drugs in the United Kingdom than in many other parts of the world and also led to the introduction of the term *atypical depression* (West and Dally 1959). Electroconvulsive therapy (ECT) has been used extensively in the United Kingdom over the years; the major controlled trials of ECT versus simulated ECT in the United Kingdom in the late 1970s and early 1980s were generated in part by public questioning of its value.

For much of the forty years, the attitude of the British drug licensing authority, the Committee on Safety of Medicines, toward the introduction of new antidepressants has been more liberal than that of the U.S. Food and Drug Administration (FDA), with some gradual convergence more recently. The main criterion has been evidence of efficacy. As a result, 28 antidepressants are currently available in the United Kingdom, including 10 tricyclic antidepressants (TCAs); five selective serotonin reuptake inhibitors (SSRIs); four other uptake inhibitors; five atypical antidepressants; and four MAOIs including moclobemide, a reversible inhibitor of MAO-A.

Despite the United Kingdom's more liberal attitude toward the introduction of new antidepressants, we tend to be conservative in practice, which means that newly licensed drugs come into widespread use slowly. SSRIs have not predominated to the same extent that they have in the United States. Figure 8–1 shows prescribing rates for antidepressants in England between 1987 and 1996. The introduction of SSRIs increased total antidepressant prescribing rates considerably but, at least up to that point, had not resulted in a decrease in TCAs.

The United Kingdom is part of the European Union, which has recently taken on wider drug licensing functions. In 1995 the European Medicines Evaluation Agency (EMEA), which is based in London, came into existence. The current licensing system in Europe is still transitional, and drugs may be licensed in three ways. A centralized procedure allows applications to be made directly to the EMEA, where they are considered by its Committee for Proprietary Medicinal Products. This route, which is optional for medicinal products, is mandatory for

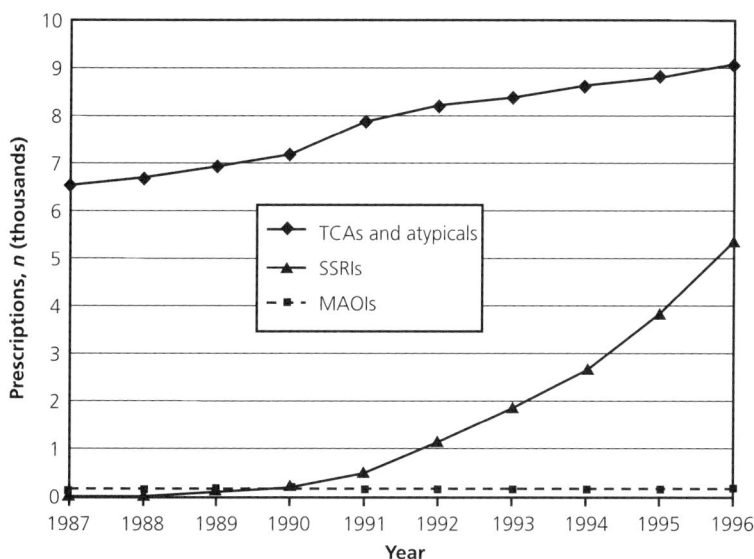

FIGURE 8–1. Prescribing rates for antidepressants in England, 1987–1996. MAOIs = monoamine oxidase inhibitors; SSRIs = selective serotonin reuptake inhibitors; TCAs = tricyclic antidepressants.
Source. Data from Department of Health, England.

biotechnology products. A second procedure allows application to national licensing authorities in accordance with a decentralized procedure whereby product licenses granted in one country receive mutual recognition in other member states, with the EMEA making a binding decision in case of disagreement. A third procedure allows application to a single licensing authority, under a national procedure whereby the product is to be marketed only in one country. The European system is being used increasingly for new antidepressants, particularly by the decentralized second route, although as with all such systems, there have been some criticisms of its transparency and rigor (Abbasi and Herxheimer 1998).

Psychotherapies

Although Freud died in London, and that city has always had a thriving and influential psychoanalytic community, psychotherapy was until the

138 Treatment of Depression: Bridging the 21st Century

1980s a minor player in the British National Health Service. A considerable change occurred in the 1980s and 1990s, particularly with a move toward briefer and more eclectic therapies, including a recent interest in interpersonal therapy (IPT). Some training in psychotherapy is now a mandatory part of the training of young psychiatrists.

For behavioral therapy, the situation has been very different. Some of the early developments were British, and thanks in part to Eysenck and his colleagues, behavioral approaches have long been used, particularly by clinical psychologists, first for phobic disorders and later for obsessive-compulsive and other disorders.

Cognitive therapy, by contrast, was more the creation of one charismatic American. Nevertheless its growth in the United Kingdom in the 1990s has been spectacular. Again it is used particularly by clinical psychologists. In the past few years general practitioners have become interested in making it available to their patients. The training experience of those who administer cognitive therapy is still quite variable, but training courses have been developed in some centers to a very high level.

The Service Context

In the British National Health Service, every member of the population is registered with a general practitioner who is the first point of contact. General practices have increasingly become larger group practices, with a primary-care team of nurses and other professionals attached.

Most depressed patients see their general practitioner for treatment, and only about 1 in 10 is referred to a psychiatrist. A similar situation exists in most of the world, and even in the highly developed specialist system of the United States, much of the care for depression is delivered by nonpsychiatrists (Schurman et al. 1985). General practitioners have been criticized for underrecognizing depression because only about 50% of cases of minor psychiatric disorder are recognized at any consultation (Goldberg and Huxley 1980), although more cases are recognized at repeat consultations in the following few months. The general practitioner's task is difficult because the diagnostic possibilities in any patient are wide, time available is limited, and presentations may be nonspecific without the patient acknowledging emotional elements. General practitioners have also been criticized for prescribing low doses of antidepressants (Johnson 1974).

Consideration of treatment in general practice is therefore important. In the 1980s my colleagues and I carried out a controlled trial to examine the efficacy of amitriptyline versus placebo in the depressive disorders seen in general practice, which are milder than those seen in the hospital (Paykel et al. 1988). We found clear evidence of efficacy, starting at a threshold severity score of 13 on the 17-item Hamilton Rating Scale for Depression; this score is a little below the threshold for major depression.

As in some other European countries, the United Kingdom has had a national campaign targeted at depression, in this case sponsored jointly by the Royal College of Psychiatrists and the Royal College of General Practitioners. The Defeat Depression Campaign (Paykel et al. 1997) ran from 1991 to 1995. One of the campaign's aims was to improve the treatment of depression in general practice through a series of guidelines, educational packages, and associated teaching activities.

Another aim of the campaign was to educate the general public. At baseline, we found that attitudes toward depression and people with depression were, on the whole, positive, but antidepressants were viewed with suspicion (Paykel et al. 1998). Although 46% of respondents to a general-population survey regarded antidepressants as effective, only 16% agreed with the statement that people with depression should be offered antidepressants; in contrast, 91% agreed that they should be offered counseling. An alarming 78% regarded antidepressants as addictive. Poor compliance is not surprising under these circumstances. Over the campaign's 5 years, attitudes became significantly more positive (Paykel et al. 1998).

Residual Depression, Relapse, and Cognitive Therapy

Since the late 1980s, after follow-up studies from the United States (Keller et al. 1984), the United Kingdom (Lee and Murray 1988), and Australia (Kiloh et al. 1988) were published that showed high rates of relapse and recurrence of depression, it has generally been recognized that improving the long-term outcome of the disorder is still a major challenge. Throughout the 1990s we carried out a series of studies aimed at investigating relapse in depression and what can be done to lessen it. The culmination of these studies has been a recently completed controlled trial of cognitive therapy that points to an increased place for this approach in the treatment of depression. In the next two sections I summarize two of these studies that are closely linked.

Residual Depression and Relapse

We first sought to establish whether the high rates of relapse that had been reported in patients originally receiving treatment in the 1970s were still present despite increased use of longer-term drug treatment. We also sought predictors of poor outcome that would identify target groups for further therapeutic efforts. We therefore undertook a systematic prospective follow-up study of 64 depressed patients admitted around 1990 to treatment facilities in Cambridge, predominantly for inpatient care. They were studied in detail at presentation and then interviewed prospectively every 3 months until a remission criterion was met or remission had failed to occur after 15 months. When remission occurred, the patients were interviewed again every 3 months for up to 15 months or until relapse, whichever came first (Hayhurst et al. 1997; Paykel et al. 1995, 1996; Ramana et al. 1995).

The findings from this study demonstrated that high relapse rates remained a problem. As in most follow-up studies, remission rates from major depression were high and remission was often rapid (Ramana et al. 1995). Only 6% of the subjects failed to achieve a remission below the research diagnostic criteria (RDC) for major depression by 15 months. However, when subjects were followed-up further, 40% of those achieving remission relapsed over the next 15 months. All the relapses had occurred by 10 months, confirming the validity of relapse as a comparatively early phenomenon.

The strongest predictor of subsequent relapse was symptomatic state at the time of remission. The remission criterion—absence of definite RDC major depression—allowed a good deal of lesser symptomatology. When ratings on the Hamilton Rating Scale for Depression at the time of remission were examined, 32% of the patients with remitting depression scored 8 or more, showing a pattern of residual symptoms. Residual symptoms were strong predictors of subsequent relapse, which occurred in 76% of these patients, in comparison with the 25% of patients without residual symptoms who experienced relapse. Figure 8–2 illustrates these findings. Partial remission of this kind has been shown to be a strong predictor of relapse (Evans et al. 1992; Faravelli et al. 1986; Georgotas et al. 1988; Mindham et al. 1973; Prien and Kupfer 1986; Simons et al. 1986). However, the frequency of partial remission has been obscured in many follow-up studies because subjects with partial remission are pooled either with those who have remitted or those who have not remitted rather than being identified separately.

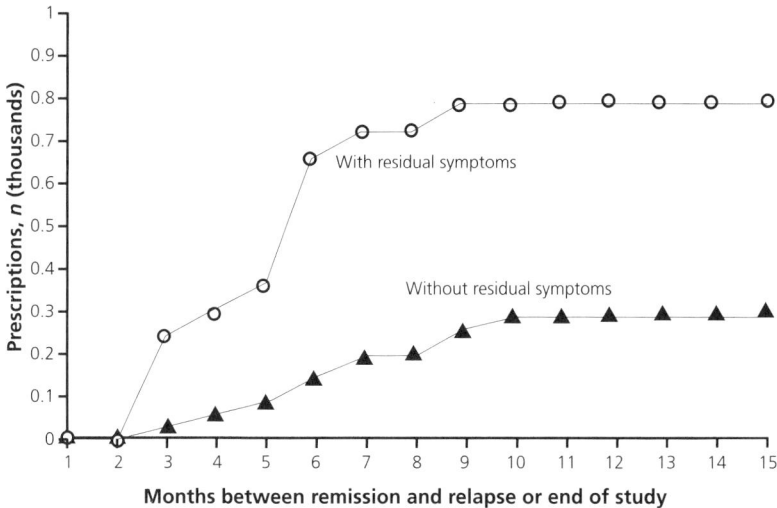

FIGURE 8–2. Survival curves for relapse in patients with and without residual symptoms at remission. Log rank statistic = 17.43, 1 df p < 0.001.
Source. From Paykel ES, Ramana R, Cooper Z, et al.: "Residual Symptoms After Partial Remission: An Important Outcome in Depression." Psychological Medicine 25:1171–1180, 1995. Used with the permission of Cambridge University Press.

Detailed examination of the characteristics of patients with residual depression revealed that in most cases they had not had preexisting dysthymic disorder nor, judging by drug treatment levels at the time of remission, were the residual symptoms mainly a consequence of inadequate drug treatment. The patients with residual symptoms tended to have received more drug treatment than did those without such symptoms, reflecting a rational therapeutic process common in naturalistic follow-up studies, whereby patients who are doing poorly are given more treatment. A common pattern in patients who remit partially and experience residual symptoms is that they receive treatment with a succession of antidepressants with limited response, often with side effects that limit very high dosages and lead to subsequent demoralization.

In a separate follow-up study of a new sample, focusing on adequacy of drug and other treatments received within 18 months after discharge from the hospital, we found further evidence that relapse was not particularly a consequence of failure to deliver appropriate drug treatment over the follow-up period (Ramana et al. 1999).

Psychologic Therapies and Relapse

The occurrence of residual depression with high relapse rates identified a target group of patients for more vigorous attempts at relapse prevention. These were patients who had not responded fully to drug treatment and whose subsequent relapse was often in spite of drugs; therefore, psychologic approaches were obviously suggested.

Two well-evaluated psychologic/psychotherapeutic approaches have been used in the treatment of depression: IPT and cognitive therapy. Evidence, although not plentiful, indicates that the effects of IPT in preventing relapse or recurrence are much weaker than in acute treatment. In the original Yale-Boston collaborative trial, in which Myrna Weissman and I were among the key participants, the precursor of IPT did not prevent relapse, although continuation antidepressants did so (Klerman et al. 1974; Paykel et al. 1975; Weissman et al. 1974). In the major controlled trial of maintenance imipramine and IPT, the effects of monthly IPT in preventing recurrence, although significant, were much weaker than those of imipramine (Frank et al. 1990). Both studies were stringent tests of IPT because they involved drug withdrawal designs with high relapse and recurrence rates subsequent to drug withdrawal in previous drug responders. More studies are required. At the time we planned our trial, evidence suggested that cognitive therapy aided in relapse prevention. The evidence has become stronger while the study has been under way.

The first evidence emerged from follow-up studies of controlled trials of antidepressants against cognitive therapy in the acute treatment of depression. Three studies showed significantly lower relapse rates after cognitive therapy (Blackburn et al. 1986; Evans et al. 1992; Simons et al. 1986). Nonsignificant trends in the same direction were found by Kovacs et al. (1981), Miller et al. (1989), and Shea et al. (1992). However, naturalistic follow-up studies of acute trials cannot be definitive. First, different kinds of patients with different prognoses for relapse may respond initially to cognitive therapy and to acute treatment with antidepressants. Second, antidepressant continuation was not always undertaken or well controlled in the follow-up studies. In one study in which it was (Evans et al. 1992), a relapse rate of 52% after antidepressant withdrawal was reduced to 32% with 1 year's maintenance, not significantly different from the 21% relapse rate after cognitive therapy, although possibly suggestive of an effect.

While our controlled trial was under way, Fava and colleagues in Bologna (Fava et al. 1994, 1996, 1998a) reported a small trial of 20 patients per group in which subjects experiencing residual depression while receiving antidepressants were given either a modified form of cognitive therapy or clinical management. Residual symptoms were relatively low, and cognitive therapy particularly targeted anxiety and irritability. In a second study, subjects with recurrent depression were randomly assigned after remission either to a much modified cognitive therapy approach including lifestyle modification and well-being therapy or to clinical management (Fava et al. 1998b). In the first study, although relapse and recurrence reduction was not significant at 2 years, it was significant at 4 years. In the second study, recurrences were significantly reduced.

In both of these studies, antidepressants were withdrawn, rendering patients highly at risk of symptom return and maximizing the possible effects of the cognitive therapy. In the more usual situation, patients will continue to receive antidepressants. Psychologic therapies require considerably more investment by the patient and are much more expensive than antidepressant treatment in terms of the therapist's time. A more realistic design for applicability in practice is to ask what a psychologic therapy can do in a group of patients who are not doing well with drug therapy and in particular to ask what it can add to the drug therapy.

Controlled Trial of Cognitive Therapy in Residual Depression

We have carried out a controlled trial of cognitive therapy in subjects with residual depression, all of whom had been given moderately high doses of antidepressants and who continued to receive them throughout the 17 months of the treatment trial and controlled follow-up period (Paykel et al. 1999). This study took place at two centers, in Cambridge and Newcastle, and my principal collaborators were Jan Scott in Newcastle and John Teasdale in Cambridge. Between the two centers, 158 unipolar depressed patients ages 21 to 65 years were included. All patients had had a previous major depression that remitted to a level below major depression but with residual symptoms (reaching 8 or more on the Ham-D and 9 or more on the Beck Depression Inventory). These criteria were modified from those for symptomatic illness and complete remission as formulated by Frank et al. (1991). All of the subjects had received antidepressants during a preliminary treatment period in which necessary doses were increased to defined adequate levels. Following randomization, subjects continued to receive the same antidepressant with dose alteration permitted only within restricted limits until the end of the study 17 months later. About 40% of subjects were receiving TCAs or atypical antidepressants at a mean dosage equivalent to 185 mg/day of amitriptyline, and about 60% were receiving SSRIs at a mean dosage equivalent to 35 mg/day of fluoxetine. Antidepressant dosages were moderately high for outpatients, particularly for Britain where dosages tend to be lower than in the United States. Approximately 15% of subjects also received lithium.

Subjects in the study were randomized into two groups: clinical management alone and clinical management with cognitive therapy. Subjects who received clinical management saw a psychiatrist every 4 weeks for 20 weeks and then every 8 weeks for another 48 weeks. They continued to take antidepressants and received supportive and assessment interviews. The other group received the same clinical management from psychiatrists in addition to 16 sessions of cognitive therapy over 20 weeks with two later booster sessions. Cognitive therapy was predominantly of the standard type for depression with an added element related to relapse prevention. Subjects in both groups were assessed regularly, using standard rating scales for symptoms and social adjustment. In addition, all treatment received from any source was documented, and at intervals special cognitive assessments were made to explore the mechanisms of cognitive therapy effects. Psychiatrists and research assistant raters were kept blind to treatment group, and patients were asked not to reveal details of their treatment.

The principal outcome measure in the study was the occurrence of a relapse, defined by two alternatives: 1) occurrence of major depressive disorder, according to the DSM-III-R criteria (American Psychiatric Association 1987), for a minimum duration of 1 month (2 weeks longer than the DSM-IIIR criterion) and two Ham-D ratings of 17 or more at least 1 week apart; and 2) persistent symptoms reaching a Ham-D score of 13 or more on two ratings 2 months apart and also at a level of distress or dysfunction at which the withholding of additional active treatment was no longer justified. This second criterion was applied only during the follow-up phase. For both types of relapse, rating by a second psychiatrist was required.

Relapse data were analyzed by Cox regression, including key predictor variables as covariates. Two analytic samples were used: intention to treat, including all patients entered into the study regardless of dropout or protocol violations; and per protocol, including only patients who satisfied protocol treatment constraints.

Cognitive therapy significantly reduced relapse rates. In the more conservative intention-to-treat analysis, the cumulative relapse rates at 68 weeks were 47% in the clinical management group and 29% in the cognitive therapy group. Cognitive therapy reduced relapses by approximately 40% of the base rate in the clinical management group, a worthwhile gain.

Further analyses are still under way. Effects on residual symptom levels were less marked than those on relapse. Examination of detailed symptom items on the Clinical Interview for Depression (Paykel 1985) showed that there were significant effects, particularly on ratings of guilt, worthlessness, and hopelessness, key targets for cognitive therapy. On social adjustment, which was evaluated by the interview version of the Social Adjustment Scale (Weissman and Paykel 1974), cognitive therapy also provided a benefit.

Overall this study has shown that adding cognitive therapy to drug treatment provided a major benefit to a group of subjects highly at risk of relapse, despite moderately high dosages of continuation and maintenance antidepressants.

Conclusion

In this chapter I have provided an overview of recent trends in the treatment of depression in the United Kingdom and discussed findings from a set of studies that focus on a well-recognized problem, that of relapse. These findings demonstrate considerable benefit from a growing treatment modality, cognitive therapy.

In general, the treatment of depression is very much the same in the United Kingdom as in the United States. Medication is used widely. ECT is used for the acute treatment of hospitalized patients more often in the United Kingdom than it is in the United States. Cost pressures exist in both countries, although the fearsome shackles of managed care have not yet been applied in the United Kingdom. Psychologic and psychotherapeutic treatments require justification in evidence that their costs are balanced by benefits. Cognitive therapy is one such treatment. Dr. Weissman and I started our research collaboration in the 1960s, undertaking a controlled trial of a psychotherapeutic modality in combination with medication. I am pleased to have journeyed back to that starting point.

References

Abbasi K, Herxheimer A: The European Medicines Evaluation Agency: open to criticism. Transparency must be coupled with greater rigour. BMJ 317:898, 1988

Ball JRB, Kiloh LG: A controlled trial of imipramine in treatment of depressive states. BMJ 2:1052–1055, 1959

Blackburn IM, Eunson KM, Bishop S: A two year naturalistic follow up of depressed patients treated with cognitive therapy, pharmacotherapy and a combination of both. J Affect Disord 10:67–75, 1986

Evans MD, Hollon SD, De Rubeis RJ, et al: Differential relapse following cognitive therapy and pharmacotherapy for depression. Arch Gen Psychiatry 49:802–808, 1992

Faravelli C, Ambonetti A, Palanti S, et al: Depressive relapses and incomplete recovery from index episode. Am J Psychiatry 49:888–891, 1986

Fava GA, Grandi S, Zielezny M, et al: Cognitive behavioral treatment of residual symptoms in primary major depressive disorder. Am J Psychiatry 151:1295–1299, 1994

Fava GA, Grandi S, Zielezny M, et al: Four-year outcome for cognitive behavioral treatment of residual symptoms in major depression. Am J Psychiatry 153:945–947, 1996

Fava GA, Rafanelli C, Grandi S, et al: Six year outcome for cognitive behavioral treatment of residual symptoms in major depression. Am J Psychiatry 155:1443–1445, 1998a

Fava GA, Rafanelli C, Grandi S, et al: Prevention of recurrent depression with cognitive behavioral therapy: preliminary findings. Arch Gen Psychiatry 55:816–820, 1998b

Frank E, Kupfer DJ, Perel JM, et al: Three year outcomes for maintenance therapies of recurrent depression. Arch Gen Psychiatry 47:1093–1099, 1990

Frank E, Prien RF, Jarrett RB, et al: Conceptualization and rationale for consensus definitions of terms in major depressive disorder: remission, recovery, relapse and recurrence. Arch Gen Psychiatry 48:851–855, 1991

Georgotas A, McCue R, Cooper TB, et al: How effective and safe is continuation therapy in elderly depressed patients: factors affecting relapse rate. Arch Gen Psychiatry 45:929–932, 1988

Goldberg DP, Huxley P: Mental Illness in the Community. London, England, Tavistock, 1980

Hayhurst H, Cooper Z, Paykel ES, et al: Expressed emotion and depression: a longitudinal study. Br J Psychiatry 171:439–443, 1997

Johnson DAW: A study of the use of antidepressant medication in general practice. Br J Psychiatry 125:186–192, 1974

Keller MB, Klerman G, Lavori PW, et al: Long-term outcome of episodes of major depression: clinical and public health significance. JAMA 252:788–792, 1984

Kiloh LG, Andrews GA, Neilson M: The long-term outcome of depressive illness. Br J Psychiatry 153:752–757, 1988

Klerman GL, DiMascio A, Weissman MM, et al: Treatment of depression by drugs and psychotherapy. Am J Psychiatry 131:186–191, 1974

Kovacs M, Rush AJ, Beck AT, et al: Depressed outpatients treated with cognitive therapy or pharmacotherapy. Arch Gen Psychiatry 38:33–41, 1981

Lee AS, Murray RM: The long-term outcome of Maudsley depressives. Br J Psychiatry 153:741–751, 1988

Miller IW, Norman WG, Keitner GI: Cognitive-behavioral treatment of depressed inpatients: six- and twelve-month follow-up. Am J Psychiatry 146:1274–1279, 1989

Mindham RH, Howland C, Shepherd M: An evaluation of continuation therapy with tricyclic antidepressants in depressive illness. Psychol Med 3:5–17, 1973

Paykel ES: The Clinical Interview for Depression: development, reliability and validity. J Affect Disord 9:85–96, 1985

Paykel ES, DiMascio A, Haskell D, et al: Effects of maintenance amitriptyline and psychotherapy on symptoms of depression. Psychol Med 5:67–77, 1975

Paykel ES, Hollyman JA, Freeling P, et al: Predictors of therapeutic benefit from amitriptyline in mild depression: a general practice placebo-controlled trial. J Affect Disord 14:83–95, 1988

Paykel ES, Ramana R, Cooper Z, et al: Residual symptoms after partial remission: an important outcome in depression. Psychol Med 25:1171–1180, 1995

Paykel ES, Cooper Z, Ramana R, et al: Life events, social support and marital relationships in the outcome of severe depression. Psychol Med 26:121–133, 1996

Paykel ES, Tylee A, Wright A, et al: The Defeat Depression Campaign: psychiatry in the public arena. Am J Psychiatry 154 (suppl 6):59–65, 1997

Paykel ES, Hart D, Priest RG: Changes in public attitudes to depression during the Defeat Depression Campaign. Br J Psychiatry 173:519–522, 1998

Paykel ES, Scott J, Teasdale JD, et al: Prevention of relapse in residual depression by cognitive therapy: a controlled trial. Arch Gen Psychiatry 56:829–835, 1999

Prien RF, Kupfer DJ: Continuous drug therapy for major depressive episodes: how long should it be maintained? Am J Psychiatry 143:18–23, 1986

Ramana R, Paykel ES, Cooper Z: Remission and relapse in major depression: a two-year prospective follow-up study. Psychol Med 25:1161–1170, 1995

Ramana R, Paykel ES, Surtees PG, et al: Medication received by depressed patients following the acute episode: adequacy and relation to outcome. Br J Psychiatry 174:128–134, 1999

Schurman RA, Kramer PD, Mitchell JB: The hidden mental health network. Arch Gen Psychiatry 42:89–94, 1985

Shea MT, Elkin I, Linber S, et al: Course of depressive symptoms over follow-up. Arch Gen Psychiatry 49:782–787, 1992

Simons AD, Murphy GE, Levine J, et al: Cognitive therapy and pharmaco-therapy of depression: sustained improvement over one year. Arch Gen Psychiatry 43:43–50, 1986

Weissman MM, Paykel ES. The Depressed Woman: A Study of Social Relationships. Chicago, IL, University of Chicago Press, 1974

Weissman MM, Klerman GL, Paykel ES, et al: Treatment effects on the social adjustment of depressed outpatients. Arch Gen Psychiatry 30:771–778, 1974

West ED, Dally PJ: Effects of iproniazid in depressive syndromes. BMJ 1:1491–1499, 1959

CHAPTER 9

Physical Treatments in Psychiatry

Advances in Electroconvulsive Therapy, Transcranial Magnetic Stimulation, and Vagus Nerve Stimulation

Harold A. Sackeim, Ph.D.

Sarah H. Lisanby, M.D.

Introduction

Despite the considerable progress that has been made in the use of pharmacologic and psychologic treatments for major depression, many patients benefit only partially or not at all (Thase and Rush 1997). The limitations of pharmacologic treatments with respect to efficacy and, in some cases, intolerable side effects have led to renewed interest in physical treatments of major depression. Electroconvulsive therapy (ECT) is the somatic treatment with the longest history of continual use in psychiatry. Transcranial magnetic stimulation (TMS) is a new technique that allows for focal, nonconvulsive stimulation of targeted brain regions (George et al. 1999). Vagus nerve stimulation (VNS) is an even

Preparation of this chapter was supported in part by grants R34 MH-35636 and R10 MH-57009 from the National Institute of Mental Health and by grants from the Magstim Company and the Cyberonics Company.

newer development that has shown efficacy in patients with treatment-resistant partial complex seizures (Schachter and Saper 1998) and is being tested for efficacy in patients with treatment-resistant major depression (Rush et al. 2000). These three techniques each involve electrical stimulation of the brain but use highly different methods. In this chapter we provide an update on the progress made in the use of ECT and discuss the potential roles of TMS and VNS in the treatment of major depression.

Electroconvulsive Therapy

Electroconvulsive therapy remains the most effective treatment available for major depression and may be of considerable benefit to patients with schizophrenia, medication-resistant acute mania, and other selective conditions (Sackeim et al. 1995; Weiner et al. 1990). In recent years the number of psychiatric patients receiving ECT in the United States has increased (Thompson et al. 1994). Moreover, during the 1990s, remarkable advances were made in the practice of ECT. This progress has changed both the way the treatment is administered and our understanding of its mechanisms of action. Our update first focuses on the advances made in stimulus dosing and optimization of the treatment. Then we provide brief updates on the prevention of relapse following response to ECT, the identification of neural systems that are responsible for the efficacy of ECT, and advances to anticipate from future ECT research.

Optimization of Electroconvulsive Therapy Administration

For decades the cardinal view of ECT was that the generalized seizure provided the necessary and sufficient conditions for efficacy (Fink 1979; Ottosson 1960). As long as generalized seizures of sufficient duration were produced, marked antidepressant effects could be expected. The dosage of electricity administered was considered irrelevant to the efficacy of the treatment but was a strong determinant of the magnitude of cognitive side effects. Consequently this fundamental view suggested that optimal treatment of depression would ensure that generalized seizures were produced at each treatment using the lowest dose of electricity possible (National Institutes of Health 1985).

Remarkably this view had never been translated into clinical practice. Until recently, standard practice had been to administer the same electrical dose to all patients. Typically this dose was close to the maximum output of the ECT device. We lacked basic information on the patient and treatment factors that determine dosing needs. For example, it was unknown whether patients have a narrow or broad range of seizure threshold, whether different electrode placements differ in dosing requirements, and the like.

Answers to these questions are now available and have had a pronounced impact on practice. The range in the minimal dose necessary to produce seizures in psychiatric patients is approximately 50-fold (Lisanby et al. 1996; Sackeim et al. 1987a, 1991). For example, generalized seizures of adequate duration can be elicited with a stimulus dose as low as 20 mC (a unit of charge) in some patients, whereas more than 1,000 mC may be required for exceptional patients with very high seizure thresholds (Lisanby et al. 1996). Almost invariably, standard practice in ECT had been to administer a high, fixed dose to all patients, and some practitioners continue to use fixed-dose techniques (Farah and McCall 1993). Consequently, many patients with low thresholds can receive electrical intensities that exceed their needs by factors of 10, 20, or more. Indeed, many of the short-term cognitive side effects that traditionally resulted from ECT were not intrinsic to the treatment but rather were outcomes of its practice (Sackeim et al. 1986).

We have also learned that factors such as gender, age, and electrode placement have substantial effects on seizure threshold (Coffey et al. 1995; Sackeim et al. 1987a, 1991). Males tend to have higher thresholds than females, threshold increases with patient age, and threshold is greater with bilateral ECT than with right unilateral ECT. The American Psychiatric Association Task Force Report on ECT strongly recommended that clinicians abandon the use of the fixed-dose approach and use methods in which electrical intensity is adjusted to the needs of individual patients (Weiner et al. 1990, 2001). One method, now in common use, is to conduct a titration procedure at the first treatment, identifying empirically the lowest amount of electricity needed to produce an adequate seizure. This method involves administering a small electrical dose that results in seizure elicitation in only a minority of patients. Under the same anesthesia, the electrical dose is progressively increased until an adequate seizure is produced. The safety of the titration method, in terms of medical and cognitive side effects, has been established (Prudic et al. 1994; Zielinski et al. 1993).

Recent studies of the efficacy of ECT administered at a low electrical dose have contradicted the fundamental premise that the generalized seizure provides the sufficient condition for efficacy. This work has also contradicted the clinical implication that the lowest possible electrical dose should always be used. A series of randomized, double-blind studies showed that depending on the electrode placement (i.e., bilateral or unilateral) and on the electrical dose, response rates to ECT in major depression vary from 17% to 70% (Sackeim et al. 1987b, 1993, 2000b). In other words, one can administer ECT and produce generalized seizures of sufficient duration at every treatment and still be giving fully inadequate treatment (comparable with placebo). This and related research has also contradicted the belief that seizure duration has a consistent relationship with efficacy (Nobler et al. 1993; Sackeim et al. 1991).

The outcome of this work has been the observation that the efficacy of right unilateral ECT is highly dependent on stimulus intensity. Right unilateral ECT has marked advantages over bilateral ECT with respect to cognitive side effects (Sackeim 1992; Sackeim et al. 1993; Weiner et al. 1986). However, the electrical dose must substantially exceed seizure threshold, probably by a factor of four or greater, in order for right unilateral ECT to exert optimal antidepressant effects (McCall et al. 2000; Sackeim et al. 2000b). The speed of clinical response to both bilateral ECT and right unilateral ECT is also influenced by the electrical dose. Higher stimulus intensity hastens clinical response (Robin and De Tissera 1982; Sackeim et al. 1993). Recently completed research has indicated that right unilateral ECT delivered at 500% above threshold (i.e., six times the threshold) is equivalent in efficacy to a robust form of bilateral ECT (150% above threshold), yet high-intensity right unilateral ECT still retains clinically significant advantages with respect to the magnitude and persistence of cognitive side effects (Sackeim et al. 2000b). Consequently, current recommendations are to use a moderately suprathreshold dose with bilateral ECT (e.g., 50% to 150% above seizure threshold) and a more marked dose increase with unilateral ECT (300%–500% above seizure threshold).

Medication Resistance and Relapse Prevention

Soon after the introduction of ECT, it was observed that between 80% and 90% of depressed patients showed marked improvement with this treatment (Kalinowsky and Hoch 1946). In general, these impressive estimates were not changed after the pharmacologic agents were introduced, and the field has assumed that the failure to respond to adequate trials of antidepressant medications has no bearing on subsequent response to ECT (Fink 1990). Indeed, the most common indication for the use of ECT in major depression has been medication resistance (Weiner et al. 1990, 2001).

Recent research has suggested that these views also require revision. The response rate to a standard course of bilateral ECT among patients who did not respond to one or more adequate trials of a tricyclic antidepressant (TCA) is impressive but substantially below that of patients who come to ECT not having received an adequate medication trial (Prudic et al. 1990). More recent work indicates that medication resistance also predicts poorer response to right unilateral ECT and that these effects hold for resistance to TCAs but not to selective serotonin reuptake inhibitors (SSRIs) (Prudic et al. 1996; Sackeim et al. 2000b). This finding does not mean that patients with medication-resistant depression will not respond to ECT. These patients often require more intensive and prolonged courses of treatment to achieve remission (Sackeim et al. 1993).

Once patients with medication-resistant depression do respond to ECT, we are faced with another dilemma: What medication should be used to prevent relapse? Unless continuation treatment follows response to ECT, we had expected that at least 50% of patients would relapse within a few months (Imlah et al. 1965; Kay et al. 1970; Seager and Bird 1962; see Sackeim 1994a for a review). Ironically, the standard practice in the field has been to use as continuation therapy the same classes of medications that did not work during treatment of the acute episode (Abrams 1997; Malcolm et al. 1991). The wisdom of this practice has been challenged.

Recent research suggests that relapse rates in the year after response to ECT are twice as high for patients who have established medication-resistant depression compared with those who come to ECT without a history of nonresponse to adequate antidepressant trials (Sackeim et al. 1990a). Traditional pharmacologic continuation therapies appear to have limited efficacy in patients with medication-resistant depression. Furthermore, in patient populations receiving ECT followed by conventional continuation therapy, the relapse rate in the first 6 months appears to be greater than 50%. Given this finding, considerable attention is now being devoted to evaluating different pharmacologic strategies to prevent relapse. In an ongoing multicenter double-blind controlled trial, patients who respond to unipolar ECT are randomized to 6 months of continuation therapy with placebo alone, nortriptyline alone, or nortriptyline combined with lithium. The randomization is stratified by pre-ECT medication resistance. The initial findings suggest an 87% relapse rate with placebo, a 61% relapse rate with nortriptyline alone, and a 41% relapse rate with the combination of nortriptyline and lithium (Sackeim 1997). In this preliminary work, virtually no patient receiving the combination treatment has relapsed 5 or more weeks after completing ECT.

Until this new information is established, two recommendations should be considered. First, when selecting a continuation therapy after response to ECT, it may be useful to review the classes and combinations of medications that previously proved unsuccessful in acute phase treatment of the major depression and then select a different class or combination. Augmentation with lithium may be particularly effective. Second, ECT is the only treatment in biologic psychiatry that is discontinued once it is proven effective. Clinicians are well aware that continuation or maintenance ECT can be highly effective (Clarke et al. 1989; Decina et al. 1987), and a controlled study comparing continuation ECT with combination nortriptyline-lithium continuation pharmacotherapy is in progress. It should be noted that the use of outpatient, continuation ECT is growing markedly at many centers in the United States. Various issues need to be resolved about the use of continuation ECT, particularly regarding optimal methods of administration (Sackeim 1994a).

Brain Imaging and Response to Electroconvulsive Therapy

The discovery that generalized seizures lacking therapeutic properties can be reliably produced has introduced new optimism in the search for the mechanisms of action in ECT. Previous skepticism centered on the view that generalized seizures produce so many systemic biologic changes that isolating epiphenomena from changes central to efficacy was unlikely (Kety 1974). Now the critical issue becomes identifying those biologic events that distinguish generalized seizures that have therapeutic properties from those that do not (Sackeim 1994b).

Considerable progress has been made in the area of functional brain imaging. Depressed patients who come to ECT are characterized by marked abnormalities in cerebral blood flow (CBF) and cerebral metabolic rate (CMR) (Drevets 1998; Sackeim et al. 1990b). Some of these deficits may be related to lesions in white matter and deep gray matter structures, perhaps reflecting an ischemic cerebrovascular disease process (Coffey et al. 1990; Sackeim et al. 2000a). This observation suggests that many of the patients who come to ECT have "trait," or static, brain abnormalities that are unlikely to resolve with clinical response.

Nonetheless, ECT produces a profound alteration of mood state, and concomitant changes in brain function have been observed. During the seizure, CBF and CMR increase profoundly (Ackermann et al. 1986); however, immediately after the seizure, functional activity decreases to below baseline levels (Nobler et al. 1994; Silfverskiöld and Risberg 1989). These reductions persist beyond the termination of ECT and are coupled with the development of slow-wave (delta frequency) activity in the electroencephalogram (EEG). The regions showing reduced CBF and CMR and increased EEG slow-wave activity are dependent in part on electrode placement. Despite producing a generalized seizure with right unilateral ECT, the changes following this intervention are largely confined to the right hemisphere, whereas bilateral ECT produces symmetric effects. More critically the alterations in CBF and EEG activity appear to be strongly related to clinical response (Nobler et al. 1994; Sackeim et al. 1996). Greater CBF reductions in anterior frontal cortical regions are associated with superior response to ECT (Nobler et al. 1994). Similarly the magnitude of the increase in slow-wave EEG activity in prefrontal regions also predicts the antidepressant effects of ECT (Sackeim et al. 1996). These findings raise the possibility that modulation of the functional activity of prefrontal cortex is a critical ingredient in the antidepressant effects of ECT. They also support the theory that inhibitory processes that terminate the seizure are targeted at sites of seizure initiation and that enhanced inhibition in prefrontal cortex is linked to the efficacy of ECT (Sackeim 1994a, 1999).

Future Directions

Improvements in the practice and understanding of ECT are likely to occur in several domains. The transition in the 1980s from the use of sine-wave to brief-pulse stimulation resulted in a marked decrease in the short-term cognitive side effects of ECT owing to greater efficiency in electrical stimulation (Weiner et al. 1986). Nonetheless the form of brief-pulse stimulation in current use may not be optimal because the pulse width is wide (e.g., 1 ms), grossly exceeding the chronaxie for neuronal depolarization (Sackeim et al. 1994). Of clinical and theoretic importance is the determination of whether shorter and more physiologic pulse widths preserve efficacy while reducing side effects.

Particularly promising is the use of pharmacologic agents to reduce the acute cognitive side effects of ECT. Despite a great deal of animal literature suggesting that various compounds are effective in preventing or reducing the amnestic effects of electrical seizure induction, little research has been conducted in the clinical context (Krueger et al. 1992). Because ECT offers a model system to investigate the putative efficacy of agents in reducing anterograde and retrograde amnesia, it is surprising that few clinical trials have been conducted (Prudic et al. 1999).

An area undergoing considerable rethinking is that of the diagnostic indications for the use of ECT. In particular, there is renewed interest in the role of ECT in the treatment of schizophrenia, particularly when combined with antipsychotic medication (Fink and Sackeim 1996; Krueger and Sackeim 1995). Provision of ECT earlier in the course of schizophrenia may produce long-term beneficial effects (Krueger and Sackeim 1995). With respect to the acute treatment of major depression, a key issue is improving rates of clinical response in patients with medication-resistant depression (Prudic et al. 1996). An older literature, based largely on first-line use of ECT, indicated that augmentation of ECT with antidepressant medications did not improve efficacy (Imlah et al. 1965; Kay et al. 1970; Seager and Bird 1962). However, recent studies suggest that the combination of ECT and a TCA (but not an SSRI) leads to improved short-term outcome (Lauritzen et al. 1996; Nelson and Benjamin 1989). A reevaluation is needed of the role of concomitant antidepressant medications with ECT both as a means of enhancing short-term efficacy and as a means of getting a head-start on relapse prevention.

Another development that will likely influence practice is that of new methods of treatment that no longer require direct electrical stimulation. We now know that electrical dose–response relationships exist in ECT, and brain imaging research indicates that alterations of functional activity in discrete neural systems may be tied to efficacy. Consequently, we need treatment methods that provide far greater control over stimulus dosing in the brain and over the spatial distribution of the brain tissue being stimulated. This control might be achieved by the use of repetitive magnetic stimulation as a convulsive treatment, a possibility under active investigation (Lisanby et al., in press; Sackeim 1994c).

Finally, the most pressing clinical question facing the use of ECT is the problem of rapid relapse. Although ECT can be of remarkable short-term benefit in patients with medication-resistant depression, optimal pharmacologic continuation therapy for this group is uncertain. We can anticipate that over the next several years, the strengths and limits of specific pharmacologic strategies will be better defined and an increased role for continuation ECT will be emphasized (Sackeim 1994a).

Transcranial Magnetic Stimulation

Through the principle of magnetic induction, TMS can induce current flow in spatially targeted regions of the cortex. At sufficient magnetic intensity, neurons will depolarize. After a train of stimulation and depending on its parameters, cortical regions may exhibit increased excitability or enhanced inhibition. This capacity to alter neuronal activity in a spatially targeted fashion gives TMS special promise as a probe to study brain–behavior relationships and the neural systems that regulate emotional processes and as a therapeutic tool in the treatment of neuropsychiatric illness (George et al. 1999).

When TMS pulses are delivered rhythmically and repetitively, the technique is termed *repetitive TMS* (rTMS). The ability of rTMS to stimulate brain areas noninvasively is a significant advance beyond techniques that require the invasive method of direct cortical electrical stimulation. This noninvasive ability is also an advance relative to transcranial electrical stimulation, as in ECT, because there is greater control over intracerebral induced current, both in magnitude and spatial distribution, with rTMS than with ECT. Research with this new tool has contributed to our understanding of various clinical and basic research issues (see George et al. 1999 for a review). As a therapeutic intervention, TMS has received the most attention to date for treatment of mood disorders (see George et al. [1999] and Lisanby and Sackeim [2000] for reviews).

Description of the Technique

Magnetic stimulators capitalize on the ability of time-varying magnetic fields to induce eddy currents in biologic tissue. Production of the magnetic field is accomplished by storing electrical charge in capacitors that discharge in brief pulses through a stimulating coil. The time-varying pulse produces a time-varying magnetic field around the coil, with the magnetic flux perpendicular to the current flow in the coil. When the magnetic field is near a conducting medium, such as the brain, electrical current is induced; with sufficient induced current, neurons depolarize. This technique has been used to stimulate peripheral nerves (Bickford and Fremming 1965; Polson et al. 1982) and the central nervous system (Barker et al. 1985, 1987).

The scalp and skull are transparent to the magnetic field. Thus, they do not present the impedance encountered by transcranial electrical stimulation, which means that TMS allows better control over the site and intensity of stimulation. With rTMS, the degree of focality depends on coil design, geometry, and orientation relative to neuronal fibers (Amassian et al. 1992; Cohen et al. 1990; Maccabee et al. 1993; Meyer et al. 1991; Mills et al. 1992; Rösler 1989; Roth et al. 1991). Currently, the limit in spatial resolution is about 0.5 cm, as demonstrated by the selective stimulation of cortical representations of neighboring muscle groups in the motor strip (Brasil-Neto et al. 1992). The strength of the magnetic field decreases with increasing distance from the coil. Even at high intensity, depth of stimulation is estimated to be 2 cm below the scalp, reaching the cortex near the gray-white junction (Epstein 1990; Rudiak and Marg 1994). This does not mean that rTMS does not have remote or transsynaptic effects. George et al. (1996) reported an increase in thyrotropin-stimulating hormone (TSH) after rTMS to the dorsolateral prefrontal cortex (DLPFC), indicating subcortical effects. In the first ^{15}O–positron emission tomography study combining CBF measurement during rTMS, Paus et al. (1997) found that rTMS delivered to the frontal eye field resulted in dose-dependent distal effects in superior parietal and medial parieto-occipital regions, consistent with the pattern of connectivity within the visual system.

The first magnetic stimulators delivered single magnetic pulses at slow rates of repetition (0.3 Hz). Single-pulse TMS or slow rTMS has been used to map sensorimotor cortex (Brasil-Neto et al. 1992; Wassermann et al. 1992) and selectively interrupt visual perception (Amassian et al. 1993). However, faster repetition rates are generally required to alter higher cortical functions and emotional processes (Ojemann 1993). New high-frequency repetitive magnetic stimulators achieve repetition rates up to 50 Hz. Use of stimulation frequencies above 1 Hz is referred to as *fast rTMS*.

Clinical Effects of rTMS in Mood Disorders

Recent trials suggest that rTMS has therapeutic properties in major depression. Three reports found that slow rTMS, administered at the vertex and various other locations, reduces depressive symptoms (Grisaru et al. 1994; Höflich et al. 1993; Kolbinger et al. 1995). Although left DLPFC rTMS is reported to induce transient sadness in normal (i.e., psychiatrically well) volunteers (George et al. 1996; Pascual-Leone et al. 1996b), recent studies have shown notable antidepressant effects when fast rTMS is delivered to the left DLPFC in clinical samples. An open trial found that left prefrontal rTMS exerted antidepressant effects in two of six patients with medication-resistant depression (George et al. 1995). Catalá et al. (1996) reported that daily rTMS applied to the left DLPFC improved symptoms of depression in seven patients with medication-resistant psychotic depression but that right DLPFC rTMS had no effect. Figiel et al. (1998) administered fast left DLPFC rTMS to 56 patients referred for ECT for treatment of largely medication-resistant depression. After 5 days of rTMS, Figiel et al. (1998) reported a 42% response rate, with a significant number of patients not requiring ECT. Using a different open design, Conca et al. (1996) treated depression in a cohort of patients with an SSRI alone or with an SSRI and rTMS augmentation. The rTMS group had a faster antidepressant response, suggesting that rTMS has potential as an augmentation strategy.

Grunhaus et al. (1998, 2000) conducted the first study in which patients were randomized to rTMS or ECT. In this nonblind comparison, 40 patients received either daily fast left DLPFC rTMS for 4 weeks or ECT. Among nonpsychotic patients, no difference was discerned in efficacy or speed of response between the two treatments. Both interventions had beneficial effects in psychotic depression, but ECT was superior. Similar to the Figiel et al. (1998) results, this study suggests that some patients may show the same magnitude of short-term response to rTMS as to ECT. The preliminary clinical findings are especially encouraging because this use of rTMS is nonconvulsive, does not involve exposure to anesthesia, and has no obvious adverse cognitive side effects.

The efficacy of any potential antidepressant treatment must be established using placebo-controlled or sham-controlled procedures under double-blind conditions. This is a particular problem for TMS because an investigator must administer the treatment, usually in sessions lasting about 20 minutes. This individual is not blind to treatment conditions and can have extensive, repeated contact with patients. In addition, there has been variability in the nature of the sham control contrasted with active rTMS conditions. Sham rTMS usually involves angulating the coil relative to the head so as to produce the peripheral effects of active rTMS (stimulation of peripheral muscles in the face and scalp, acoustic artifact) while minimizing induced current in the brain. Different methods of angulation have been used, and some supposed sham conditions may result in significant induced current in the brain (Lisanby et al. 1998).

A set of trials have examined the efficacy of slow and fast rTMS under quasi-blind conditions. Pascual-Leone et al. (1996a) reported that 5 days of left DLPFC rTMS exerted marked antidepressant effects in 11 of 17 patients with medication-resistant psychotic depression. Right DLPFC rTMS, vertex rTMS, and left and right DLPFC sham rTMS produced no change. The magnitude of therapeutic effect in this study was remarkable, with 50% reductions in Hamilton Rating Scale for Depression scores obtained after 5 days of fast left DLPFC rTMS. In contrast, in another blind, sham-controlled trial, George et al. (1997) found that daily left DLPFC rTMS for 2 weeks had statistically significant but clinically unimpressive antidepressant activity in outpatients with major depression.

The reason for the discrepancy in the magnitude of therapeutic effects in these studies is unknown but may relate to the specific stimulation parameters used. A recent sham-controlled study of slow rTMS delivered with a nonfocal, round coil over the right hemisphere in 71 patients with major depression found robust antidepressant effects with the active condition (Klein et al. 1999). This finding is of particular importance because the major safety risk of fast rTMS is the induction of a seizure (Wassermann 1998). Slow rTMS appears to lack this risk. Tormos et al. randomized depressed patients to 2 weeks of treatment with fast left DLPFC rTMS, slow left DLPFC rTMS, slow right DLPFC rTMS, and sham stimulation (personal communication, A. Pascual-Leone, March 1998). Both fast left and slow right DLPFC rTMS exerted marked antidepressant effects, with little change in the slow right and sham conditions. Fast rTMS is believed to result in a net excitatory effect, whereas the neurophysiologic changes following slow rTMS may reflect increased inhibition (George et al. 1999). The Tormos et al. findings, in line with other studies, suggest that increased excitation in left prefrontal regions or increased inhibition in right prefrontal regions is associated with antidepressant effects.

Future Directions

It is far from established that rTMS will have a significant clinical role in the treatment of major depression. As noted previously, initial studies of rTMS have been characterized by disparate effect sizes for therapeutic properties and methodologic limitations regarding the nature of sham control and the adequacy of the blind. It appears that rTMS can exert antidepressant effects; however, we lack information about the longevity of these effects and the characteristics of the patients most likely to benefit. A fundamental question when considering the role of rTMS is whether its therapeutic properties are potent in patients with medication-resistant (and ECT-resistant) depression, or whether the patients most likely to benefit from rTMS are those whose depression has responded to other somatic treatments. The initial studies have suggested that clinical improvement with rTMS occurs rapidly; therefore, even if rTMS is most suitable for the patient subgroups that ordinarily would receive pharmacologic treatment, rTMS might be used as an augmentation agent to accelerate antidepressant response (Conca et al. 1996).

The antidepressant effects of rTMS appear to be highly contingent on the site and parameters of stimulation. Available evidence suggests that fast rTMS to the left DLPFC and slow rTMS to the right DLPFC both have significant therapeutic properties. This observation raises critical questions about the neural circuitry involved in reversing the symptoms of major depression and the nature of physiologic alterations that sustain antidepressant effects. The coupling of rTMS treatment studies with brain imaging investigation should prove fertile in advancing understanding of the mechanisms of action of this intervention (George et al. 1999).

Vagus Nerve Stimulation

Vagus nerve stimulation (VNS) using the Neurocybernetic Prosthesis (NCP) developed by Cyberonics (Webster, TX) was approved by the U.S. Food and Drug Administration in 1997 for the treatment of medically resistant partial complex seizures. VNS involves the surgical implantation of a battery-operated stimulator on the upper left side of the patient's chest. Leads ending in helical electrodes are tunneled from the stimulator to the left vagus nerve. The stimulation parameters are programmable and allow control over output current (0–4 mA), pulse frequency (1–145 Hz), pulse width (130–1,000 ms), signal-on time (7–270 s), and signal-off time (0.2–180 min) (Schachter and Saper 1998).

An external magnet placed against the chest can be used to provide additional stimulation. In some cases this additional stimulation may interrupt or weaken a seizure (Hammond et al. 1992).

Approximately 80% of fibers in the vagus nerve are afferent to higher brain centers, providing visceral feedback from the head, neck, thorax, and abdomen (Agostini et al. 1957). Early research demonstrated that VNS in animals can lead to marked changes in the EEG, including the induction of highly desynchronized or synchronized cortical activity, depending on stimulation parameters (Zanchetti et al. 1952). The primary output of the vagus nerve is to the nucleus of the solitary tract (NTS). The NTS has three primary projections: 1) autonomic preganglionic and related motor neurons in the medulla and spinal cord, involved in the regulation of heart rate, blood pressure, and respiration; 2) reticular formation in the medulla, which modulates arousal and autonomic reflexes; and 3) the widespread areas in the forebrain, principally via projections of the parabrachial nucleus to intralaminar thalamic nuclei (Ruggiero et al. 1989; Saper 1987). Based on the physiologic consequences of VNS, especially desynchronization of cortical rhythms, and its accessibility as a means of altering widespread functional brain activity, animal studies were conducted that established the anticonvulsant properties of VNS (McLachlan 1993; Zabara 1992).

The animal work was followed by large-scale clinical trials in patients with treatment-resistant complex partial seizures. The clinical trials used multicenter, double-blind, randomized, parallel group, active control designs. The NCP system was implanted in all subjects, who were randomly assigned to low- or high-intensity stimulation conditions (Ben-Menachem et al. 1994; Ramsay et al. 1994; Vagus Nerve Stimulation Study Group 1995). Overall the findings indicated that high-intensity VNS resulted in greater improvement in seizure frequency than did low-intensity stimulation. An unusual aspect of the findings with VNS is that efficacy in control of seizures appears to improve with time. Instead of developing tolerance, VNS patients appear to experience further reductions in seizure frequency at long-term follow-up (Salinsky et al. 1996). The principle side effects of VNS are hoarseness, throat pain, coughing, dyspnea, and altered pitch of the voice.

Although VNS appears to be a valuable intervention for patients with treatment-resistant epilepsy, whether it will be of benefit for those with treatment-resistant major depression is uncertain. The rationale for testing its efficacy in mood disorders is based on several indirect observations. First and most critically, significant overlap exists between the anticonvulsant medications used to control epilepsy and the mood stabilizers commonly used to treat affective disorders. Furthermore, ECT, a highly effective antidepressant and antimanic treatment, has profound anticonvulsant effects (Sackeim 1999; Sackeim et al. 1983). Second, several investigators in the epilepsy trials claimed that VNS was associated with mood elevation, possibly independent of seizure control. Unfortunately, formal assessment of mood change was not conducted. Third, VNS is known to act on the central neurotransmitter systems implicated in the pathophysiology of major depression. For instance, in animal models, lesioning of the locus coeruleus reverses the anticonvulsant properties of VNS, suggesting a role for norepinephrine release (Krahl et al. 1998). In humans, VNS has been shown to produce increased cerebrospinal fluid levels of 5-hydroxyindoleactic acid, the major metabolite of serotonin. Finally, functional imaging studies during VNS suggest widespread modulation of cerebral activity, including regions dysregulated in major depression (e.g., Henry et al. 1998).

A preliminary study has suggested that VNS is effective in the treatment of unipolar and bipolar major depression (Rush et al. 2000). Because this intervention involves surgery, perioperative risks, and a potentially significant side effect burden, its role will likely be limited to those patients who have exhausted established somatic treatments for major depression owing to intolerance or lack of response. What is particularly intriguing about VNS is that the preliminary evidence from trials in epilepsy shows progressive improvement in seizure control with time. Given that patients with treatment-resistant major depression often have highly recurrent or chronic presentations, there may be a role for a treatment that by its very nature ensures compliance and long-term benefit in mood regulation. In the next few years, further research will determine whether VNS can fulfill this role.

References

Abrams R: Electroconvulsive Therapy, 3rd Edition. New York, Oxford University Press, 1997

Ackermann RF, Engel J Jr, Baxter L: Positron emission tomography and auto-radiographic studies of glucose utilization following electroconvulsive seizures in humans and rats. Ann N Y Acad Sci 462:263–269, 1986

Agostini E, Chinnock JE, Daly MD, et al: Functional and histological studies of the vagus nerve and its branches to the heart, lungs, and abdominal viscera in the cat. J Physiol 135:182–205, 1957

Amassian VE, Eberle L, Maccabee PJ, et al: Modelling magnetic coil excitation of human cerebral cortex with a peripheral nerve immersed in a brain-shaped volume conductor: the significance of fiber bending in excitation. Electroencephalogr Clin Neurophysiol 85:291–301, 1992

Amassian VE, Cracco RQ, Maccabee PJ, et al: Unmasking human visual perception with the magnetic coil and its relationship to hemispheric asymmetry. Brain Res 605:312–316, 1993

Barker AT, Jalinous R, Freeston IL: Non-invasive magnetic stimulation of human motor cortex. Lancet 1:1106–1107, 1985

Barker AT, Freeston IL, Jalinous R, et al: Magnetic stimulation of the human brain and peripheral nervous system: an introduction and the results of an initial clinical evaluation. Neurosurgery 20 (suppl 1):100–109, 1987

Ben-Menachem E, Mañon-Espaillat R, Ristanovic R, et al: Vagus nerve stimulation for treatment of partial seizures, 1: a controlled study of effect on seizures. First International Vagus Nerve Stimulation Study Group. Epilepsia 35:616–626, 1994

Bickford RG, Fremming BD: Neuronal stimulation by pulsed magnetic fields in animals and man. Digest of the 6th International Conference on Medical Electronics and Biological Engineering, 1965, p 112

Brasil-Neto JP, McShane LM, Fuhr P, et al: Topographic mapping of the human motor cortex with magnetic stimulation: factors affecting accuracy and reproducibility. Electroencephalogr Clin Neurophysiol 85:9–16, 1992

Catalá M, Rubio B, Pascual-Leone A: Lateralized effect of rapid-rate transcranial magnetic stimulation (rTMS) of dorsolateral prefrontal (DLPF) cortex on depression. Neurology 46:A325, 1996

Clarke TB, Coffey CE, Hoffman GW, et al: Continuation therapy for depression using outpatient electroconvulsive therapy. Convulsive Therapy 5:330–337, 1989

Coffey CE, Figiel GS, Djang WT, et al: Subcortical hyperintensity on magnetic resonance imaging: a comparison of normal and depressed elderly subjects. Am J Psychiatry 147:187–189, 1990

Coffey CE, Lucke J, Weiner RD, et al: Seizure threshold in electroconvulsive therapy, I: initial seizure threshold. Biol Psychiatry 37:713–720, 1995

Cohen LG, Roth BJ, Nilsson J, et al: Effects of coil design on delivery of focal magnetic stimulation: technical considerations. Electroencephalogr Clin Neurophysiol 75:350–357, 1990

Conca A, Koppi S, Konig P, et al: Transcranial magnetic stimulation: a novel antidepressive strategy? Neuropsychobiology 34:204–207, 1996

Decina P, Guthrie EB, Sackeim HA, et al: Continuation ECT in the management of relapses of major affective episodes. Acta Psychiatr Scand 75:559–562, 1987

Drevets WC: Functional neuroimaging studies of depression: the anatomy of melancholia. Annu Rev Med 49:341–361, 1998

Epstein CM: Localizing the site of magnetic brain stimulation in humans. Neurology 40:666–670, 1990

Farah A, McCall WV: Electroconvulsive therapy stimulus dosing: a survey of contemporary practices. Convuls Ther 9:90–94, 1993

Figiel GS, Epstein C, McDonald WM, et al: The use of rapid-rate transcranial magnetic stimulation (rTMS) in refractory depressed patients. J Neuropsychiatry Clin Neurosci 10:20–25, 1998

Fink M: Convulsive Therapy: Theory and Practice. New York, Raven Press, 1979

Fink M: How does ECT work? Neuropsychopharmacology 3:77–82, 1990

Fink M, Sackeim HA: Convulsive therapy in schizophrenia? Schizophr Bull 22:27–39, 1996

George MS, Wassermann EM, Williams WA, et al: Daily repetitive transcranial magnetic stimulation (rTMS) improves mood in depression. Neuroreport 6:1853–1856, 1995

George MS, Wassermann EM, Williams WA, et al: Changes in mood and hormone levels after rapid-rate transcranial magnetic stimulation (rTMS) of the prefrontal cortex. J Neuropsychiatry Clin Neurosci 8:172–180, 1996

George MS, Wassermann EM, Kimbrell TA, et al: Mood improvement following daily left prefrontal repetitive transcranial magnetic stimulation in patients with depression: a placebo-controlled crossover trial. Am J Psychiatry 154:1752–1756, 1997

George MS, Lisanby SH, Sackeim HA: Transcranial magnetic stimulation: applications in psychiatry. Arch Gen Psychiatry 56:300–311, 1999

Grisaru N, Yarovslavsky U, Abarbanel J, et al: Transcranial magnetic stimulation in depression and schizophrenia. Eur Neuropsychopharmacol 4:287–288, 1994

Grunhaus L, Dannon P, Schrieber S: Effects of transcranial magnetic stimulation on severe depression: similarities with ECT. Biol Psychiatry 43:76S, 1998

Grunhaus L, Dannon PN, Schreiber S, et al: Repetitive transcranial magnetic stimulation is as effective as electroconvulsive therapy in the treatment of nondelusional major depressive disorder: an open study. Biol Psychiatry 47:314–324, 2000

Hammond EJ, Uthman BM, Reid SA, et al: Electrophysiological studies of cervical vagus nerve stimulation in humans, I: EEG effects. Epilepsia 33:1013–1020, 1992

Henry TR, Bakay RA, Votaw JR, et al: Brain blood flow alterations induced by therapeutic vagus nerve stimulation in partial epilepsy, I: acute effects at high and low levels of stimulation. Epilepsia 39:983–990, 1998

Höflich G, Kasper S, Hufnagel A, et al: Application of transcranial magnetic stimulation in treatment of drug-resistant major depression: a report of two cases. Human Psychopharmacology 8:361–365, 1993

Imlah NW, Ryan E, Harrington JA: The influence of antidepressant drugs on the response to electroconvulsive therapy and on subsequent relapse rates. Neuropsychopharmacology 4:438–442, 1965

Kalinowsky LB, Hoch PH: Shock Treatments and Other Somatic Procedures in Psychiatry. New York, Grune & Stratton, 1946

Kay DW, Fahy T, Garside RF: A seven-month double-blind trial of amitriptyline and diazepam in ECT-treated depressed patients. Br J Psychiatry 117:667–671, 1970

Kety S: Biochemical and neurochemical effects of electroconvulsive shock, in Psychobiology of Convulsive Therapy. Edited by Fink M, Kety S, McGaugh J, et al. Washington, DC, VH Winton & Sons, 1974, pp 285–294

Klein E, Kreinin I, Chistyokov A, et al: Therapeutic efficacy of right prefrontal slow repetitive transcranial magnetic stimulation in major depression: a double-blind controlled study. Arch Gen Psychiatry 56:315–320, 1999

Kolbinger H, Höflich G, Hufnagel A, et al: Transcranial magnetic stimulation (TMS) in the treatment of major depression: a pilot study. Human Psychopharmacology 10:305–310, 1995

Krahl SE, Clark KB, Smith DC, et al: Locus coeruleus lesions suppress the seizure-attenuating effects of vagus nerve stimulation. Epilepsia 39:709–714, 1998

Krueger RB, Sackeim HA: Electroconvulsive therapy and schizophrenia, in Schizophrenia. Edited by Hirsch SR, Weinberger D. Oxford, Blackwell Scientific, 1995, pp 503–545

Krueger RB, Sackeim HA, Gamzu ER: Pharmacological treatment of the cognitive side effects of ECT: a review. Psychopharmacol Bull 28:409–424, 1992

Lauritzen L, Odgaard K, Clemmesen L, et al: Relapse prevention by means of paroxetine in ECT-treated patients with major depression: a comparison with imipramine and placebo in medium-term continuation therapy. Acta Psychiatr Scand 94:241–251, 1996

Lisanby SH, Sackeim HA: TMS in major depression, in Transcranial Magnetic Stimulation (TMS): Applications in Neuropsychiatry. Edited by George MS, Belmaker RH. Washington, DC, American Psychiatric Press, 2000, pp 185–200

Lisanby SH, Devanand DP, Nobler MS, et al: Exceptionally high seizure threshold: ECT device limitations. Convuls Ther 12:156–164, 1996

Lisanby SH, Luber B, Schroeder C, et al: Intracerebral measurement of rTMS and ECS induced voltage in vivo. Biol Psychiatry 43:100S, 1998

Lisanby S, Luber B, Finck A, et al: Deliberate seizure induction with repetitive transcranial magnetic stimulation. Arch Gen Psychiatry, in press

Maccabee PJ, Amassian VE, Eberle LP, et al: Magnetic coil stimulation of straight and bent amphibian and mammalian peripheral nerve in vitro: locus of excitation. J Physiol (Lond) 460:201–219, 1993

Malcolm K, Dean J, Rowlands P, et al: Antidepressant drug treatment in relation to the use of ECT. J Psychopharmacol 5:255–258, 1991

McCall WV, Reboussin DM, Weiner RD, et al: Titrated moderately suprathreshold vs fixed high-dose right unilateral electroconvulsive therapy: acute antidepressant and cognitive effects. Arch Gen Psychiatry 57:438–444, 2000

McLachlan RS: Suppression of interictal spikes and seizures by stimulation of the vagus nerve. Epilepsia 34:918–923, 1993

Meyer BU, Britton TC, Kloten H, et al: Coil placement in magnetic brain stimulation related to skull and brain anatomy. Electroencephalogr Clin Neurophysiol 81:38–46, 1991

Mills KR, Boniface SJ, Schubert M: Magnetic brain stimulation with a double coil: the importance of coil orientation. Electroencephalogr Clin Neurophysiol 85:17–21, 1992

National Institutes of Health: Consensus conference: electroconvulsive therapy. JAMA 254:2103–2108, 1985

Nelson JP, Benjamin L: Efficacy and safety of combined ECT and tricyclic antidepressant drugs in the treatment of depressed geriatric patients. Convuls Ther 5:321–329, 1989

Nobler MS, Sackeim HA, Solomou M, et al: EEG manifestations during ECT: effects of electrode placement and stimulus intensity. Biol Psychiatry 34:321–330, 1993

Nobler MS, Sackeim HA, Prohovnik I, et al: Regional cerebral blood flow in mood disorders, III. treatment and clinical response. Arch Gen Psychiatry 51:884–897, 1994

Ojemann GA: Functional mapping of cortical language areas in adults: intra-operative approaches, in Electrical and Magnetic Stimulation of the Brain and Spinal Cord. Edited by Devinsky BD. New York, Raven Press, 1993, pp 155–163

Ottosson J-O: Experimental studies of the mode of action of electroconvulsive therapy. Acta Psychiatr Scand 145(suppl):1–141, 1960

Pascual-Leone A, Catalá MD, Pascual-Leone Pascual A: Lateralized effect of rapid-rate transcranial magnetic stimulation of the prefrontal cortex on mood. Neurology 46:499–502, 1996a

Pascual-Leone A, Rubio B, Pallardo F, et al: Rapid-rate transcranial magnetic stimulation of left dorsolateral prefrontal cortex in drug-resistant depression. Lancet 348:233–237, 1996b

Paus T, Jech R, Thompson CJ, et al: Transcranial magnetic stimulation during positron emission tomography: a new method for studying connectivity of the human cerebral cortex. J Neurosci 17:3178–3184, 1997

Polson MJR, Barker AT, Freeston IL: Stimulation of nerve trunks with time-varying magnetic fields. Med Biol Eng Comput 20:243–244, 1982

Prudic J, Sackeim HA, Devanand DP: Medication resistance and clinical response to electroconvulsive therapy. Psychiatry Res 31:287–296, 1990

Prudic J, Sackeim HA, Devanand DP, et al: Acute cognitive effects of subconvulsive electrical stimulation. Convuls Ther 10:4–24, 1994

Prudic J, Haskett RF, Mulsant B, et al: Resistance to antidepressant medications and short-term clinical response to ECT. Am J Psychiatry 153:985–992, 1996

Prudic J, Fitzsimons L, Nobler MS, et al: Naloxone in the prevention of the adverse cognitive effects of ECT: a within-subject, placebo controlled study. Neuropsychopharmacology 21:285–293, 1999

Ramsay RE, Uthman BM, Augustinsson LE, et al: Vagus nerve stimulation for treatment of partial seizures, 2: safety, side effects, and tolerability. First International Vagus Nerve Stimulation Study Group. Epilepsia 35:627–636, 1994

Robin A, De Tissera S: A double-blind controlled comparison of the therapeutic effects of low and high energy electroconvulsive therapies. Br J Psychiatry 141:357–366, 1982

Rösler KM: Significance of shape and size of the stimulating coil in magnetic stimulation of the human motor cortex. Neurosci Lett 100:347–352, 1989

Roth BJ, Saypol JM, Hallett M, et al: A theoretical calculation of the electric field induced in the cortex during magnetic stimulation. Electroencephalogr Clin Neurophysiol 81:47–56, 1991

Rudiak D, Marg E: Finding the depth of magnetic brain stimulation: a re-evaluation. Electroencephalogr Clin Neurophysiol 93:358–371, 1994

Ruggiero DA, Cravo SL, Arango V, et al: Central control of the circulation by the rostral ventrolateral reticular nucleus: anatomical substrates. Prog Brain Res 81:49–79, 1989

Rush AJ, George MS, Sackeim HA, et al: Vagus nerve stimulation (VNS) for treatment-resistant depressions: a multicenter study. Biol Psychiatry 47:276–286, 2000

Sackeim HA: The cognitive effects of electroconvulsive therapy, in Cognitive Disorders: Pathophysiology and Treatment. Edited by Moos WH, Gamzu ER, Thal LJ. New York, Marcel Dekker, 1992, pp 183–228

Sackeim HA: Central issues regarding the mechanisms of action of electroconvulsive therapy: directions for future research. Psychopharmacol Bull 30:281–308, 1994a

Sackeim HA: Continuation therapy following ECT: directions for future research. Psychopharmacol Bull 30:501–521, 1994b

Sackeim HA: Magnetic stimulation therapy and ECT. Convuls Ther 10:255–258, 1994c

Sackeim HA: What's new with ECT. American Society of Clinical Psychopharmacology Progress Notes 8:27–33, 1997

Sackeim HA: The anticonvulsant hypothesis of the mechanisms of action of ECT: current status. J ECT 15:5–26, 1999

Sackeim HA, Decina P, Prohovnik I, et al: Anticonvulsant and antidepressant properties of electroconvulsive therapy: a proposed mechanism of action. Biol Psychiatry 18:1301–1310, 1983

Sackeim HA, Portnoy S, Neeley P, et al: Cognitive consequences of low-dosage electroconvulsive therapy. Ann N Y Acad Sci 462:326–340, 1986

Sackeim HA, Decina P, Kanzler M, et al: Effects of electrode placement on the efficacy of titrated, low-dose ECT. Am J Psychiatry 144:1449–1455, 1987a

Sackeim HA, Decina P, Prohovnik I, et al: Seizure threshold in electroconvulsive therapy: effects of sex, age, electrode placement, and number of treatments. Arch Gen Psychiatry 44:355–360, 1987b

Sackeim HA, Prohovnik I, Moeller JR, et al: Regional cerebral blood flow in mood disorders, I: comparison of major depressives and normal controls. Arch Gen Psychiatry 47:60–70, 1990a

Sackeim HA, Prudic J, Devanand DP, et al: The impact of medication resistance and continuation pharmacotherapy on relapse following response to electroconvulsive therapy in major depression. J Clin Psychopharmacol 10:96–104, 1990b

Sackeim HA, Devanand DP, Prudic J: Stimulus intensity, seizure threshold, and seizure duration: impact on the efficacy and safety of electroconvulsive therapy. Psychiatr Clin North Am 14:803–43, 1991

Sackeim HA, Prudic J, Devanand DP, et al: Effects of stimulus intensity and electrode placement on the efficacy and cognitive effects of electroconvulsive therapy. N Engl J Med 328:839–846, 1993

Sackeim HA, Long J, Luber B, et al: Physical properties and quantification of the ECT stimulus, I: basic principles. Convuls Ther 10:93–123, 1994

Sackeim HA, Devanand DP, Nobler MS: Electroconvulsive therapy, in Psychopharmacology: The Fourth Generation of Progress. Edited by Bloom F, Kupfer D. New York, Raven, 1995, pp 1123–1142

Sackeim HA, Luber B, Katzman GP, et al: The effects of electroconvulsive therapy on quantitative electroencephalograms: relationship to clinical outcome. Arch Gen Psychiatry 53:814–824, 1996

Sackeim HA, Lisanby SH, Nobler MS, et al: MRI hyperintensities in major depression: the meaning of encephalomalacia, in Advances in Psychiatry. Edited by Andrade C. New Delhi, Oxford University Press, 2000a, pp 73–116

Sackeim HA, Prudic J, Devanand DP, et al: A prospective, randomized, double-blind comparison of bilateral and right unilateral electroconvulsive therapy at different stimulus intensities. Arch Gen Psychiatry 57:425–434, 2000b

Salinsky MC, Uthman BM, Ristanovic RK, et al: Vagus nerve stimulation for the treatment of medically intractable seizures: results of a 1-year open-extension trial. Vagus Nerve Stimulation Study Group. Arch Neurol 53:1176–1180, 1996

Saper CB: Diffuse cortical projections systems: anatomical organization and role in cortical function, in Handbook of Physiology: The Nervous System, Vol 5. Edited by Plum F. Bethesda, MD, American Physiological Society, 1987, pp 169–210

Schachter SC, Saper CB: Vagus nerve stimulation. Epilepsia 39:677–686, 1998

Seager CP, Bird RL: Imipramine with electrical treatment in depression: a controlled trial. J Ment Sci 108:704–707, 1962

Silfverskiöld P, Risberg J: Regional cerebral blood flow in depression and mania. Arch Gen Psychiatry 46:253–259, 1989

Thase ME, Rush AJ: When at first you don't succeed: sequential strategies for antidepressant nonresponders. J Clin Psychiatry 58(suppl 13):23–29, 1997

Thompson JW, Weiner RD, Myers CP: Use of ECT in the United States in 1975, 1980, and 1986. Am J Psychiatry 151:1657–1661, 1994

Vagus Nerve Stimulation Study Group: A randomized controlled trial of chronic vagus nerve stimulation for treatment of medically intractable seizures. Neurology 45:224–230, 1995

Wassermann EM: Risk and safety of repetitive transcranial magnetic stimulation: report and suggested guidelines from the International Workshop on the Safety of Repetitive Transcranial Magnetic Stimulation, June 5–7, 1996. Electroencephalogr Clin Neurophysiol 108:1–16, 1998

Wassermann EM, McShane LM, Hallett M, et al: Noninvasive mapping of muscle representations in human motor cortex. Electroencephalogr Clin Neurophysiol 85:1–8, 1992

Weiner RD, Rogers HJ, Davidson JR, et al: Effects of stimulus parameters on cognitive side effects. Ann N Y Acad Sci 462:315–325, 1986

Weiner RD, Fink M, Hammersley D, et al: The Practice of Electroconvulsive Therapy: Recommendations for Treatment, Training, and Privileging. Washington, DC, American Psychiatric Press, 1990

Weiner RD, Coffey CE, Fochtmann L, et al: The Practice of Electroconvulsive Therapy: Recommendations for Treatment, Training, and Privileging, 2nd Edition. Washington, DC, American Psychiatric Press, 2001

Zabara J: Inhibition of experimental seizures in canines by repetitive vagal stimulation. Epilepsia 33:1005–1012, 1992

Zanchetti A, Wang SC, Moruzzi G: The effect of vagal stimulation on the EEG pattern of the cat. Electroencephalogr Clin Neurophysiol 4:357–361, 1952

Zielinski RJ, Roose SP, Devanand DP, et al: Cardiovascular complications of ECT in depressed patients with cardiac disease. Am J Psychiatry 150:904–909, 1993

10

Achieving Better Treatment Outcomes in Early Onset Depression

David A. Brent, M.D.

Overview

Early onset depression, or depression that has its onset prior to age 18 years, is common, recurrent, impairing, and has long-term consequences into adult life. Epidemiologic studies indicate that approximately 2% of prepubertal children have a major mood disorder, with the prevalence increasing to 5%–8% in adolescents (Fleming and Offord 1990; Lewinsohn and Hops 1993). Early onset depression is often both a chronic and a recurrent condition. In clinical samples an episode lasts 6–8 months, and the rate of relapse after symptomatic improvement is around 40% (Birmaher et al. 2000; Emslie et al. 1997; Kovacs et al. 1984a; Wood et al. 1996). A high rate of recurrence has been documented, with approximately 40% experiencing a recurrence within 2 years, nearly 75% in 5 years, and almost all experiencing another episode of depression sometime during adult life (Harrington et al. 1990;

Preparation of this chapter was supported by NIMH grants MH-46500 and MH-55123. Ms. Vanessa Ash's assistance in preparing the manuscript was greatly appreciated.

Kovacs et al. 1984b). Impairment has been well documented during the episode as a "scar" of the episode, and over the long run, consisting of an increased risk of poor performance in school and work, impaired interpersonal relationships, personality disorder, legal problems, substance abuse, suicide attempts, and completed suicide (Brent et al. 1993a; Kandel and Davies 1982; Kovacs et al. 1993; Lewinsohn et al. 1997, 1998; Rohde et al. 1994; Shaffer et al. 1996). In sum, early onset depression has long-term functional implications that interfere with the optimal developmental trajectory into adult life. Therefore, the proper treatment of this condition is of great public health interest.

Review of Extant Clinical Trials for Early-Onset Depression

Clinical trials for early onset depression can be divided into three types: clinical trials with symptomatic volunteers, clinical psychotherapy trials with clinically referred subjects, and clinical psychopharmacologic trials with clinically referred subjects.

Studies of symptomatic volunteers in general have shown that cognitive-behavioral therapy (CBT), usually delivered in a group format, was superior to a wait-list control condition (Kahn et al. 1990; Lewinsohn et al. 1990; Reynolds and Coats 1986; Stark et al. 1987). A meta-analysis showed that the effect sizes for these contrasts ranged between $d = 0.4$ and $d = 1.8$, with an average of around 1.0 (Reinecke et al. 1998). Evidence indicates persistence of treatment effects at follow-up, with a median effect size of $d = 0.6$ (Reinecke et al. 1998). However, for studies that also included an alternative psychosocial intervention (e.g., supportive group treatment, relaxation therapy), with one exception (Lerner and Clum 1990), no significant differences were found between CBT and the alternative treatments (Kahn et al. 1990; Reynolds and Coats 1986; Stark et al. 1987).

Studies of psychotherapy in clinical populations have been relatively few. A comparison of six to nine sessions of CBT with supportive therapy for the treatment of child and adolescent mood disorders found no difference; both groups showed a relatively high rate of relapse (Vostanis et al. 1996a, 1996b). Harrington et al. (1998) found that a brief family intervention was no better than treatment as usual for depressed, suicidal adolescents, although the family intervention was efficacious in reducing suicidality in the nondepressed subgroup. Wood et al. (1996) found that five to eight sessions of individual CBT was superior to relaxation therapy for child and adolescent mood disorders, but that by 6-month follow-up, the CBT group had relapsed and the relaxation therapy group had continued to recover, so that the two groups converged over time. Brent et al. (1997) compared CBT, family therapy, and supportive therapy and found that CBT resulted in more rapid and complete symptomatic improvement in major depression than either of the other two treatments. All three groups had a fairly high rate of relapse of around 30% at 2-year follow-up. Only 60% of the CBT group could be considered recovered at the end of treatment, leaving a substantial proportion of patients who were at least partially symptomatic.

Only one study of clinically referred adolescents has used group treatment. A comparison of two types of group therapy (therapeutic group support and social skills) found therapeutic group support to be superior to social skills therapy for the treatment of adolescent depression (Fine et al. 1991). Although the differences were statistically significant, they were not clinically significant, and the two treatments appeared equivalent at 9-month follow-up (Fine et al. 1991).

Clinical trials of psychopharmacologic treatment for child and adolescent depression focused primarily on the use of tricyclic antidepressants but have consistently failed to find a difference between drug and placebo, both in individual studies and on meta-analysis (Birmaher et al. 1998; Geller et al. 1990, 1992; Hazell et al. 1995; Kutcher et al. 1994; Puig-Antich et al. 1987). However, two studies have shown that selective serotonin reuptake inhibitors (SSRIs) are superior to placebo for the treatment of adolescent depression. First, Emslie et al. (1997) showed that fluoxetine was superior to placebo for the treatment of major depression. Even so, only 56% of the active drug group responded to treatment, and only 31% of the patients were considered recovered at the end of the 8-week trial. Second, a large, multicenter acute study compared the efficacy of paroxetine, imipramine, and placebo for adolescent major depression, and found that although paroxetine was superior to placebo, imipramine was not. This study was the first with adequate power to accept the null hypothesis that imipramine was not better than placebo (Keller et al. 1998).

Critique of Extant Trials

The studies in symptomatic volunteers can be criticized insofar as it is uncertain how volunteers are representative of patients seen in clinical settings. In addition, most of the studies of symptomatic volunteers compared treatment with a wait-list control condition, which does not control for the attention and support that is part of any intervention. Moreover, in several of these studies, when an alternative treatment was available, substantial differences were not found between the experimental and control treatments, undercutting somewhat the conclusions of efficacy for CBT. The greater endurance of treatment effects and relatively nonspecific response to treatment in these studies of symptomatic volunteers stands in contrast to the results of studies in clinically referred samples.

Treatment studies in patients can also be criticized with respect to the sampling frame because many clinical studies rely on advertising to obtain a sufficient number of subjects. As we discuss later in this chapter, subjects who are found through advertisements may respond to treatment differently than do clinically referred patients. Moreover, the inclusion and exclusion criteria for most clinical trials may make it difficult to generalize the results to patients seen in the real world (Weisz et al. 1995).

Perhaps the biggest weakness of all the extant clinical trials is that an intrinsic mismatch exists between the duration of treatment (5–16 weeks) and the duration of the depressive episode (6–8 months). The high rate of relapse—around 30%–40% in 6-month to 2-year follow-ups—in both psychosocial and pharmacologic trials, supports the view that the duration of acute treatment studies in these trials is simply too brief (Birmaher et al. 2000; Brent et al. 1999; Emslie et al. 1998; Vostanis et al. 1996b; Wood et al. 1996). Furthermore, naturalistic and quasiexperimental studies support the role of continuation treatment for both fluoxetine and CBT in preventing depressive relapse (Emslie et al. 1998; Kroll et al. 1996). In a 1-year naturalistic follow-up study, Emslie et al. (1998) found that patients who discontinued fluoxetine were 2.3 times more likely to relapse than those who discontinued medication. Kroll et al. (1996) found that depressed patients who received six monthly booster sessions of CBT after acute treatment had a relapse rate of 20%, compared with a 50% relapse rate among a previous cohort of control subjects receiving only acute CBT.

A related issue is that although symptomatic improvement is a necessary endpoint, the high rate of nonresponse and low rate of complete recovery indicate that this endpoint is not sufficient. It is unclear to what extent the high rate of partial response and nonresponse is a result of the brevity of these trials. A longer duration of treatment may be required for more complete symptomatic relief and functional improvement. Identification of a profile of patients who are unlikely to respond to brief intervention may be helpful in terms of both planning treatment and designing treatments to target resistant depression.

Dropout

Dropout from treatment is a potentially serious outcome; patients who drop out tend to be at greatest risk for prolonged depression and suicidal behavior. In one study, dropout was associated with greater hopelessness, which is a risk factor for suicidal behavior (Brent et al. 1998; Kazdin et al. 1983).

Treatment Nonresponse

Although there is extensive literature on the pharmacotherapy of adult depression with regard to when one can declare someone a treatment nonresponder (Thase et al. 1997), this work has not yet been performed in juvenile populations. The consensus in the adult literature is that one can declare a patient a nonresponder after 4–6 weeks of adequate pharmacotherapy and after 8–10 weeks of psychotherapy. Emslie et al. (1998) noted continual recovery after the completion of an 8-week trial of fluoxetine for those who continued treatment. In our psychotherapy study, we found that lack of response by 6 weeks was indicative of treatment failure, but beyond that the degree of partial response was not predictive of outcome at the end of 12–16 weeks (Brent et al. 1998). The pattern of treatment response in early onset depression is an important area of further inquiry.

Several studies have examined predictors of failure to respond to either pharmacologic or psychosocial treatment. Later age at onset or at presentation predicted worse outcome in two studies (Emslie et al. 1998; Jayson et al. 1998). This is a curious finding, because some longitudinal and family genetic studies have found that earlier age at onset is associated with a poorer prognosis and greater family loading for mood disorder (Kovacs and Devlin 1998; Kovacs et al. 1984a, 1984b). Other predictors of poor outcome included greater depression severity and poor functional status at intake and the presence of comorbid conditions, especially anxiety, greater cognitive distortion, and double depression (i.e., depression comorbid with dysthymia) (Brent et al. 1998; Clarke et al. 1992; Emslie et al. 1997; Jayson et al. 1998). One finding that should be investigated further is the role of parental depression on outcome. We found that in the presence of maternal depressive symptoms, the superior efficacy of CBT over other credible psychosocial treatments vanished (Brent et al. 1998) (Figure 10–1). These findings are consistent with naturalistic, longitudinal studies showing that comorbid conditions, dysthymic disorder, and exposure to parental depression all are associated with increased episode length (Kovacs et al. 1984a; Sanford et al. 1995; Warner et al. 1992).

One domain that deserves greater attention is the source of referral. Subjects who entered a clinical psychotherapy trial for the treatment of depression via an advertisement had much better outcomes than did those who came through clinical referral, despite overall similarity in depression severity at intake (Brent et al. 1998) (Figure 10–2). This difference was partially mediated by the fact that subjects coming to the study via advertisements were less hopeless than the clinically referred group (Brent et al. 1998) (Figure 10–3). The rank order in treatment efficacy was the same in the advertising and clinically referred groups, but the overall rate of depression at the end of the trial was four to eight times higher in the clinical group than in the advertising group. This finding should sound a cautionary note for investigators who rely heavily on advertising to recruit adequate numbers of subjects for clinical trials. Our findings are also consistent with the findings in studies of symptomatic volunteers, which report more enduring effects of treatment and higher response rates to nonspecific interventions than do studies of clinically referred subjects.

Rapid Response

In contrast to those patients who are not likely to respond to a brief course of either CBT or medication, some patients may respond to pla-

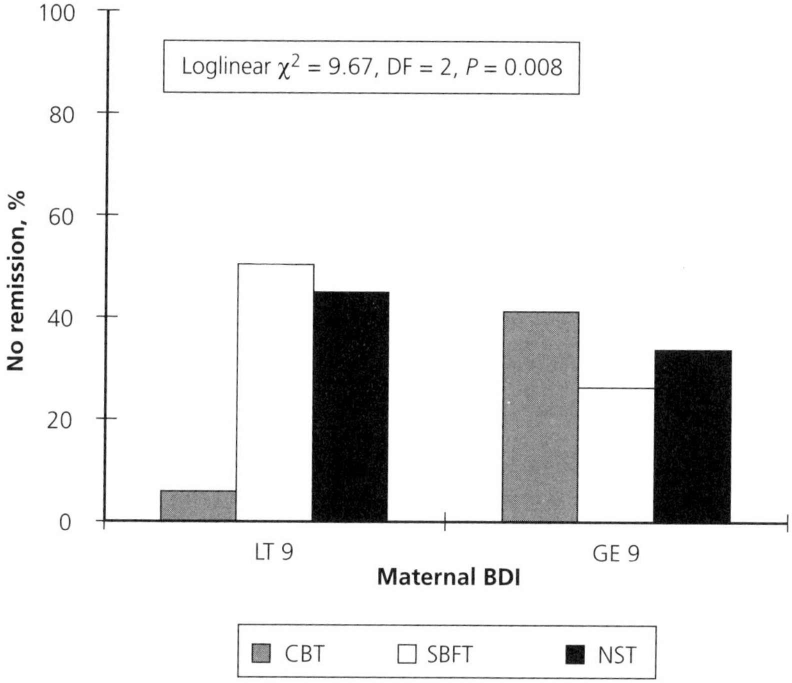
100
80
60
40
20
0
No remission, %
Loglinear χ^2 = 9.67, DF = 2, P = 0.008
LT 9
GE 9
Maternal BDI
CBT
SBFT
NST

FIGURE 10–1. Failure to achieve remission as a function of self-reported maternal depression. BDI = Beck Depression Inventory; CBT = cognitive-behavioral therapy; GE = greater than or equal to; LT = less than; NST = nondirective supportive therapy; SBFT = systemic-behavioral therapy.
Source. Brent DA, Kolko D, Birmaher B, et al.: "Predictors of Treatment Efficacy in a Clinical Trial of Three Psychosocial Treatments for Adolescent Depression." *J Am Acad Child Adolesc Psychiatry* 37(9):906–914, 1998.

cebo, education, or very brief, supportive intervention. According to Rintelmann et al. (1996), depressed patients who responded during the placebo washout period and were subsequently excluded from the Emslie et al. (1997) randomized clinical trial of fluoxetine for juvenile depression were younger and had better levels of overall function than did those who were placebo nonresponders. In our psychotherapy clinical trial, 31% of 100 depressed adolescents showed at least a 50% improvement on the Beck Depression Inventory by the beginning of the second treatment session (Renaud et al. 1998). Moreover, this group of rapid responders had a much higher rate of recovery and a lower rate

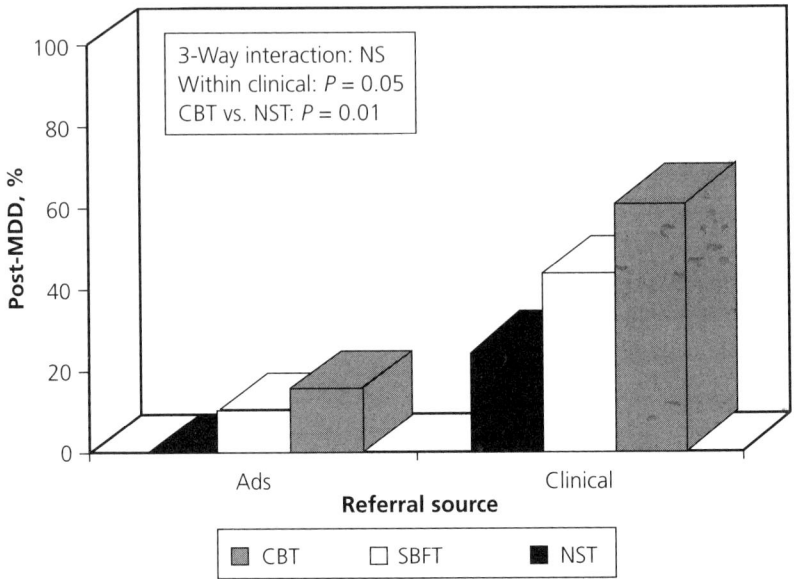

FIGURE 10-2. Rate of major depressive disorder at the end of treatment (post–major depressive disorder [post-MDD]) among treatment groups, by referral source. CBT = cognitive-behavioral therapy; NS = not significant; NST = nondirective supportive therapy; SBFT = systemic-behavioral therapy. *Source.*   Brent DA, Kolko D, Birmaher B, et al.: "Predictors of Treatment Efficacy in a Clinical Trial of Three Psychosocial Treatments for Adolescent Depression." *J Am Acad Adolesc Psychiatry* 37(9):906–914, 1998.

of recurrence of depression at follow-up compared with those who did not respond as rapidly. The rapid responder group was not markedly different than the other subjects and was not easily identified ahead of time. The rapid responders were characterized by a higher rate of one-parent families, lower self-reported (but not interview-rated) depression, lower hopelessness, and higher rate of maternal substance abuse compared with the rest of the samples. Perhaps this group was reacting to difficult family circumstances and therefore responded to support alone, given that 100% of the rapid responders in the supportive cell achieved clinical recovery. This finding suggests that a subgroup of depressed adolescents may not require a full "dose" of acute psychotherapy or pharmacotherapy, thereby conserving some resources for those

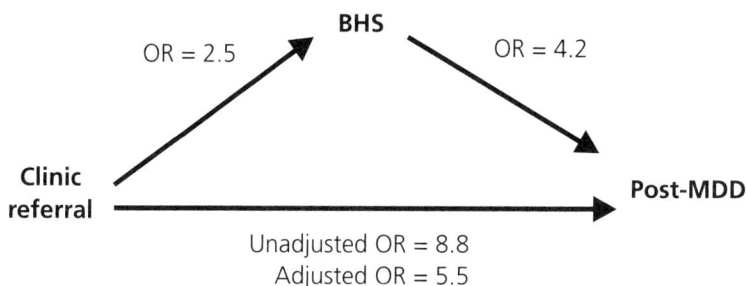

FIGURE 10–3. Tests of mediation: clinic referral (versus referral via advertisement) as a predictor of major depressive disorder at the end of treatment (post-MDD), mediated by Beck Hopelessness Scale (BHS; cutpoint = 13). OR = odds ratio.
Source. Brent DA, Kolko D, Birmaher B, et al.: "Predictors of Treatment Efficacy in a Clinical Trial of Three Psychosocial Treatments for Adolescent Depression." *J Am Acad Child Adolesc Psychiatry* 37(9):906–914, 1998.

patients with refractory depression who may require longer or more intense courses of treatment.

From the Laboratory to the Clinic

How well do acute treatments tested in the "laboratory" of the university setting transfer to real-world settings? Weisz et al. (1995) have observed that real-world patients often have greater clinical complexity, which may render them less responsive to treatments that have been shown to be efficacious under more controlled conditions. One can model how treatments may work for patients with greater clinical complexity by stratifying cases according to the number of adverse predictors of outcome. Cases with more adverse predictors of outcome are more like those seen under real-world conditions. A treatment intervention that is robust even with greater clinical complexity is likely to transfer well to real-world conditions, as it appears that CBT may do for adolescent depression (Brent et al. 1998) (Figure 10–4).

Relapse and Recurrence

Relatively few treatment studies have examined the long-term predictors of course. Two studies suggest that continuation of either CBT or

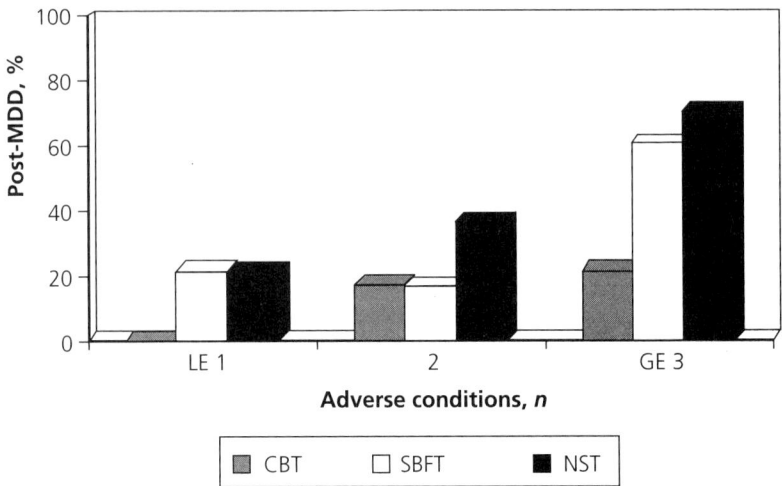

FIGURE **10–4.**   Rate of major depressive disorder at the end of treatment (post-MDD) as a function of the number of adverse conditions (i.e., comorbid anxiety, clinical source of referral, high cognitive distortion, and hopelessness). CBT = cognitive-behavioral therapy; GE = greater than or equal to; LE = less than or equal to; NST = nondirective supportive therapy; SBFT = systemic-behavioral therapy.

Source.   Brent DA, Kolko D, Birmaher B, et al.: "Predictors of Treatment Efficacy in a Clinical Trial of Three Psychosocial Treatments for Adolescent Depression." *J Am Acad Child Adolesc Psychiatry* 37(9):906–914, 1998.

fluoxetine decreases the relapse rate, although neither study used a randomized continuation–discontinuation design (Emslie et al. 1998; Kroll et al. 1996). Our data suggest that depression severity at intake, failure to recover after acute treatment, and family discord all predict recurrence and persistent depression (Birmaher et al. 2000). Because many of the patients who did not recover had subsyndromal depression, these findings are also consistent with the finding that treatment of subsyndromal depression results in a lower risk of the development of full-blown major depression (Clarke et al. 1995).

Predictors of Additional Service Use

Another way to assess the adequacy of a treatment package is to examine the additional services that are requested by families or recommended by treating clinicians. In our clinical psychotherapy trial of adolescent depression, we found that slightly more than half of the sample required additional services over the treatment period and subsequent 2-year follow-up (Brent et al. 1999). In the acute phase, the need for additional services was predicted by double depression, insofar as few patients with this condition responded to acute treatment. About half of patients with double depression eventually recovered, after a median of 10 months, with a combination of medication and psychotherapy. In the continuation phase of treatment, additional service use was predicted by three sets of problems: recurrence or relapse of depressive symptoms, behavioral problems, and family discord. The high rate of relapse and recurrence of depression and the additional services required to treat these relapses and recurrences provide additional evidence that 12–16 weeks of treatment may be too brief for many patients with early onset depression to stay depression free. The high prevalence of use of a combination of medication and psychotherapy for depression that is refractory to psychotherapy alone suggests that the combination of medication and psychotherapy deserves more careful evaluation for chronic depression. Behavioral difficulties and family discord were the two strongest predictors for inpatient hospitalization, indicating that treatment of depression alone was not sufficient to deal with these other, frequently co-occurring domains of difficulty.

Recommendations

Improving Compliance and Decreasing Dropout Rates

A consistent finding across almost all studies of chronic disease management is the importance of patient activation through education (Von Korff et al. 1997). In open trials of CBT, we found the dropout rate to be 40%. Once we added a psychoeducational component for the patient and family, the dropout rate (admittedly in the context of a clinical trial) was only 10% (Brent et al. 1993b). Psychoeducation, a critical element to be included in all interventions for depression, helps families know what to expect from treatment and how to monitor for treatment response, adverse side effects, and depressive relapse. If a patient has a profile consistent with treatment-resistant depression (e.g., double depression, comorbidity, parental depression), then the patient and family should be advised that the course of treatment will most likely be more protracted and that some trial and error may be needed to find the proper medication. In order to preserve the alliance with the patient and family, the clinician must inform them of these caveats *before* treatment begins.

Our findings about the prediction of early dropout and about the superior response in study subjects who responded to advertisements have a common thread related to hope and hopelessness. Study subjects who dropped out of treatment were more hopeless than those who stayed in treatment. Some of the greater efficacy of treatment in patients who responded to advertisements was explained by lower levels of hopelessness, despite similar depression severity (Brent et al. 1998). Therefore, at the initial phase of treatment, capitalizing on the motivation of the patient and family, instillation of hope that the treatment will work, and discussion of thoughts of hopelessness about the treatment are critical, both to prevent dropout and to boost outcome. Investigators should report results of clinical trials stratified by referral source, because the admixture of clinically referred subjects and those responding to advertisements may create substantial heterogeneity in treatment response.

Boosting the Efficacy of Acute Treatment

In their longitudinal follow-up study, Emslie et al. (1998) suggested that the rate of recovery improves with the length of treatment, although more work is needed to define when a patient can be termed a nonresponder. Predictors of poor response to either pharmacotherapy or cognitive therapy are convergent: chronicity of depression, severity of depression, comorbid condition, and family difficulties (Brent et al. 1998; Clarke et al. 1992; Emslie et al. 1998). These predictors are similar to predictors of treatment failure reported in the adult literature (Hirschfeld et al. 1995).

A critical component for improving outcome for the acute treatment of depression is having a strategic approach to chronic depression, which in patients with early onset depression most often takes the form of double depression. First, patients and their families should be apprised of the hope for eventual recovery and the realistic expectation that a chronic condition will take longer to respond and that treatment will probably involve some degree of trial and error. Second, given the low rate of response to psychotherapy alone and new data showing that a combination of CBT and an antidepressant is superior to either monotherapy in adult chronic depression, patients with double depression should receive combined treatment. Third, as discussed later in this chapter, this group of patients is at high risk for relapse and recurrence, necessitating a careful long-term strategy for continuation and maintenance therapy.

The treatment of more severe depression requires further empiric work in the juvenile age group. Data from the adult multicenter collaborative study on depression indicate that imipramine was superior to CBT, but not to interpersonal therapy, for treatment of more severe depression (Elkin et al. 1989). Other studies have indicated that CBT and antidepressants both have an incomplete response to treatment of more severe depression (Thase et al. 1992, 1997). The role of the combination of medication and psychotherapy in severe early onset depression certainly merits further study.

Comorbid anxiety was a strong predictor of poor response to psychotherapy in two studies. In one study of symptomatic volunteers, comorbid anxiety predicted a poor response to group CBT (Clarke et al. 1992), whereas in a study of referred patients, it predicted a *poorer* outcome for family and supportive therapy but a *better* response to individual CBT (Brent et al. 1998). Our clinical impression is that problems with comorbid anxiety are overshadowed by the acute presentation of depression, but these difficulties reassert themselves as the depression begins to lift. Because anxiety disorders are a significant source of impairment and frequently co-occur with depression (Angold and Costello 1993), these conditions must be assessed and targeted as an integral component of the treatment of depression.

The presence of significant maternal depressive symptoms moderated the efficacy of CBT. Specifically, in the presence of these symptoms, CBT was no more efficacious than either family or supportive treatment, whereas in the absence of maternal depression, CBT was significantly better than the other two treatments (Brent et al. 1998). This finding is unlikely to be caused by genetic factors, because the lifetime rates of maternal (and paternal) depression were unrelated to outcome; only current maternal symptomatology was related to outcome. This finding suggests that treatment of maternal depression in this sample might have improved the outcome of CBT, and it is certainly consistent with naturalistic, longitudinal observations (Warner et al. 1992). We offered parents free treatment, but only a small proportion availed themselves of this service. Perhaps if parental treatment had been presented as part of the package required to help the identified patient (i.e., the child) get well, more parents would have been amenable to this intervention. To our knowledge, the impact of parental depression on outcome in pharmacotherapy has not been assessed.

Based on our data, almost one-third of depressed adolescents showed a greater than 50% decrease in the severity of depressive symptoms within one to two sessions of intake (Renaud et al. 1998). Follow-up of this subgroup of rapid responders showed that they continued to have a much more benign course than the rest of the depressed cohort, with a much greater rate of recovery and substantially lower rates of relapse and recurrence. To conserve resources for patients who may require intensive or long-term treatment, we recommend that all patients and their families receive psychoeducation and then a brief follow-up assessment. Patients who show an improvement of greater than 50% should be followed-up without further intervention.

Continuation Treatment

A major theme throughout the treatment literature is the high rate of relapse and recurrence once the acute treatment is withdrawn (Emslie et al. 1998; Vostanis et al. 1996b; Wood et al. 1996). Quasiexperimental studies indicate that continuation treatment may convey protection against relapse of depression (Emslie et al. 1998; Kroll et al. 1996). In our study of additional service use, we found a dramatic increase in additional service use about 3 months after the end of acute treatment, again suggesting the need for some kind of continuation treatment during the period of vulnerability to relapse (Brent et al. 1999). Therefore, continuation treatment with either psychotherapy or medication is recommended for at least 3–6 months after symptomatic recovery.

The role of symptomatic recovery in prediction of eventual course is a critical one. We and others have found that patients who continue to evince subsyndromal levels of depression are at risk for recurrence and persistence of depression (Clarke et al. 1995). Therefore, aggressive treatment of subsyndromal depression, perhaps with combination treatment, is recommended (Fava et al. 1998).

We found a strong and important relationship between family discord and both recurrence and persistence of depression (Birmaher et al. 2000). In our psychotherapy trial, family conflict was a strong predictor of relapse or recurrence and was particularly high in patients who were persistently depressed over the follow-up period. What is intriguing is that family conflict was not predictive of response to acute treatment and had the most effects only in prolonging the time to full recovery. This finding suggests a strategy that considers both the importance of family intervention and the sequence of the family intervention in relation to other interventions.

We recommend that family interventions be limited during the acute phase to psychoeducation and assessment and treatment of parental psychopathology unless family discord is an explicit complaint by the family or the adolescent. We base this recommendation on the relative resistance that families of depressed adolescents have to family treatment and on the superiority of CBT to family therapy for the acute relief of depressive symptoms (Brent et al. 1997). Moreover, in our measure of parent satisfaction with treatment, both family and supportive treatments deteriorated over time compared with CBT (Brent et al. 1997). Follow-up analyses showed that when discord was prominent, families were quite satisfied with family treatment, but when reported conflict was low, families became dissatisfied with this form of intervention (Stein et al., in press).

If the clinician has helped the adolescent achieve a modicum of symptom relief from depression, the alliance with the family and the patient should be relatively good. If evidence of significant family problems is still present at the end of acute treatment, this is a logical time to begin a second phase of psychoeducation and to recontract for additional services by discussing with the family what strategies would best help their adolescent to recover completely or stay well. Continuation of acute treatment (e.g., with medication or booster CBT sessions) should constitute one component of this phase of intervention. However, if significant family problems remain or emerge, it is reasonable to inform the family that these difficulties will likely interfere with the long-term chances of their adolescent staying depression free and to offer a series of sessions to target the identified family problems. Naturally this intervention requires empiric evaluation.

Future Research

In addition to testing the potential efficacy of these recommendations for the treatment of depression and the prevention of relapse, other areas require further attention. First, additional research is needed to address the treatment of depression in real-world settings, such as community mental health centers, primary care, or school settings, to determine whether the acute treatments that are efficacious in the university setting also help in the real world. Second, we now a have reasonable profile of patients who will not respond to acute monotherapy. We need to develop and test treatments for patients with treatment-resistant depression. This need extends to the treatment of comorbid conditions, such as the combination of mood disorder and anxiety, attention-deficit/hyperactivity disorder, conduct disorder, and substance abuse. Third, we need to develop and test maintenance interventions for patients who have chronic and recurrent depression, as has been outlined in adult depression (Kupfer 1999). Fourth, as we learn more about the genetics of depression and related conditions, we may be able to use genetic markers to predict treatment response and, hence, to target treatments more precisely and even to develop pharmacologic interventions that will be more efficacious for a genetic subgroup (Smeraldi et al. 1998). Finally, given that depressive episodes leave psychosocial scars, prevention—perhaps targeting youth whose parents have early onset depression—may be the most cost-effective strategy.

References

Angold A, Costello EJ: Depressive comorbidity in children and adolescents: empirical, theoretical, and methodological issues. Am J Psychiatry 150:1779–1791, 1993

Birmaher B, Waterman GS, Ryan ND, et al: Randomized, controlled trial of amitriptyline versus placebo for adolescents with "treatment-resistant" major depression. J Am Acad Child Adolesc Psychiatry 37:527–535, 1998

Birmaher B, Brent DA, Kolko D, et al: Clinical outcome after short-term psychotherapy for adolescents with major depressive disorder. Arch Gen Psychiatry 57:29–36, 2000

Brent DA, Perper JA, Moritz G, et al: Psychiatric risk factors of adolescent suicide: a case control study. J Am Acad Child Adolesc Psychiatry 32:521–529, 1993a

Brent DA, Poling K, McKain B, et al: A psychoeducational program for families of affectively ill children and adolescents. J Am Acad Child Adolesc Psychiatry 32:770–774, 1993b

Brent DA, Holder D, Kolko D, et al: A clinical psychotherapy trial for adolescent depression comparing cognitive, family, and supportive treatments. Arch Gen Psychiatry 54:877–885, 1997

Brent DA, Kolko D, Birmaher B, et al: Predictors of treatment in efficacy in a clinical trial of three psychosocial treatments for adolescent depression. J Am Acad Child Adolesc Psychiatry 37:906–914, 1998

Brent DA, Kolko D, Birmaher B, et al: A clinical trial for adolescent depression: predictors of additional treatment in the acute and follow-up phases of the trial. J Am Acad Child Adolesc Psychiatry 38:263–270, 1999

Clarke G, Hops H, Lewinsohn PM, et al: Cognitive-behavioral group treatment of adolescent depression: prediction of outcome. Behav Ther 23:341–354, 1992

Clarke GN, Hawkins W, Murphy M, et al: Targeted prevention of unipolar depressive disorder in an at-risk sample of high school adolescents: a randomized trial of group cognitive intervention. J Am Acad Child Adolesc Psychiatry 34:312–321, 1995

Elkin I, Shea T, Watkins JT, et al: National Institute of Mental Health Treatment of Depression Collaborative Research Program: general effectiveness of treatments. Arch Gen Psychiatry 46:971–982, 1989

Emslie G, Rush JA, Weinberg WA, et al: A double-blind, randomized placebo-controlled trial of fluoxetine in depressed children and adolescents. Arch Gen Psychiatry 54:1031–1037, 1997

Emslie GJ, Rush AJ, Weinberg WA, et al: Fluoxetine in child and adolescent depression: acute and maintenance treatment. Depression and Anxiety 7:32–39, 1998

Fava GA, Rafanelli C, Cazzaro M, et al: Well-being therapy: a novel psychotherapeutic approach for residual symptoms of affective disorders. Psychol Med 28:475–480, 1998

Fine S, Forth A, Gilbert M, et al: Group therapy for adolescent depressive disorder: a comparison of social skills and therapeutic support. J Am Acad Child Adolesc Psychiatry 30:79–85, 1991

Fleming JE, Offord DR: Epidemiology of childhood depressive disorders: a critical review. J Am Acad Child Adolesc Psychiatry 29:571–580, 1990

Geller B, Cooper MA, Graham DL, et al: Double-blind placebo-controlled study of nortriptyline in depressed adolescents using a "fixed plasma level" design. Psychopharmacol Bull 26:85–90, 1990

Geller B, Cooper TB, Graham DL, et al: Pharmacokinetically designed double-blind placebo-controlled study of nortriptyline in 6- to 12-year-olds with major depressive disorder. J Am Acad Child Adolesc Psychiatry 31:34–44, 1992

Harrington R, Fudge H, Rutter M, et al: Adult outcomes of childhood and adolescent depression, I: psychiatric status. Arch Gen Psychiatry 47:465–473, 1990

Harrington R, Kerfoot M, Dyer E, et al: Randomized trial of a home-based family intervention for children who have deliberately poisoned themselves. J Am Acad Child Adolesc Psychiatry 37:512–518, 1998

Hazell P, O'Connell D, Heathcote D, et al: Efficacy of tricyclic drugs in treating child and adolescent depression: a meta-analysis. BMJ 310:897–901, 1995

Hirschfeld RMA: Psychosocial predictors of outcome in depression, in Psychopharmacology: The Fourth Generation of Progress. Edited by Bloom, FE, Kupfer, DJ. New York, Raven, 1995, pp 1113–1121

Jayson D, Wood A, Kroll L, et al: Which depressed patients respond to cognitive-behavioral treatment? J Am Acad Child Adolesc Psychiatry 37:35–39, 1998

Kahn JS, Kehle TJ, Jenson WR, et al: Comparison of cognitive-behavioral relaxation, and self-modeling interventions for depression among middle-school students. School Psychology Review 19:196–211, 1990

Kandel DB, Davies M: Epidemiology of depressive mood in adolescents: an empirical study. Arch Gen Psychiatry 39:1205–1212, 1982

Kazdin AE, French NH, Unis AS, et al: Hopelessness, depression, and suicidal intent among psychiatrically disturbed inpatient children. J Consult Clin Psychol 51:504–510, 1983

Keller MB, Ryan N, Birmaher B, et al: Paroxetine and imipramine in the treatment of adolescent depression. Data presented at the 151st annual meeting of the American Psychiatric Association, Toronto, Ontario, Canada, May 1998

Kovacs M, Devlin B: Internalizing disorders in childhood. J Child Psychol Psychiatry 39:47–63, 1998

Kovacs M, Feinberg TL, Crouse-Novak MA, et al: Depressive disorders in childhood, I: a longitudinal study of characteristics and recovery. Arch Gen Psychiatry 41:229–237, 1984a

Kovacs M, Feinberg T, Crouse-Novak M, et al: Depressive disorders in childhood: II. a longitudinal study of the risk for a subsequent major depression. Arch Gen Psychiatry 41:643–649, 1984b

Kovacs M, Goldston D, Gatsonis C: Suicidal behaviors and childhood-onset depressive disorders: a longitudinal investigation. J Am Acad Child Adolesc Psychiatry 32:8–20, 1993

Kroll L, Harrington R, Jayson D, et al: Pilot study of continuation cognitive-behavioral therapy for major depression in adolescent psychiatric patients. J Am Acad Child Adolesc Psychiatry 35:1156–1161, 1996

Kupfer DJ: Research in affective disorders comes of age. Am J Psychiatry 156:165–167, 1999

Kutcher S, Boulos C, Ward B, et al: Response to desipramine treatment in adolescent depression: a fixed-dose, placebo-controlled trial. J Am Acad Child Adolesc Psychiatry 33:686–694, 1994

Lerner MS, Clum GA: Treatment of suicide ideators: a problem-solving approach. Behavior Therapy 21:403–411, 1990

Lewinsohn PM, Hops H: Adolescent psychopathology: I. prevalence and incidence of depression and other DSM-III-R disorders in high school students. J Abnorm Psychol 102:133–144, 1993

Lewinsohn PM, Clarke GN, Hops H, et al: Cognitive-behavioral treatment for depressed adolescents. Behavior Therapy 21:385–401, 1990

Lewinsohn PM, Rohde P, Seeley JR, et al: Axis II psychopathology as a function of Axis I disorders in childhood and adolescence. J Am Acad Child Adolesc Psychiatry 36:1752–1759, 1997

Lewinsohn PM, Rohde P, Seeley JR: Major depressive disorder in older adolescents: prevalence, risk factors, and clinical implications. Clin Psychol Rev 18:765–794, 1998

Puig-Antich J, Perel JM, Lupatkin W, et al: Imipramine in prepubertal major depressive disorders. Arch Gen Psychiatry 44:81–89, 1987

Reinecke MA, Ryan NE, DuBois L: Cognitive-behavioral therapy of depression and depressive symptoms during adolescence: a review and meta-analysis. J Am Acad Child Adolesc Psychiatry 37:26–34, 1998

Renaud J, Brent DA, Baugher M, et al: Rapid response to psychosocial treatment for adolescent depression: a two-year follow-up. J Am Acad Child Adolesc Psychiatry 37:1184–1190, 1998

Reynolds WM, Coats KI: A comparison of cognitive-behavioral therapy and relaxation training for the treatment of depression in adolescents. J Consult Clin Psychol 54:653–660, 1986

Rintelmann JW, Emslie GJ, Rush AJ, et al: The effects of extended evaluation on depressive symptoms in children and adolescents. J Affect Disord 41:149–156, 1996

Rohde P, Lewinsohn PM, Seeley JR: Are adolescents changed by an episode of major depression? J Am Acad Child Adolesc Psychiatry 33:1289–1298, 1994

Sanford M, Szatmari P, Spinner M, et al: Predicting the one-year course of adolescent major depression. J Am Acad Child Adolesc Psychiatry 34:1618–1628, 1995

Shaffer D, Gould MS, Fisher P, et al: Psychiatric diagnosis in child and adolescent suicide. Arch Gen Psychiatry 53:339–348, 1996

Smeraldi E, Zanardi R, Benedetti F, et al: Polymorphism within the promoter of the serotonin transporter gene and antidepressant efficacy of fluvoxamine. Mol Psychiatry 3:508–511, 1998

Stark KD, Reynolds WM, Kaslow NJ: A comparison of the relative efficacy of self-control therapy and a behavioral problem-solving therapy for depression in children. J Abnorm Child Psychol 15:91–113, 1987

Stein D, Brent DA, Bridge J, et al: Parent-rated credibility in a clinical psychotherapy trial of adolescent depression: mediators and moderators. J Psychother Pract Res, in press

Thase ME, Howland RH: Refractory depression: relevance of psychosocial factors and therapies. Psychiatr Ann 24:232–239, 1994

Thase ME, Simons AD, McGeary J, et al: Relapse after cognitive behavior therapy of depression: potential implications for longer courses of treatment. Am J Psychiatry 149:1046–1052, 1992

Thase ME, Greenhouse JB, Frank E, et al: Treatment of major depression with psychotherapy or psychotherapy-pharmacotherapy combinations. Arch Gen Psychiatry 54:1009–1015, 1997

Von Korff M, Gruman J, Schaefer JH, et al: Collaborative management of chronic illness. Ann Intern Med 127:1097–1102, 1997

Vostanis P, Feehan C, Grattan E, et al: Treatment for children and adolescents with depression: lessons from a controlled trial. Clinical Child Psychology and Psychiatry 1:199–212, 1996a

Vostanis P, Feehan C, Grattan E, et al: A randomised controlled outpatient trial of cognitive-behavioural treatment for children and adolescents with depression: 9-month follow-up. J Affect Disord 40:105–116, 1996b

Warner V, Weissman MM, Fendrich M, et al: The course of major depression in the offspring of depressed parents: incidence, recurrence and recovery. Arch Gen Psychiatry 49:795–801, 1992

Weisz JR, Donenberg GR, Han SS, et al: Bridging the gap between laboratory and clinic in child and adolescent psychotherapy. J Consult Clin Psychology 63:688–701, 1995

Wood A, Harrington R, Moore A: Controlled trial of a brief cognitive-behavioral intervention in adolescent patients with depressive disorders. J Child Psychol Psychiatry 37:737–746, 1996

CHAPTER 11

New Ideas for Testing Treatments — What's Wrong and How to Fix It

Impaired Discovery and Fact-Poor Practice

Donald F. Klein, M.D.

Introduction

Initially my plan was to indicate (once again; see Klein 1993, 1996) that much of psychiatric clinical practice is not based on firm knowledge derived from systematic observation or experimental science. Then I would proceed to demonstrate that clinical trials could be made substantially more effective and meaningful by various technical improvements such as proper diagnosis using semistructured interviews; experienced, well-trained diagnosticians and evaluators; monitoring of clinical procedures to confirm diagnostic and management skills, thus allowing ongoing concurrent attention to quality control; use of well-developed self-rating scales, both as dependent variables and to calibrate the tendency to grade inflation during clinical interviews done to

This chapter was supported in part by PHS grant MH-30906, MHCRC-New York State Psychiatric Institute.

attempts to ensure an adequate flow of subjects; audio-recording and analysis of all patient contacts by an independent team; measurement of patient functioning in daily living, work, interpersonal relationships, and leisure time; measurement of health service use; broadening of symptomatic and behavioral sources of information to include knowledgeable informants; use of daily patient reports provoked by random beepers and linked with automated telephone interactive query systems; attention to the enhancement of positive motivations of both patients and investigators; and provision of a psychotherapeutic context for medication trials to diminish attrition and more closely reflect clinical practice.

Many other technical and analytic suggestions are possible (Klein 1999a, 1999b, 1999c). However, I realized that practically all clinical trials do not address important clinical questions: How does this regimen compare with alternative treatments regarding speed of onset, breadth of effect, and cost? Given treatment failure, or partial response, what next—adjunctive treatments or switch treatments, and how to do it? What is the pattern of relapse? Is maintenance treatment indicated, and if so, what frequency of contact, dosage, regimen, laboratory testing, and the like are needed?

With these issues in mind, I decided to switch gears and consider the institutional changes necessary to accelerate the process of psychotropic drug discovery and to afford a rational base for clinical practice.

Cultural Lag

The spurt in development of effective pharmacologic agents is essentially a post–World War II phenomenon. With sudden innovations, a period of cultural lag occurs during which research; production; marketing mechanisms; and social, legislative, and regulatory practices slowly come to grips with such developments. New drugs have clearly demonstrated their worth but raise clinical and toxicologic concerns that have not been adequately addressed. This is true of pharmacology in general but is specially true of psychopharmacology because of our lack of objective psychiatric diagnostic methods and the relatively primitive state of our understanding of the pathophysiology of psychiatric disease. This is of particular importance because the discovery and development of methods appropriate to our relatively advanced understanding of the pathophysiology of hypertension, allergy, and the like, which led to the development of specific receptor agonists and antagonists, are being uncritically applied to psychiatry.

Drug Discovery

Walkup et al. (1998) present the conventional view of drug development:

> Progress in drug development has occurred in four phases. After the phase of discovery by pure serendipity, the second phase included the use of animal models to test drug effects to identify potential therapeutic candidates. Predictable animal models of drug response were used to standardize the process. Basic scientific knowledge derived from animal models led to the third phase. Advances in molecular biology in combination with sophisticated computer programs allow for new molecules to be designed based on knowledge of the structure of receptors, neurotransmitters, and other neuropeptides. Medications will not only target the cell surface but may ultimately be able to be sent into cells to act directly on the pathologic mechanism. (p. 1265)

The problem with this idealization is that our animal models of schizophrenia, bipolar disorder, major depressive disorder, panic disorder, obsessive-compulsive disorder, and the like are conspicuously poor. (I believe this is because the major psychotropic drugs normalize deranged circuitry, which makes searching for pharmacodynamic effects on normal animals unrewarding [Klein 1978, 1988a, 1988b, 1991a, 1991b].) Animal models have been predictive only in the generalized anxiety states, which are closely linked to ordinary fear.

The Federation of American Societies for Experimental Biology (FASEB) released a report titled "Federal Funding for Biomedical and Related Life Sciences Research FY 2000 Recommendation" (FASEB 1999). Although FASEB's recommendations are largely sensible, their understanding of clinical research is that it "applies the understanding gained from basic research to problems of human health." In the area of psychiatry this conclusion is premature because of insufficient knowledge of both physiology and pathophysiology. Even for general medicine this conclusion is somewhat forced. According to FASEB (1999), "The 1998 Nobel Prize was awarded to NIH funded researchers for their work showing how nitric oxide regulates blood vessels and blood flow to different organs. This discovery helped in the development of the anti-impotence drug Viagra." However, the recognition of Viagra's erectile benefit was a serendipitous discovery made during the investigation of Viagra as an antihypertensive drug. Once the clinical discovery was made, basic research was required for understanding the mechanism. The problematic reality is that every major psychotropic drug advance has been due to serendipity.

The Fostering of Serendipity for Psychotropic Agents

Serendipitous observations of unexpected clinical benefits are fostered by an environment in which patient symptomatology is easily observed and beneficial effects are quick and unmistakable. This was the case for phenothiazine, antipsychotics, and tricyclic antidepressants and anti-panic agents. However, in more subtle, inherently fluctuating diseases in which medication effects may be more modest, the likelihood of serendipitous observation is curtailed and becomes easily contaminated by false-positive, clinically misleading reports.

A recent case in point is the unfortunate side effect of sexual inhibition caused by the selective serotonin reuptake inhibitors. This common effect was not noted by the industry in its initial descriptions of the efficacy of these drugs. After the effect became clinically obvious, many anecdotes of supposedly beneficial adjunctive medications were reported. Nonetheless, to this day no large-scale case series or controlled treatment study has examined this important treatment-impairing side effect. Perhaps the pharmaceutical industry has avoided such studies because an open admission of the importance of this side effect might have negative repercussions on marketing. Clinical anecdotal reports often come from private practice or settings that do not foster the development of detailed case series, let alone controlled evaluations. Academia has not seen such studies as an important goal.

The Current State of Psychiatry

An unblinking look at the state of patient-oriented research in psychiatry must recognize several problematic facts. Psychiatric diagnosis is still at a descriptive syndromal level because objective, specific, diagnostic tests of almost all psychiatric diseases are not available. Therefore, our syndromal categories include many phenocopies with diverse etiologies and pathophysiologies (Klein 1998).

Our pathophysiologic theories are poorly supported and have a bad historical record. Few have survived pointed tests. The conventional wisdom about the mechanism of action of both the psychotherapies and the pharmacotherapies is superficial. Rarely has this wisdom been put to the test, and when tested it has proven lacking. Basic research has been beneficial by critiquing some of our simplistic pathophysiologic notions, as by the demonstration via knockout mice that neither serotonin nor dopamine are crucial to cocaine effects. The hopes that genetic research will sharply delineate psychiatric diseases have floundered amid the problems of complex genetics, polygenetic determinism, and multiple phenocopies. Genomic research will also require careful delineation of pathophysiologic mechanisms and distinctions among phenocopies. Even though a specific genetic mechanism was isolated in Huntington disease 15 years ago and the protein in question has been determined, translation into therapeutic interventions has not occurred. This is probably because of the tremendous—still largely unknown—epigenetic cascade between gene, gene product, and clinical pathophysiology.

Because the major advances in psychiatry have been serendipitous, one would think that our scientific leadership should have focused on developing clinical contexts that foster serendipity. "Chance and the prepared mind" requires the clinical opportunity for discovery.

The Need for an Illness Focus

If we had detailed knowledge of normal psychologic and brain physiologic functions, then the evaluation of psychiatric dysfunction would be a relatively straightforward deduction. Attempting to evaluate dysfunction without a prior basic understanding of normal functioning seems misguided and bound to be incomplete at best and entirely erroneous at worst. This stand would seem even more self-evident if dysfunction was only an arbitrary evaluation of deviant but normal functioning (as antinosologists frequently claim) (Klein 1999).

However, the organism, and particularly the brain, is fantastically complex. The past half century has given us a mind-boggling glimpse of the unplumbed complexities that lie ahead. To seriously hope that we will soon be able to deductively understand brain dysfunctions from our deep grasp of normal functions or genetic predispositions seems wishful thinking. Fortunately, the history of medical advances has not depended on correctly understanding normal functioning but rather has focused on illness, which illuminates impaired functions, highlights pathogenic processes, and allows empiric determinations of the means for repair or compensation.

The development of antipsychotics, antidepressants, and anxiolytics fostered the neurosciences. The development of vaccines and antibiotics fostered immunology. The treatment of scurvy, pellagra, and beriberi led to an awareness of the importance of vitamins, which in turn illuminated enzymatic cofactors. It follows that in psychiatry, given our inadequate grasp of pathophysiology and etiology, a major research focus should be the detailed, imaginative study of the therapeutic impact on illness. Such a strong focus on understanding the processes that underlie effective treatment of psychiatric illness, from the point of view of repairing or compensating for hypothesized dysfunctions, is a good bet for advancing both pathophysiology and clinically useful understanding.

The Need for Large, Long-Term Clinical Research Facilities

It is no accident that the early serendipitous psychopharmacologic observations occurred in the context of long-term inpatient care. These patients were well known to staff, so substantial clinical changes were obvious. Furthermore, in those days hospitalization was not sharply curtailed, meaning that the maintenance of clinical gains and the management of side effects could be assessed.

Because of economic constraints, the average length of a hospital stay has been drastically shortened so that psychiatric wards are now often crisis decompression centers rather than initiators of effective care. Clinicians simply cannot be certain in less than 1 week whether a newly instituted medication will be specifically beneficial for the patient or even if acute benefits will be maintained after discharge. Therefore, high patient transience destroys the opportunity for making serendipitous clinical observations. That aftercare is radically divorced from the inpatient staff further degrades the possibility of clinical discovery.

A recent report by the National Advisory of Mental Health Council's Clinical Treatment and Services Research Workgroup (1998) addressed the need to generate information to better enable people with mental illnesses to receive optimal care. Of the 49 recommendations, two seem particularly relevant.

> Recommendation 31: NIMH [the National Institute of Mental Health] should revise and renew public announcements (PAs) in the spirit of the Public-Academic (PAL) Program to maintain and promote existing partnerships between academic researchers and public care systems, health plans, both carve-outs and health maintenance organizations (HMOs) and employers providing health benefits and their representative groups.

> Recommendation 32: NIMH research centers, which demonstrate great potential to secure partnerships with service delivery systems and to utilize these systems to conduct intervention research, should be supplemented to develop, implement, and sustain such partnerships.

The workgroup recognized the necessity for somehow bridging academic research and actual treatment programs but envisioned this process only in terms of so-called partnerships. It is my belief that this approach will succeed only rarely and that a far more radical reconstruction yielding large, research-oriented treatment facilities is necessary for knowledge generation.

Treatment-Refractory Depression

I have presented elsewhere an analysis demonstrating that carrying out effectiveness studies in the context of the usual clinical setting is simply too difficult, is resistant to randomization, yields unreliable measurements, and is open to multiple confounded explanations (Klein and Smith 1999). Yet one needs to evaluate and provide improved treatment for patients with the more usual but more complicated illnesses. I suggest developing large, multisite, research-oriented, treatment-developing demonstration clinics. I focus in this section on the problem of adequate care for patients with treatment-refractory depression.

To address the major clinical problem of treatment-resistant depression, a recent Request for Proposals from the NIMH (RFP# NIMH-99-DS-0003) advertised a 5-year cost reimbursement contract with the option of an additional 5 years. The NIMH noted that

> Despite the enormous public health significance of the problem of treatment resistant depression, systematic research on this topic has been very difficult. The major research questions to be addressed in this study include the following: for a person with depression who has not responded adequately, at what point should the diagnosis of treatment resistance be made, and when should treatment be changed in order to optimize outcome? How should the type of depression (melancholic, atypical, minor) influence the optimal point at which treatment has changed? How does the type of the initial treatment determine the optimal point at which treatment is changed? Does the optimal point at which treatment is changed vary among various populations (age, gender, race, and ethnicity)? How does the presence of medical comorbidity influence the optimal point at which treatment is changed? How does the present psychiatric comorbidity (substance abuse, axis II, other diagnoses) influence the optimal point at which treatment is changed?
>
> Underlying this contract is a dilemma that confronts the field concerning the practical limitations of designing trial treatment approaches to treatment-resistant depression. A large number of treatment options are currently in use as secondary therapy including numerous augmentation and drug-switching strategies. Comparisons of these treatment modalities having adequate statistical power would require large numbers of people. This problem is compounded by the fact that using stringent criteria for the definition of treatment resistance, subject recruitment is a limiting factor. Selecting the key questions to be addressed in designing a trial with sufficient external validity and statistical power would likely require a major consensus development effort to identify critical treatment options.

Consensus development is required because insufficient systematic clinical data have accumulated to allow a data-based, substantive selection of likely hypotheses concerning what to do when the first or second treatment fails. Such data are not available because research-oriented clinical facilities that could generate such data do not exist. Thus, obtaining a consensus of experts is the best that can be done currently, but it should be clear that this contract proposes a very large Phase III study, without systematic Phase II data.

This contract facilitates putting together an ad hoc multisite group of academic centers exhorted to somehow engage community clinical facilities: "The contractor should provide an outreach plan for recruiting practitioner sites that have not been involved in previous treatment trials, particularly ones in managed care or public mental health settings. Inclusions of more representative trials sites also facilitate translation of study results into clinical practice."

One wonders how this "outreach plan" can be effectively done given that such practitioner sites have no experience in systematic behavioral observation or in reliable recording of clinical data. Clearly the academic sites will have to supplement the practitioner sites with research-trained personnel for both diagnosis and monitoring, thus radically modifying the practitioner sites. Furthermore, any consensus agreement concerning a staged treatment algorithm must profoundly alter the usual treatment procedures indigenous to those sites.

My belief is that in pursuing the entirely desirable goal of extending treatments and treatment evaluations to broader patient populations, the institutional problems have not been adequately addressed. Without the development of research-oriented clinics to provide a database that will lead to fruitful large-scale comparative trials, one will always be stuck with such a top-down a priori approach.

Generating Treatment Outcome Data for Patients with Treatment-Refractory Disorders

How could consensus have had more data to build on, given that efforts at improving care should focus on those who respond partially or not at all? I propose that in all research-oriented effectiveness clinics a second tier of expert clinicians review all such cases. If a particular treatment course has not gone well, would switching or adding an adjunctive treatment be best? For certain groups with a defined level of nonresponse, one could identify such patients and have an exploratory fixed algorithm specifying the next level of adjunctive or substitute treatment programs, thus yielding actuarial outcome data. Explanatory hypotheses and promising treatment plans should be stipulated, carried out, and monitored. Apparently beneficial treatment protocols would be systematically administered to patients with similarly refractory cases. If a treatment appears frequently beneficial, this forms the Phase II discovery basis for an efficacy trial. Pharmacologic, psychosocial, and combination interventions could be assessed.

I estimate that three expert reviews of new treatment-refractory cases each week would require about 1,000 patients entering treatment per year. Reviewing accumulated treatment-refractory cases would consume much expert time. A centrally administered network of several high-volume effectiveness clinics could systematically investigate and develop testable treatment plans for difficult cases. Patients with treatment-refractory illnesses place disproportionate burdens on the treatment system; however, without such a comprehensive approach, treatment efforts are piecemeal and ineffective.

Predictive assessments are needed to identify patients who are likely to respond poorly to standard interventions, thus allowing earlier alternative treatment approaches. Continued positive clinical experience across sites lays the groundwork for proper efficacy trials. When such patients continue to do poorly, further treatment development by clinical exploration is clearly needed.

Institute of Medicine Report

An important document addressing the operations of the National Institutes of Health (NIH) was produced by the Institute of Medicine Committee on the NIH Research Priority-Setting Process (1998) to deal with various extra-scientific attempts to modify the NIH structure and priority-setting mechanism. In particular, some members of Congress believe there should be more of a correlation between research funding and the distribution of disease burdens and costs in the population. Also, disease-specific interest groups have campaigned for allocations of NIH research funding for particular diseases, which may deprive other research areas of funds. For instance, a campaign advocating increased research on Parkinson disease led to the Senate authorizing a $100,000,000 program in the FY 1998 appropriations bill. Some members of Congress and the NIH leadership objected to this micromanagement, calling for an Institute of Medicine report.

The Institute of Medicine report essentially says that the NIH criteria for funding research are scientifically sound but could be improved and better accepted if the public had more say. Currently, the various pressure groups have an undifferentiated urge for more funding in a particular area but do not press for revisions in the clinical infrastructure that would allow for the systematic accumulation of hypothesis-relevant clinical data. I believe that these groups have not understood the importance of such a development. Nothing in the Institute of Medicine report recognizes a need for developing research-oriented clinical facilities.

Socioeconomic Problems in the Development of Research-Oriented Clinics

Research-oriented clinics will incur increased costs by requiring good, educated personnel; continued training; reliable, frequent patient measurements; and expert consultations to which the ordinary community clinic does not aspire. These innovations may produce a competitive tension between community clinics and research clinics. Research-effectiveness clinics will provide services that will certainly be more costly than in community clinics but may well produce superior results. At the very least, their system of meticulous, multidimensional outcome evaluations will present a challenge to conventional facilities to provide comparable diagnostic and outcome data.

Realistic Prospects

Utopian projections of ideal systems fail regularly. Similar recommendations for research-oriented psychiatric clinical facilities were made by

Reiling (1899) and more recently by Klein (1970) and have been reiterated in several different contexts. The reasons they remain hoped-for goals rather than actual accomplishments are plain. Socioeconomic development is the outcome of a clash of interests between various stakeholders as well as the stakeholders' developing conceptions of what is in their interest. To date, none of the important stakeholders has viewed the development of research-effectiveness clinics as a tool that would advance their goals. Indeed, the stakeholders concerned with profitable clinical care may see such developments as directly competitive.

I have actively participated in scientific advisory committees in the area of patient advocacy for anxiety and depressive disorders and have reviewed the work of the foremost nonfederal psychiatric research support group, NARSAD (National Alliance for Research on Schizophrenia and Depression). It seems plain that these groups attempt to foster research that fits within the current structure of clinical care and research support. Furthermore, approaches that emphasize brain imaging, receptorology, and genetics or simple clinical trials have been the focus of their research attention. One must look for those whose interests directly support such developments in systematic clinical discovery, although they may not as yet have recognized this fact. In my view, new critical views on research must rely primarily on a deepening understanding of the therapeutic development process on the part of the psychiatric patient advocacy groups and those who support psychiatric research.

Support from industry may develop now that the 1997 Food and Drug Administration (FDA) Modernization and Accountability Act has provided major incentives (6 months of additional marketing exclusivity) for pediatric studies. This extremely encouraging development indicates that Congress recognizes unmet treatment needs and can develop incentives for industry to address them. Currently, industry is still wrestling with the problem of how these incentives should modify their research programs. In fiscal year 1998, the total budget of all NIH incentives amounted to $13.6 billion. In contrast, the pharmaceutical industry spends approximately $19 billion annually and the biotechnology industry approximately $8 billion annually. To put these resources to work in a broader framework than the current short-term, acute treatment clinical trials focused on FDA approval would be a real advance.

Federal legislation giving incentives or mandating via the FDA that industrial medication trials be carried out in psychiatric patients with defined comorbidities (e.g., substance abuse) and that postmarketing longitudinal studies be done to demonstrate maintained benefits and a lack of long-term toxicity could provide the finances necessary to support the suggested research clinical structures. Patient advocacy groups and the research community should clarify for Congress that such a development would accelerate both clinical and basic psychopharmacologic research while drastically improving clinical practice.

Social Problems and Process

The strength of the democratic system is in how it deals with social problems. However, the system's methods are often neither swift nor accurate. Therefore, the situation often has to get pretty bad before it can get better, when adaptive and corrective mechanisms are finally put into place. We may be getting to that point owing to the concurrent crises in clinical care and clinical research.

Recent changes in clinical care have been made in an effort to save money rather than to improve quality. Improvement in care is obviously called for, as shown by recent studies indicating that currently available knowledge is not effectively applied by clinicians in all fields of medicine. It remains an open question whether improving care will save or cost money or whether our society can see the necessity for the improvement of medical care on the basis of noneconomic social values.

Another looming problem is the diminishing supply of physician-scientists who study patients and their diseases, taking their observations to systematic case series and clinical trials. Relatively fewer first-time physician-investigators have applied for NIH awards over the past several years. Clinically trained researchers are at risk, without support for training or career development. Research-effectiveness clinics would provide a natural home for the training and career development of physician-scientists.

The new Intervention Research Centers (IRC) promulgated by the NIMH may be a step in this direction, but it is doubtful that any of the current IRC proposals include large-scale clinical facilities, if for no other reason than that the grant funds allocated are insufficient. Funding these clinics is obviously a major issue. Some imaginative combination of federal, industrial, academic, and service funds will be required. Such funding may be possible once it is realized that this innovation is in the interest of all the stakeholders in the psychiatric arena.

References

FASEB (Federation of American Societies for Experimental Biology): Federal Funding for Biomedical and Related Life Sciences Research FY 2000 Recommendations. Bethesda, MD, 1999. Available online at http://www.faseb.org/opar/fund2000

Institute of Medicine Committee on the NIH Research Priority-Setting Process: Improving Priority Setting and Public Input at the National Institutes of Health. Copyright 1998. Available online at http://www.nap.edu/readingroom/books/nih

Klein DF: Constraints on psychiatric treatment research produced by the organization of clinical services, in Nonscientific Constraints on Medical Research. Edited by Merlis S, New York, Raven, 1970, pp 69–90

Klein DF: A proposed definition of mental illness, in Critical Issues in Psychiatric Diagnosis. Edited by Spitzer R, Klein DF. New York, Raven, 1978, pp 41–71

Klein DF: Cybernetics, activation, and drug effects. Acta Psychiatr Scand (The Netherlands) 77:126–137, 1988a

Klein DF: Rheostat and cybernetic issues: comments on "The Current Status of the Dopamine Hypothesis of Schizophrenia." Neuropsychopharmacology 1:187–188, 1988b

Klein DF: Improvement of Phase III psychotropic drug trials by intensive Phase II work. Neuropsychopharmacology 4:251–258, 1991a

Klein DF: Reply to commentaries: improvement of Phase II psychotropic drug trials by intensive Phase II work. Neuropsychopharmacology 4:269–271, 1991b

Klein DF: Clinical psychopharmacologic practice: the need for developing a research base. Arch Gen Psychiatry 50:491–494, 1993

Klein DF: Preventing hung juries about therapy studies. J Consult Clin Psychol 64:81–87, 1996

Klein DF: Panic and phobic anxiety: phenotypes, endophenotypes, and genotypes. Am J Psychiatry 155:1147–1149, 1998

Klein DF: A checklist for developing and reviewing comparative treatment evaluations in the areas of psychotherapy and pharmacotherapy, in Psychotherapy Indications and Outcomes. Edited by Janowsky DS. Washington, DC, American Psychiatric Press, 1999a, pp 367–381

Klein DF: The current utility and future development of algorithms, in Textbook of Treatment Algorithms in Psychopharmacology. Edited by Fawcett J. Chichester, U.K., Wiley, 1999b, pp 33–36

Klein DF: Studying the respective contributions of pharmacotherapy and psychotherapy: toward collaborative controlled studies, in Psychiatry in the New Millennium. Edited by Weissman S, Sabshin M, Eist H. Washington, DC, American Psychiatric Press, 1999c, pp 217–235

Klein DF: Harmful dysfunction, disorder, disease, illness, and evolution. J Abnorm Psychol 108:421–429, 1999

Klein DF, Smith, LB: Organizational requirements for effective clinical effectiveness studies. Prevention and Treatment. http://journals.apa.org/prevention/volume2/pre0020002a.html, posted March 21, 1999

National Advisory of Mental Health Council's Clinical Treatment and Services Research Workgroup, NIH/NIMH: Bridging Science and Service. Updated January 14, 1998, www.nimh.nih.gov/research/bridge.htm

Reiling J (ed): JAMA 100 years ago. JAMA 32:434, 1899

Walkup JT, Cruz K, Kane S, et al: The future of pediatric psychopharmacology. Child and Adolescent Psychopharmacology 45:1265–1278, 1998

CHAPTER 12

Practice Guidelines and Algorithms

A. John Rush, M.D.

Introduction

Until the early 1980s, the medication management of severe and persistent mental illnesses was relatively straightforward and uncomplicated, with only a limited range of treatment options. There were two classes of antidepressant drugs (monoamine oxidase inhibitors and tricyclic antidepressants); one class of antipsychotic agents (the classic neuroleptics); and one medication (lithium) for the treatment of bipolar disorder. Since then, 10 new antidepressant medications, one new

The work reported herein was supported by a grant from the National Institute of Mental Health (MH-53799) and by funding from the Robert Wood Johnson Foundation; the Meadows Foundation; the Moody Foundation; the Nannie Hogan Boyd Charitable Trust; the Texas Department of Mental Health and Mental Retardation; the Center for Mental Health Services; and Mental Health Connections, a partnership between Dallas County Mental Health and Mental Retardation and the Department of Psychiatry, University of Texas Southwestern Medical Center, which receives funding from the Texas State Legislature and the Dallas County Hospital District. In addition, unrestricted educational grants were provided by Abbott Laboratories; Bristol-Myers Squibb Company; Eli Lilly and Company; Forest Laboratories; Glaxo-Wellcome, Inc.; Janssen Pharmaceutica; Novartis Pharmaceuticals Corporation; Pfizer, Inc.; and Wyeth-Ayerst Laboratories.

antimanic medication (sodium divalproex), and several new atypical antipsychotic agents have been approved for use by the U.S. Food and Drug Administration. Fortunately, since 1980, diagnostic reliability has also improved markedly—making a match between diagnosis and pharmacotherapeutic treatment(s) feasible (American Psychiatric Association 1980, 1987, 1994a).

In the 1990s, wide variations in physician practices were recognized, particularly in general medicine (Gafni and Birch 1993; Kissick 1994; Welch et al. 1993) and in psychiatry. In response to these wide practice variations and the increasing number of available options, treatment guidelines have been developed both for psychiatric care providers (major depressive disorder [American Psychiatric Association 1993], bipolar disorder [American Psychiatric Association 1994b; Bauer et al. 1999; Dennehy and Suppes 1999; Kahn et al. 1996; Suppes et al. 1998], schizophrenia [American Psychiatric Association 1997; Chiles et al. 1999, McEvoy et al. 1996, 1999; Miller et al. 1999]) and for primary care providers (Depression Guideline Panel 1993a, 1993b).

An important additional force hastening guideline development has been demands by patients and families for high-quality, predictable pharmacotherapeutic and psychosocial treatments. This growing emphasis is based in part on a paradigm shift that entails defining the quality of care not only by the processes involved but also by the clinical outcomes achieved (Rush et al. 1998). Furthermore, with the emphasis on health care cost containment, the separation of behavioral health from general health care is becoming less common. Furthermore, provider-driven care has become more patient driven. As a result of new medications, the emphasis has shifted from humane custodial care to care aimed at symptom remission, restoration of function, and recovery.

Another force, the development of managed medicine, has led administrators to seek methods to ensure the most efficient use of resources—providing the maximum value for the health care dollar (Woolf 1990). As a result, many managed care organizations have developed implicit or explicit guidelines, sometimes called disease management protocols, for primary care (e.g., asthma, diabetes, arthritis) and specialty care settings (Brown et al. 1995). Thus a growing range of treatment options, wide variation among practitioners in implementing these options, demands by patients and families for better treatment, and the

need to improve efficiencies in care have led to the development of
more specific treatment recommendations.

Options, Guidelines, Algorithms, Disease Management Protocols, and Clinical Pathways

Various terms and concepts have been used to specify and characterize
various clinical procedures used to define treatments of different disorders (Institute of Medicine Committee to Advise the Public Health Service on Clinical Practice Guidelines 1990). *Treatment options* specify
alternative available treatments based on expert opinion—such as those
enumerated in textbooks of medicine. More recently, with the development of evidence-based medicine (Haynes et al. 1977; Rosenberg and
Sackett 1996; Sackett 1997; Sackett and Rosenberg 1995), *practice
guidelines* present treatment options along with the scientific evidence
that supports each. Evidence-based clinical practice guidelines are ex-
emplified by the American Psychiatric Association (1993, 1994a, 1997)
guidelines and by the U.S. Department of Health and Human Services
Agency for Health Care Policy and Research (AHCPR) guidelines (Depression Guideline Panel 1993a, 1993b).

In essence, practice guidelines attempt to distill an evolving scientific
database into clinically useful recommendations, with the hope of rapidly
informing practitioners of critical research findings that affect care. The Institute of Medicine (1990) defined clinical practice guidelines as "systematically developed statements to assist practitioner and patient decisions
about appropriate health care for specific clinical circumstances" (p. 8). Appropriate health care, as defined by Park et al. (1986), occurs "when the
clinical benefit obtained outweighs the harm and cost involved." Woolf
(1990) defines practice guidelines as "the official statements or policies of
major organizations and agencies on the proper indications for performing
a procedure or treatment or the proper management for specific clinical
problems" (p. 1812). The American Psychiatric Association (1993) views
guidelines as patient care strategies developed to assist clinicians and clinical decision making. The Institute of Medicine (1990) assisted the AHCPR
in developing the first eight of the following nine attributes of practice
guidelines (Clinton et al. 1994). Paraphrased, the attributes include:

- *Validity.* Quality scientific and clinical evidence leads to the guidelines, which lead to projected outcomes.
- *Reliability/reproducibility.* Two groups of experts distill the same evidence to arrive at the same guidelines; recommendations are then interpreted and applied consistently in practice.
- *Clinical applicability.* The intended patient population is stated explicitly.
- *Clinical flexibility.* Guidance is provided regarding variability among treatment options given patient factors; guideline exceptions are specified.
- *Clarity.* Recommendations are stated clearly and are easy to follow.
- *Multidisciplinary process.* Key affected groups participate in guideline development.
- *Documentation.* The procedures used to develop the guidelines are specified.
- *Scheduled review.* A specific time frame for future review and possible revision is stated clearly.
- *Empirically tested.* Guidelines are empirically evaluated prospectively to assess their effect on patient outcomes.

Algorithms, clinical pathways, or *disease management protocols* are more specific than guidelines. They recommend specific treatments and sequences for their implementation. They specify the *strategies* (i.e., which treatments to use, in what order, and in what sequence) and often the *tactics* (i.e., how to use each of the treatment options chosen). Algorithms are viewed as cognitive tools intended to assist, but not limit, clinical decision-making (Jobson 1997; Kasper and Jobson 1997; Trivedi et al. 1998). A clinical algorithm often provides a flowchart to specify the clinical processes that might follow based on a patient's clinical status and prior treatment response. To develop these more specific recommendations, both scientific evidence (typically used to recommend strategies) and clinical judgment (often used to specify the tactics) are used.

Most guidelines attempt to recommend preferred care—that is, care that is good for most individuals. Because guidelines are based on group data, however, they can only make group-based recommendations. To define *optimal* care for an individual, practitioners must appropriately adapt and tailor guideline recommendations to each individual patient—transforming preferred care (for a group) into optimal care (for an individual) (see Rush and Prien 1995).

The development of evidence-based guidelines entails a shift in emphasis from expert opinions to a distillation of scientific information to make recommendations. However, research findings and scientific evidence typically lag behind or only partly address questions confronting clinicians on a daily basis. Simply put, most randomized clinical trials are conducted for regulatory review or approval. They define the comparative safety, tolerability, and efficacy of diverse treatments for groups of patients. However, they rarely provide definitive evidence in sufficient detail on when to choose or how to optimally implement a treatment option with individual patients. Consequently, the more specific the recommendations (i.e., algorithms versus guidelines), the greater the present need to supplement scientific evidence with clinical consensus. The following discussion will use the term *guidelines* to refer to the whole group of treatment recommendations, ranging from specific algorithms to disease management protocols.

Rationale for Guidelines

There are both clinical and administrative reasons to develop and use guidelines (Table 12–1). First, the major aim is to improve clinical decision making (i.e., the quality of care), which should in turn improve clinical outcomes, make more efficient use of resources, or both. Second, as the lengths of stay in various settings (e.g., hospitals, day treatment centers) shrink, patients who begin a treatment (e.g., medication) in one venue often do not remain long enough to determine whether the treatment produces the desired results. Therefore, treatment plans must be consistent across both settings and clinicians so that a treatment trial (which may last 4–12 weeks) is consistently conducted—both well enough and long enough—so that a patient's response can be accurately gauged and revisions can be made when needed.

Finally, guidelines or algorithms can provide a benchmark to define the clinical outcomes that follow from a particular treatment plan. When a new treatment becomes available, we typically do not know where this treatment fits in the sequence of available options. For example, if a new atypical antipsychotic agent becomes available, should

TABLE 12–1.   *Rationale for developing and using guidelines*

Clinical	Administrative
Facilitate clinical decision making	Improve cost efficiency of treatment
Improve quality of care	Make costs more predictable
Improve clinical outcomes	Define costs related to specific treatments or outcomes
Make treatment plans consistent across sites and providers	Provide a basis for defining when new medications are cost effective
Conveniently list options for appropriately tailoring treatment to individuals	Define where new treatments fit for optimal clinical outcomes
Provide adequate clinical documentation	Provide adequate clinical documentation

Source. Rush et al. 1998. This material is in the public domain and can be reproduced without permission, but appropriate citation is required.

it be inserted after one or after two trials with other atypical agents? Does the new agent benefit patients who have not benefited from previously available agents? If an algorithm exists, the new treatment can be inserted into the algorithm at one step or another to determine empirically where it fits best. In essence, for both clinicians and patients, the hopes are that algorithms will produce 1) a more rapid response, 2) a more complete response (i.e., symptom reduction, functional restoration), 3) lower patient attrition, or 4) lower side effect burdens for more patients than usual care. Administrators hope that algorithms will serve to make optimal use of finite resources (i.e., improve the cost efficiency of treatment) and to make costs more predictable. Algorithms can also provide information by which to relate costs to specific treatments or to particular outcomes. With the insertion of a new treatment into an established stepwise sequence of care at various points, one can also gauge the cost benefit of the new treatment.

Figure 12–1 provides a system (administrative) perspective of the potential benefits of guidelines that improve the quality of care and clinical outcomes. Because better or preferred care—perhaps facilitated by algorithms—should reduce symptoms and improve function, it should result in less disability and, secondarily, reduced use of hospital, crisis,

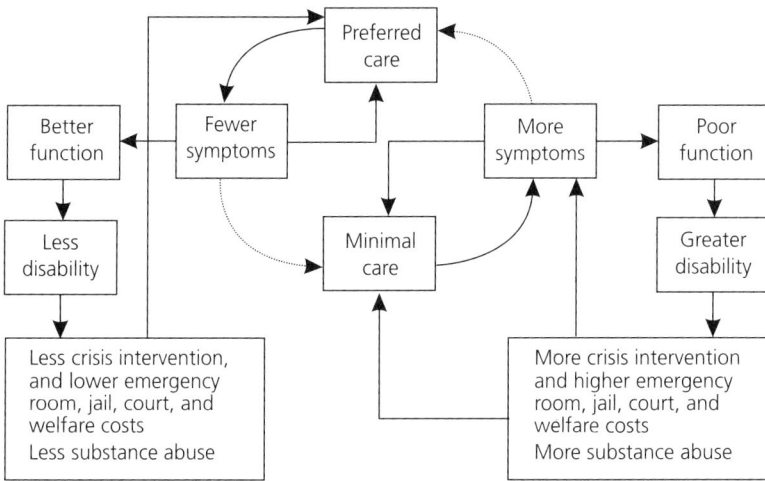

FIGURE 12–1. Consequences of preferred versus minimal care.
Source.   Rush et al. 1999b. This material is in the public domain and can be reproduced without permission.

and emergency services (as well as courts, jails, prisons, and the welfare system) and reduce the risk of chronicity and secondary complications.

   These hypothetical clinical and administrative benefits of practice guidelines have yet to be empirically established in psychiatry. Furthermore, such guidelines have inherent risks:

- Treatment recommendations may simply be wrong (i.e., recommendations, even if supported by randomized clinical trials, may not produce better outcomes than usual care). For example, subjects used in scientific studies may differ from patients seen in routine care, or clinical consensus used to develop treatment recommendations where scientific gaps exist may be flawed, and so on.
- Alternatively, because most psychiatric disorders are heterogeneous, treatment recommendations may be useful for only a subset of affected patients.
- Treatment recommendations may increase cost with or without improving outcomes.

Procedures Used to
Define Guidelines or Algorithms

Gilbert et al. (1998) reviewed the range of procedures used to develop guidelines and algorithms. The methods vary according to how they address the following issues: 1) topic selection, 2) participants in the algorithm development, 3) evaluation of the quality of the scientific literature used to construct the algorithms, 4) filling gaps in research evidence when constructing the algorithms, 5) development of consensus, 6) consideration of the tradeoffs between cost and clinical effectiveness, and 7) the role of expert clinical judgment.

Methods for guideline development include 1) informal consensus, 2) formal consensus, 3) evidence-based guideline development, and 4) explicit guideline development (Woolf 1990, 1991). *Informal consensus* relies on an expert panel reaching a consensus through open discussion. Basically, participants simply decide on what to recommend. Eddy (1992) notes that this "global subjective judgment" may yield poor quality.

Formal consensus, which was pioneered by the National Institutes of Health Consensus Development Program, uses an expert panel to make recommendations based on a consensus reached during a structured, 2½-day conference (Martin 1981; Perry and Kalberer 1980). Initially, experts present the evidence followed by open discussion during a plenary session. Thereafter, an invited panel produces the guidelines during a closed session followed by a presentation of the panel's recommendations to an audience of the panelists' peers.

A variant of this formal consensus method, introduced by the RAND Corporation, has recently been used in a modified form by the Tri-University consortium (Kahn et al. 1997). In this method, an expert panel is provided with background articles that review existing scientific evidence relevant to the topic of the guideline to be developed, followed by a two-step process using the Delphi technique (Jones and Hunter 1995; Linston and Turoff 1975). Before the first meeting, each panelist assesses the appropriateness of several possible procedures for each of a series of indications, using a nine-point score. The panel then meets and uses the scores to identify areas of disagreement. After thorough discussion, the panel rescores the evidence based on this discussion. This method can produce a long list of appropriateness scores, which according to Woolf (1990, 1991) can be a problem because it is difficult for clinicians to apply the results in practice.

Evidence-based guidelines grade the strength of recommendations based on the quality of the evidence, with rules for grading established a priori (see Table 12–2 for a list of commonly used levels of evidence). Practitioners are provided with weighted guidance as to the expected effectiveness of each step in an algorithm. This approach has increased the scientific rigor of guidelines, but it has often been unable to produce recommendations given the frequent gaps in the scientific literature (Woolf 1990, 1991). Thus neutral recommendations—neither for nor against a treatment—are often issued. The American Psychiatric Association (1993, 1994b, 1997) uses a modification of this approach, whereby levels of scientific credibility are denoted for each recommendation, but a panel of experts reviews the evidence and designs the guideline.

TABLE **12–2.** *Types of evidence*

Clinical opinion

Case reports

Consecutive case series

Effectiveness trials

Open comparative trials

Randomized controlled trials (masked)

Randomized controlled trials (not masked)

Source. Data from the Texas Medication Algorithm Project (Rush et al. 1999b). This material is in the public domain and can be reproduced without permission, but appropriate citation is required.

Work by Eddy (1990a, 1990b, 1990c, 1991) has led to the use of more explicit methods for guideline development. These guideline developers specify the benefits, harms, and costs of potential interventions and derive explicit estimates of the probability of each outcome. Some critics argue that this method is too complex and requires too much time to develop the guidelines.

Principles Used to Define Algorithms

No matter the degree of specificity nor the level of acceptable evidence, virtually all treatment plans are based on key underlying assumptions or values that should be made explicit and that guide how to formulate, revise, and specify the recommendations (Cook and Giacomini 1999; Shaneyfelt et al. 1999). For example, one might suggest that staging treatments within an algorithm should begin with the simplest, least complicated treatments and move to more complicated treatment combinations only when patients have failed to respond to prior, less complicated interventions. An alternative principle could be to start with medications that are least costly on a per-pill basis (often disregarding longer-term overall costs of managing the illness).

The following assumptions were used in developing the Texas Medication Algorithm Project (TMAP) algorithms (Chiles et al. 1999; Crismon et al. 1999; Dennehy and Suppes 1999; Miller et al. 1999; Rush et al. 1998, 1999a, 1999b).

- Only include treatment strategies with demonstrated efficacy.
- Only use expert consensus when gaps exist in the scientific literature.
- Include clinicians, patients and their families, advocates, administrators, and other decision makers in the development of the algorithms.
- Incorporate patient preference if treatments have similar efficacy and safety profiles (assumes patients' adherence increases if preference is exercised).
- Provide clinicians with choices among otherwise equivalent treatments.
- Employ a consultation/support system to respond to clinicians' questions and concerns during algorithm implementation.
- Use symptom ratings at key decision points to increase consistency in assessing outcomes at each algorithm stage.
- Provide patients and their families with education (e.g., describe the disorder, specific medications, side effects, and expected outcomes).
- Ensure that clinicians have adequate visit time and visit frequency to implement the plan based on guideline recommendations of visit frequency, length of an appointment, and clinical staffing needed to implement the plan.

- Test the feasibility of initial recommendations, make appropriate revisions based on this evaluation, and then implement the plan more widely.
- Initial treatments should be less complex, easier to implement, and safer than those at later stages.
- Symptom response (as well as side effect) assessments and the time in the treatment stage dictate when and whether to proceed to the next stage.
- Tactics are suggested (not required) when appropriate to ensure applicability to a wide range of patients.
- Costs should be assessed in relation to patient outcomes (i.e., to specify the benefits accrued and associated costs). This information is important so that program managers can make budget decisions that center on the purchase of patient outcomes.
- Patients may enter at any stage depending on treatment history, which may recommend entry at later (more complex) stages.
- The clinician can choose to skip one or more strategic steps, or even not to use the algorithm, depending on the patient's treatment history and general medical health, associated comorbidities, patient preference, and other factors.
- Concise but informative chart documentation of treatment strategies, tactics, and patient outcomes ensures continuity of care across treatment environments and providers.

Issues in Guideline Development

Once the principles and procedures used to develop guidelines have been specified, substantial tensions (philosophical complexities) must be addressed and agreed on to frame and specify guidelines or algorithms (Table 12–3)—a task further complicated by the wide audience for guidelines (Table 12–4).

Nomothetic (Group) Data Versus Idiographic (Individual) Decisions

As detailed elsewhere (Rush and Prien 1995), scientific studies produce data for groups of patients. As a result, guidelines (algorithms) provide group-based recommendations. However, clinicians provide treatment

TABLE 12–3.   *Tensions in guideline development*

Nomothetic (group) evidence versus idiographic (individual) decisions

Clinical consensus versus scientific evidence	General versus specific
Disorder specific versus practice specific	When to revise
Defining the role of patient preference	Preferred versus reimbursable practices
Textbook versus cookbook format	Cost driven versus outcome driven

Source. Data from the Texas Medication Algorithm Project (Rush et al. 1999b). This material is in the public domain and can be reproduced without permission, but appropriate citation is required.

TABLE 12–4.   *Audiences for guidelines*

Patients/families	Payors
General practitioners	Purchasers
Specialists	Educators
Researchers	Students/trainees
Quality assurers	Lawyers
Antipsychiatry proponents	Politicians

Source. Data from the Texas Medication Algorithm Project (Rush et al. 1999b). This material is in the public domain and can be reproduced without permission, but appropriate citation is required.

to one patient at a time. They attempt to select and apply relevant group-based information to individuals. In some cases, this approach requires that group data are either modified or entirely ignored to provide optimal care to an individual. Thus a major tension inherent in all guidelines is between the desire to provide specific guidance and the limitations of information based on groups of patients.

With more specific recommendations, the level of guidance increases, but the certainty that each particular recommendation applies to every individual is reduced. When plans are more specific (i.e., algorithms as opposed to guidelines), users must decide even more often and carefully whether and how to adapt or ignore these group-based suggestions. The more specific the recommendations, the greater the need for more sophisticated basic knowledge (e.g., pharmacologic principles) and for more extensive clinical experience.

General Versus Specific

Another major tension is the need to balance specificity with flexibility. Recommended strategies (what to do) without salient tactical suggestions (how to do it) are often insufficiently specific. For example, appropriate medication(s) may be recommended, but if not used at the proper doses for proper lengths of time, the recommendations will not produce the desired outcome. Thus, some tactical recommendations must be included for algorithms to be useful in diverse clinical situations. Yet these more specific tactical recommendations are often based as much on clinical experience as on scientific evidence. Furthermore, tactical recommendations must still retain substantial flexibility so that practitioners can tailor them to individual patients (e.g., the doses and rates of dose increases for the elderly often differ from those for younger, less medically fragile patients). If a guideline is overly specific, it will be suitable for very few patients. If the guideline is too general, it will fail to provide useful guidance.

One approach is to provide a range of treatment options for each treatment step (increasing flexibility and applicability to a large number of patients) and to give parameters that might specify tactical variations. For example, some tactical recommendations are relatively specific (e.g., the minimally effective therapeutic dose), whereas others are more general (e.g., a response is expected between 4 and 8 weeks at the recommended therapeutic doses).

Disorder-Specific Versus Practice-Specific

Another issue in guideline development is whether to make different treatment recommendations depending on where patients are seen (e.g., specialty versus primary care settings). Settings often differ in various elements of care (e.g., length of visits, amount of time for diagnostic evaluation, visit frequency), all of which affect outcome. In general medicine, primary care patients should receive the same type and quality of treatment as provided by specialty sectors. When necessary treatment elements are not available in primary care settings—because of procedural or incentive obstacles or because the needed procedure exceeds provider skills—then specialty care is recommended. Discussion and resolution of this controversy for mental illnesses is needed. Otherwise, the same patient with the same illness would receive different care depending on the type of provider or setting rather than on what is best.

Assuming that the disorder and not the setting determines the treatment recommendations, one must still define the population for which treatments are recommended. Is the treatment for all patients, the so-called average patient, or specific subgroups? In general, the choice of target populations aims at the average patient who may also present with additional disorders (comorbidities).

For some conditions, a different set of guidelines is provided for distinct diagnostic subtypes. For example, in major depressive disorder, the guidelines recommend different treatments for patients with and without psychotic features because evidence suggests that an antidepressant combined with an antipsychotic is more effective than an antidepressant alone in treating psychotic depressions (American Psychiatric Association 1993; Crismon et al. 1999; Depression Guideline Panel 1993b).

Clinical Consensus versus Scientific Evidence

Scientific evidence almost always has significant gaps. Science has not answered all of the key clinical questions needed to guide treatment. Whether and how these information gaps are filled must be specified. For example, both the AHCPR and the American Psychiatric Association guidelines relied heavily on the available scientific evidence. They then specified (with appropriate notation) where inferences, logic, or clinical opinion or consensus was used to complete the recommendations.

When to Revise

Because guidelines and algorithms go beyond listing treatment options to make more-specific recommendations, more frequent revisions are needed than when less-specific recommendations are made. As scientific evidence becomes available—especially where previously there was little or none—revisions are clearly indicated. But how much evidence is sufficient to recommend revisions? What kinds of evidence (e.g., clinical impression versus scientific evidence) are required? How much and what types of scientific evidence; whose clinical impression? For example, when a new antidepressant or antipsychotic agent (or a new psychotherapy) becomes available, how many patients should be exposed to it before including it in algorithm revisions? If included, at what step should it be included in the algorithm? Algorithms often recommend multiple medication steps, but science rarely defines more than the first two. What kinds of evidence are needed to revise recommendations for subsequent treatment steps, those typically defined based on logic, pharmacologic theories, and clinical impressions?

Defining the Role of Patient Preference

Guidelines often recommend that patient preference play a determining role in selecting among otherwise medically equivalent treatments (i.e., those that are equally effective, safe, and tolerable) (e.g., Crismon et al. 1999; Hlatky 1995; Schulberg et al. 1998, 1999). Some treatments are associated with particular side effects, whereas other equally effective and safe treatments have different side effects. Some patients may prefer to risk certain types of side effects (e.g., sexual dysfunction), but for others this risk is not acceptable. Patient participation in selecting among otherwise equal treatments that differ in side effects should increase patient adherence.

Preferred Versus Reimbursable Practices

Reimbursement for the treatment of mental illnesses has become more restrictive over the past decade. Caps on the number of outpatient visits and hospital days, reduced access to providers with more advanced training (M.D.s, Ph.D.s), restricted formularies, and incentives to gatekeepers to deny specialty care can lead to practices without scientific support or can preclude practices that have scientific support. When formulating guidelines or algorithms, developers must decide whether to adapt evidence-based recommendations to the realities of current practice or to make recommendations that are based on the evidence— without regard to whether changes in selected health care practices or in reimbursement environments are clearly indicated. To date, most guidelines have chosen to follow the evidence rather than tailor recommendations to specific environments because 1) the ranges of environments often change and 2) improved patient care rather than environmental acceptability is the aim (e.g., American Psychiatric Association 1993; Crismon et al. 1999; Depression Guideline Panel 1993a, 1993b). Specific treatment settings are ultimately responsible for adapting the guidelines to their specific reimbursement environments (Cook and Giacomini 1999).

Textbook Versus Cookbook Format

The form and format of guidelines play a key role in whether they have credibility and whether they can be implemented. An enumeration of options with or without evidence may affect practice modestly. Although more specific recommendations provide greater guidance, they are more intrusive, which may lead to rejection of the guidance altogether. Therefore, guidelines (e.g., Depression Guideline Panel 1993a, 1993b) and algorithms (e.g., Crismon et al. 1999) must be digested, further modified, and made specific by those who are to provide the care. In this way the recommendations will be assimilated and understood and are more likely to be implemented, thereby avoiding the cookbook approach.

Cost-Driven Versus Outcome-Driven

Even if guidelines improve the quality of treatment and clinical outcomes, costs may increase or decrease (i.e., guidelines may increase cost but also increase value) (Institute of Medicine 1990). Guideline developers will often confront a tension between cost-based recommendations and guidance aimed at optimizing clinical outcomes, especially in care systems that already lack sufficient resources. For example, guidelines might recommend outpatient visits every 7–10 days for unstable patients undergoing medication adjustments, yet the system norm may be visits every 14–21 days. If more frequent visits are provided, more patients may remain in treatment and better outcomes may ensue, but the cost of care (i.e., more visits, more medication) will increase. Patients receiving such treatment should have better work performance; fewer sick days; and less overall functional impairment, pain, and suffering. Cost offsets may or may not be sufficient to compensate for the increased costs associated with better outcomes (Katon et al. 1995; Von Korff et al. 1998). If one chose to guide treatment based only on costs to the treatment system, then the "less care is better" and "no care is best" approaches would prevail.

Furthermore, few prospective empiric studies have gauged the clinical and functional benefits that result from more intensive or extensive care for mental illnesses. Thus the actual value, for example, of increasing the use of more expensive medication (on a per-pill basis) or more intensive or frequent treatments (e.g., medication plus psychotherapy) is not clearly articulated. Without information on value, clinical outcomes must be the guiding force for developing guidelines. Once guidelines are established and implemented, then the cost of guideline-driven care can be identified. Thereafter, studies of portions of the recommendations could reveal the effects on cost and clinical outcomes.

Guideline Implementation

A chronic disease management program must include four essential elements: 1) practice design revisions, 2) patient education, 3) expert care, and 4) information systems (Gilbert et al. 1998; Katon et al. 1997; Rush et al. 1999a, 1999b; Von Korff et al. 1998). *Practice design revisions* include appropriate appointment setting, reminders to patients to keep appointments, follow-up procedures for missed appointments, and specification of roles for diverse providers in a multidisciplinary team. *Patient education* involves developing skills in self-management, behavioral change, use of social supports, and, most important, development of a clinician–patient partnership to manage the condition. *Expert care* requires education and decision support for clinicians and easy access to consultation if problems or obstacles are encountered. *Information systems* are needed to provide reminders and feedback to both clinicians and patients (e.g., a simplified outcome measure for providers and patients that facilitates care plan revisions, rapid access to new research that affects treatment decisions, and systems to reduce paperwork burden).

Both *intelligent adherence* and *appropriate deviation* by clinicians are needed to implement any guideline or algorithm. First, the plan must be both credible and understandable. Second, it must be agreed to by the responsible clinicians. Third, administrative obstacles must be removed and incentives put in place (e.g., clinicians must have sufficient time and staff support to implement them). Fourth, patients and families or significant others must be informed about, commit to, and participate as partners in the plan itself. Finally, simple, efficient quality assurance procedures are needed to ensure appropriate implementation.

Credible, Practical Guidelines

Guidelines must be both credible and practical—with a sufficient range of options and enough flexibility so that practitioners can tailor the options to each individual (e.g., considering the patient's treatment history, age, concomitant psychiatric or general medical conditions, and concomitant medications). Treatment options at various stages allow applicability to a wider range of patients; yet if too general, algorithms provide little useful guidance. They should not be so complex that few clinicians are able to conceptualize or understand them.

The guidelines must also be credible. Whenever possible, scientific evidence should form the basis for recommendations. When scientific evidence is insufficient, clinical consensus established in an open, formal, and replicable way (e.g., Kahn et al. 1996; McEvoy et al. 1996) is needed to fill critical information gaps so that the guidelines can clearly specify care in most clinical situations. In essence, guidelines must have both clinical and scientific credibility.

Providers

Treatment guidelines are not substitutes for clinical judgment. Instead, they represent a problem-solving aid for clinicians when making optimal clinical decisions. Each decision point in the guideline requires professional judgment. In general, the degree of specificity provided by guidelines should suit the users' needs.

Clinicians must be skilled in diagnosis, the recognition and interpretation of side effects, the assessment of response versus nonresponse, drug interactions, and the like. Furthermore, clinicians must know when various clinical factors call for a need to either deviate from the algorithm or disregard it entirely.

Because guidelines provide only a framework for clinical decision making, clinicians who are not trained in basic pharmacology, physiology, and pathology or who are clinically inexperienced may misconstrue the apparent transparency of treatment guidelines for simplicity of implementation. Many experienced providers, however, may be unfamiliar with using algorithms or even specific medications within the plan. Thus, even experienced clinicians often need assistance (training, ongoing technical support, or consultation) initially. Furthermore, administrators may incorrectly decide that less experienced or knowledgeable personnel should implement guidelines, thereby leading to poor or even tragic outcomes.

Engaging clinicians in the development of guidelines that they are expected to use is extremely useful (Crismon et al. 1999; Rush et al. 1998, 1999a, 1999b). Certain care systems or specific populations (e.g., public sector or primary care patients or the elderly) may require modifications of elements in guidelines to ensure compatibility with system policies, patient populations, and provider types and settings. Conversely, system policies may also need to be changed to implement the guidelines.

Clinicians vary in how they judge whether a response has occurred and in when they make these judgments. They are often unfamiliar with standard symptomatic assessment and with the intricacies of patient education. Initial didactic educational efforts must be followed by ongoing consultation to assist clinicians in implementation. Clinicians are more likely to follow the recommendations if user-friendly feedback and prompts are provided to assist them in recognizing key decision points and in considering various treatment options in a timely fashion (Crismon et al. 1999; Rush et al. 1998, 1999a, 1999b).

My experience with TMAP suggests that clinician education should include information on the overall algorithm, each medication, patient education procedures and materials, symptom assessment, and problem-solving strategies when treatment obstacles or undesired outcomes are encountered. Education should include didactic presentations, consultation on demand, feedback on algorithm adherence, and intermittent conferences to discuss guideline revisions (Rush et al. 1998, 1999a, 1999b). More consistent implementation across providers is facilitated by these efforts.

Administrators

Because guidelines may shift budget requirements (e.g., to formulary from other sources, to increased visit frequency or length, or to other practice redesigns noted earlier), administrative and budget officers must understand and act (e.g., by shifting budgets and personnel or by creating incentives) to support implementation of these plans. When administrators are asked to support algorithms that recommend more expensive medications (on a per-pill basis) at earlier steps, they confront budgetary problems. Administrators need education and specific reasons for why these recommendations are being made and their potential clinical and budgetary benefits and disadvantages.

Administratively, a major benefit of guidelines is that they provide predictable and documentable outcomes—both clinical (e.g., symptoms, disability) and budgetary (e.g., costs, health care use)—because they must defend these plans and find resources to implement them. However, depending on routine practices, these plans may or may not reduce overall treatment system costs or even societal costs.

Patients and Families

Patient education markedly improves appointment attendance, medication adherence, attainment of therapeutic blood levels, and clinical outcomes (Basco and Rush 1995; Haynes et al. 1996; Kelly et al. 1990; Melinkow and Kiefe 1994; Robinson et al. 1997). Much as in the management of diabetes or other chronic general medical conditions, depressed patients and their families must learn how to recognize symptoms and side effects, when and how to seek clinician assistance, and how to detect early relapses or recurrences.

The principles underlying patient and family education are to 1) reiterate key points, 2) deliver less complex information early and more complex messages when patients are more stable, and 3) emphasize patients' participation in their own treatment. Initial education consists of explicit information about the symptoms of the illness and the medications prescribed. Patients may learn how to self-monitor their symptoms and side effects. Once they become less symptomatic, patients need to know about overall prognosis, how to detect symptom worsening, and whether to begin psychosocial treatments. With further improvement, patients must plan for longer-term issues (e.g., pursuit of employment, management of interpersonal relationships, intercurrent life events, general medical conditions, pregnancy). Information can be delivered individually or in a group format (as patients improve) (Rush et al. 1998,

1999b). Referral to support groups may also be helpful (Rush et al. 1999b).

In sum, education aims at increasing adherence, early side effect and relapse detection, optimal symptom resolution, and optimal reduction in disability, all of which help to enhance safety and clinical benefit.

Methods to Ensure
Appropriate Implementation (and Deviations)

Consensus is needed on several elements essential to the proper implementation of guidelines: 1) a consistent method for clinicians to gauge clinical benefit associated with each treatment step, 2) an agreed-upon window of time (critical decision point) during which these evaluations occur, 3) a uniform charting system to make apparent to other clinicians what clinical decisions were made based on what information, and 4) simple methods to check whether recommended practices were followed.

Clinical impression indicates that some clinicians may accept a modest treatment response, whereas others may not. Some clinicians pursue the next treatment step, whereas others do not. Some clinicians change treatments prematurely, before full benefits can occur, whereas others inappropriately persist when changes are needed. Reaching a consensus as to what is a sufficient level of treatment response, when it is expected, and how to gauge it should reduce inappropriate variations between providers.

Careful reviews of most medication records frequently reveal that much essential information is not recorded (Clark et al. 1996; Fowles et al. 1995; Kashner 1998; Kashner et al. 1999). It is often difficult to discern 1) how well or how poorly the patient was doing, 2) the level of side effect burden, 3) why a decision was made to change (or not change) the treatment, or 4) why a particular adjunctive medication was used to control side effects such as anxiety. A more uniform, short, standard chart entry (much like recording anticoagulant doses and prothrombin times or insulin recommendations and glucose levels) would make more explicit the "how" and "why" of clinical decision making.

Let us assume that the first three issues have been resolved and that chart notes provide the needed information. We now must decide how to measure the degree to which a clinician is adhering to the algorithm. The fewer the options, the easier it is to measure adherence. However, most useful algorithms must be flexible. Practitioners often have to skip treatment steps based on the patient's treatment history, clinical presentation, medical status, and the like. Tactics must also be flexible (e.g., a seemingly subtherapeutic medication dose may be justified in a 75-year-old patient who has several concurrent general medical conditions). Treatment that in some situations is entirely appropriate could be viewed as inappropriate in other settings.

One approach is to specify algorithm steps (with several therapeutically equivalent options at each step) and only a few essential tactics (e.g., minimal dosages, minimal treatment duration before evaluating response). The comparative frequencies with which practitioners are within or outside of these recommendations can then be identified.

However, we are not sure which tactical or strategic deviations affect clinical outcomes. Some deviations may matter more for some patient populations or practice settings and less for others. Some deviations (e.g., skipping a stage) are not true deviations per se. Unlike in the management of diabetes, in which objective intermediate outcomes (e.g., blood glucose or carboxyhemoglobin) are used, we have no laboratory measures for psychotropic medication management. We have only symptomatic or functional changes by which to guide treatment. Therefore, greater clinical judgment is needed to implement the recommendations.

Clinical Implications

If treatment guidelines are implemented, several new issues will be confronted. In theory, both quality of care and clinical outcome should improve, with costs either going up or down. If costs go up, then we confront the value issue. That is, if better outcomes are attained, are they worth the cost? Only two studies to date have prospectively evaluated the clinical and economic effects of using treatment guidelines (for depression in the primary care setting) to find substantially better outcomes but at greater costs (Katon et al. 1995; Von Korff et al. 1998). These studies also strongly suggested a need for specific practice design revisions. The ongoing TMAP project addresses similar issues in a specialty-care public-sector population (Crismon et al. 1999; Gilbert et al. 1998; Rush et al. 1998, 1999a, 1999b).

An overemphasis on cost is extremely dangerous because it can often lead to the assumption that only those treatments that reduce costs or that have been proven to increase work attendance or productivity are worth it. Saving treatment costs will—with many psychiatric patients—cause care to shift to jails and prisons, thus increasing the costs to society. Alternatively, these emphases deny care to the retired and others for whom we do not yet have highly effective treatments (e.g., patients with Alzheimer's disease).

Guidelines provide a basis for creating a solid and scientifically supportable level of care that, if properly developed, puts patient welfare first. Making care explicit, logical, and consistent across providers should increase accountability, ensure coordination of care, and produce cost-appropriate efficiencies. Therefore, guidelines must 1) be of the highest quality, 2) undergo timely revisions, 3) be driven by long-term patient benefits (not short-term budgets or profits), and 4) be supported by administrative efforts to provide the time and resources for proper implementation.

Research Implications

Many major questions remain unanswered and deserve further study. Do treatment guidelines for mental illnesses produce better clinical outcomes than usual care and, if so, at what cost? Are they worth it? Are they especially cost effective for particular groups of patients, clinicians, disorders, or clinical settings (e.g., primary versus specialty care)? Which are the active ingredients in a guideline? What are the most cost-efficient ways to implement guidelines (e.g., education, chart audits, prompts, economic incentives, computer platform)? When should guidelines be revised? What level of evidence is needed to make revisions?

Finally, and perhaps most important, we need a much more solid evidence base to recommend treatment options and steps if the first treatment does not produce a satisfactory response (e.g., If one atypical antipsychotic fails to work, will the next one work? Does failure with one selective serotonin reuptake inhibitor recommend for or against another? Where does psychotherapy fit into these treatment plans?).

Answers to these and other key questions have major health care policy, administrative, clinical practice, and public health implications. These kinds of questions are the logical product of the remarkable advances made over the past several decades in mental illness research with regard to improved diagnostic methods, cutting-edge pathobiologic discoveries, and the availability of an ever-expanding therapeutic armamentarium. Perhaps clinical practice guidelines can help to ensure that patients will have access to these advances in a predictable way.

Acknowledgments

The author thanks David Savage and Fast Word, Inc., Dallas, for their secretarial support and Kenneth Z. Altshuler, M.D., Stanton Sharp Distinguished Chair and Professor and Chairman, Department of Psychiatry, University of Texas Southwestern Medical Center, for administrative support.

References

American Psychiatric Association: Diagnostic and Statistical Manual of Mental Disorder, 3rd Edition. Washington, DC, American Psychiatric Association, 1980

American Psychiatric Association: Diagnostic and Statistical Manual of Mental Disorders, 3rd Edition, Revised. Washington, DC, American Psychiatric Association, 1987

American Psychiatric Association: Practice guideline for major depressive disorder in adults. Am J Psychiatry 150(suppl):1–26, 1993

American Psychiatric Association: Diagnostic and Statistical Manual of Mental Disorders, 4th Edition. Washington, DC, American Psychiatric Association, 1994a

American Psychiatric Association: Practice guideline for the treatment of patients with bipolar disorder. Am J Psychiatry 151(suppl):1–36, 1994b

American Psychiatric Association: Practice guideline for the treatment of patients with schizophrenia. Am J Psychiatry 154(suppl):1–63, 1997

Basco MR, Rush AJ: Compliance with pharmacotherapy in mood disorders. Psychiatr Ann 25:269–270, 278–279, 1995

Bauer MS, Callahan AM, Jampala C, et al: Clinical practice guidelines for bipolar disorder from the Department of Veterans Affairs. J Clin Psychiatry 60:9–21, 1999

Brown JB, Shye D, McFarland B: The paradox of guideline implementation: how AHCPR's depression guideline was adapted at Kaiser Permanente northwest region. Jt Comm J Qual Improv 21:5–21, 1995

Chiles JA, Miller AL, Crismon ML, et al: The Texas Medication Algorithm Project: development and implementation of the schizophrenia algorithm. Psychiatr Serv 50:69–74, 1999

Clark RE, Ricketts SK, McHugo GJ: Measuring hospital use without claims: a comparison of patient and provider reports. Health Serv Res 31:153–169, 1996

Clinton JJ, McCormick K, Besteman J: Enhancing clinical practice: the role of practice guidelines. Am Psychol 49:30–33, 1994

Cook D, Giacomini M: The trials and tribulations of clinical practice guidelines. JAMA 281:1950–1951, 1999

Crismon ML, Trivedi M, Pigott TA, et al: The Texas Medication Algorithm Project: report of the Texas Consensus Conference Panel on Medication Treatment of Major Depressive Disorder. J Clin Psychiatry 60:142–156, 1999

Dennehy EB, Suppes T: Medication algorithms for bipolar disorder. Journal of Practical Psychiatry and Behavioral Health 5:142–152, 1999

Depression Guideline Panel: Clinical practice guideline number 5, in Depression in Primary Care, Vol 1: Detection and Diagnosis. Rockville, MD, U.S. Department of Health and Human Services, Public Health Service, Agency for Health Care Policy and Research. AHCPR Publication No. 93-0550, 1993a

Depression Guideline Panel: Clinical practice guideline number 5, in Depression in Primary Care, Vol 2: Treatment of Major Depression. Rockville, MD, U.S. Department of Health and Human Services, Public Health Service, Agency for Health Care Policy and Research. AHCPR Publication No. 93-0551, 1993b

Eddy DM: Guidelines for policy statements: the explicit approach. JAMA 263:2239–2240, 1990a

Eddy DM: Practice policies: what are they? JAMA 263:877–880, 1990b

Eddy DM: Practice policies: where do they come from? JAMA 263:1265–1275, 1990c

Eddy DM: A Manual for Assessing Health Practices and Designing Practice Policies. Philadelphia, PA, American College of Physicians, 1991

Fowles JB, Lawthers AG, Weiner JP, et al: Agreement between physicians' office records and Medicare part B claims data. Health Care Financing Review 16:189–199, 1995

Gafni A, Birch S: Guidelines for the adoption of new technologies: a prescription for uncontrolled growth in expenditures and how to avoid the problem. Can Med Assoc J 148:913–917, 1993

Gilbert DA, Altshuler KZ, Rago WV, et al: Texas Medication Algorithm Project: definitions, rationale and methods to develop medication algorithms. J Clin Psychiatry 59:345–351, 1998

Haynes RB, McKibbon KA, Kanani R: Systematic review of randomized trials of interventions to assist patients to follow prescriptions for medications. Lancet 348:383–386, 1996

Haynes RB, Taylor DW, Sackett DL: Compliance in Health Care. Baltimore, MD, Johns Hopkins University, 1977

Hlatky MA: Patient preferences and clinical guidelines. JAMA 273:1219–1220, 1995

Institute of Medicine Committee to Advise the Public Health Service on Clinical Practice Guidelines: Clinical Practice Guidelines: Directions for a New Program. Edited by Field MJ, Lohr KN. Washington, DC, National Academy Press, 1990

Jobson K: International Psychopharmacology Algorithm Project: algorithms in psychopharmacology. Int J Psychiatry Clin Pract 1(suppl):S3, 1997

Jones J, Hunter H: Consensus methods for medical and health services research. BMJ 311:376–380, 1995

Kahn DA, Carpenter D, Docherty JP, et al: The Expert Consensus Guideline Series. Treatment of bipolar disorder. J Clin Psychiatry 57(suppl):3–88, 1996

Kahn D, Docherty J, Carpenter D, et al: Consensus methods in practice guideline development: a review and description of a new method. Psychopharmacol Bull 33:631–639, 1997

Kashner TM: Agreement between administrative files and written medical records: a case of the Department of Veterans Affairs. Med Care 36:1324–1336, 1998

Kashner TM, Suppes T, Rush AJ, et al: Measuring use of outpatient care among mentally ill individuals: a comparison of self reports and provider records. Evaluation and Program Planning 22:31–39, 1999

Kasper S, Jobson K: First European Meeting for Algorithms on the Psychopharmacology of Psychiatric Disorders. International Journal of Psychiatry in Clinical Practice 1(suppl):S1, 1997

Katon W, Von Korff M, Lin E, et al: Collaborative management to achieve treatment guidelines; impact on depression in primary care. JAMA 273:1026–1031, 1995

Katon W, Von Korff M, Lin E, et al: Population-based care of depression: effective disease management strategies to decrease prevalence. Gen Hosp Psychiatry 19:169–178, 1997

Kelly GR, Scott JE, Mamon J: Medication compliance and health education among outpatients with chronic mental disorders. Med Care 28:1181–1197, 1990

Kissick WL: Medicine's Dilemmas: Infinite Needs versus Finite Resources. New Haven, CT, Yale University Press, 1994

Linstone HA, Turoff M: The Delphi Method: Techniques and Applications. Reading, MA, Addison-Wesley, 1975

Martin DL: Health technology evaluation in the U.S.: the NIH Consensus Development Program. Dimens Health Serv 58:9, 1981

McEvoy JP, Weiden PJ, Smith TE, et al: The Expert Consensus Guideline Series. Treatment of schizophrenia. J Clin Psychiatry 57(suppl):3–58, 1996

McEvoy JP, Scheifler PL, Frances A: Treatment of schizophrenia 1999. The Expert Consensus Guideline Series. Treatment of schizophrenia 1999. J Clin Psychiatry 60(suppl):3–80, 1999

Melinkow J, Kiefe C: Patient compliance and medical research: issues in methodology. J Gen Intern Med 9:96–105, 1994

Miller AL, Chiles JA, Chiles JK, et al: The Texas Medication Algorithm Project (TMAP) schizophrenia algorithms. J Clin Psychiatry 60:649–657, 1999

Park RE, Fink A, Brook RH, et al: Physician ratings or appropriate indications for six medical and surgical procedures. Am J Public Health 76:766–772, 1986

Perry S, Kalberer JT Jr: The NIH consensus-development program and the assessment of health-care technologies: the first two years. N Engl J Med 303:169–172, 1980

Robinson P, Katon W, Von Korff M, et al: The education of depressed primary care patients: what do patients think about interactive booklets and a video? J Fam Pract 44:562–571, 1997

Rosenberg WM, Sackett DL: On the need for evidence-based medicine. Therapie 51:212–217, 1996

Rush AJ, Prien R: From scientific knowledge to the clinical practice of psychopharmacology: can the gap be bridged? Psychopharmacol Bull 31:7–20, 1995

Rush AJ, Crismon ML, Toprac MG, et al: Consensus guidelines in the treatment of major depressive disorder. J Clin Psychiatry 59(suppl):73–84, 1998

Rush AJ, Crismon ML, Toprac MG, et al: Implementing guidelines and systems of care: experiences with the Texas Medication Algorithm Project (TMAP). Journal of Practical Psychiatry and Behavioral Health 5:75–86, 1999a

Rush AJ, Rago WV, Crismon ML, et al: Medication treatment for the severely and persistently mentally ill: the Texas Medication Algorithm Project. J Clin Psychiatry 60:284–291, 1999b

Sackett DL: Evidence-Based Medicine. How to Practice and Teach EBM. New York, Churchill Livingstone, 1997

Sackett DL, Rosenberg WM: The need for evidence-based medicine. J R Soc Med 88:620–624, 1995

Schulberg HC, Katon W, Simon GE, et al: Treating major depression in primary care practice; an update of the Agency for Health Care Policy and Research practice guidelines. Arch Gen Psychiatry 55:1121–1127, 1998

Schulberg HC, Katon W, Simon GE, et al: Best clinical practice: guidelines for managing major depression in primary medical care. J Clin Psychiatry 60(suppl):19–26, 1999

Shaneyfelt TM, Mayo-Smith MF, Rothwangle J: Are guidelines following guidelines? the methodological quality of clinical practice guidelines in the peer-reviewed medical literature. JAMA 281:1900–1905, 1999

Suppes T, Rush AJ Jr, Kraemer HC, et al: Treatment algorithm use to optimize management of symptomatic patients with a history of mania. J Clin Psychiatry 59:89–96, 1998

Trivedi MH, DeBattista C, Fawcett J, et al: Developing treatment algorithms for unipolar depression in cyberspace: International Psychopharmacology Algorithm Project (IPAP). Psychopharmacol Bull 34:355–359, 1998

Von Korff M, Katon W, Bush T, et al: Treatment costs, cost offset, and cost-effectiveness of collaborative management of depression. Psychosom Med 60:143–149, 1998

Welch WP, Miller ME, Welch HG, et al: Geographic variation in expenditures for physicians' services in the United States. N Engl J Med 328:621–627, 1993

Woolf SH: Practice guidelines: a new reality in medicine, I: recent developments. Arch Intern Med 150:1811–1818, 1990

Woolf SH: Manual for Clinical Practice Guideline Development. Rockville, MD, Agency for Health Care Policy and Research. AHCPR Publication 91-0007, 1991

Psychotherapy and Evolving Health Care

Introduction

William C. Sanderson, Ph.D.

Changes in the United States health care system, set in full motion during the 1990s, are influencing every area of health care. These changes have a profound impact on the practice of psychotherapy. This section of the book deals with the current status of the health care system and what must be accomplished if psychotherapy is to survive the evolving health care system in the 21st century (Sanderson 1995).

The introduction of managed care (or any other system that monitors the use and cost of services, such as health maintenance organizations) is reshaping the way in which psychotherapy is practiced. In the traditional fee-for-service model, decisions about the cost and length of treatment were choices made primarily by the doctor and the patient. The cost of psychotherapy was of little concern to the clinician. The fee-for-service model encouraged service because more service created more income. However, in response to the increased costs of psychotherapy, and in particular to the perceived endless nature of psychotherapy, managed care organizations are pressuring clinicians to allocate decreasing (less than usual) amounts of service.

Although to date the focus of managed care organizations' cost cutting has been almost entirely on limiting the number of therapy sessions, managed care organizations will ultimately have to focus on quality and efficacy in order to compete. Managed care organizations are clearly motivated to cut costs; however, they must also satisfy the consumer (i.e., patient) and the payer (e.g., the employer providing health benefits). Therefore, they have to balance cost cutting with patient outcome. Simply reducing the length of treatment may not accomplish this goal, because most psychotherapists are trained in long-term therapeutic interventions that require more sessions than managed care organizations are willing to cover. Reducing the length of therapies devised to take place over a longer period of time may result in ineffective outcomes, leading both to consumer dissatisfaction and to increased costs down the road if the disorder becomes more severe or less responsive to treatment. Thus, concern for the effectiveness of an intervention will eventually temper managed care organizations' focus on economics (Bennett 1992).

Another force that will have a significant impact on the practice of psychotherapy is the establishment of clinical practice guidelines and treatment consensus statements (Chapter 12). In all medical fields, significant variability exists in the treatments delivered to patients. Patients are not necessarily receiving the most effective treatments. Thus, to ensure that patients uniformly receive the optimal intervention—whether a type of medication, surgical procedure, or psychotherapy—clinical practice guidelines are being developed that usually rely on systematic evaluation of scientific and clinical data.

The Agency for Health Care Policy and Research (AHCPR) and the Public Health Service (Depression Guideline Panel 1993) have been developing practice guidelines that consider only treatments with efficacy demonstrated in randomized, controlled trials. For an intervention to be included as a first-line treatment, research evidence attesting to its efficacy must be available.

The recommendations of the clinical practice guidelines for psychotherapy are quite clear (Depression Guideline Panel 1993). When psychotherapy is selected as the sole treatment, the guideline states:

> Psychotherapy should generally be time-limited, focused on current problems, and aimed at symptom resolution rather than personality change as the initial target. Since it has not been established that all forms of psychotherapy are equally effective for major depression, if one is chosen as the sole treatment, it should have been studied in randomized controlled trials. (p. 84)

In addition to endorsing specific psychologic treatments for depression—cognitive-behavioral therapy (Chapter 13) and interpersonal psychotherapy (Chapter 14), both of which have efficacy data—the report goes on to state: "Long-term therapies are not currently indicated as first-line acute phase treatments" (p. 84). Thus, the paradox between clinicians' current training in long-term psychotherapy and the guideline recommendation is obvious (Chapter 15).

Clinical guidelines and treatment consensus statements have a significant impact on the way that clinicians practice psychotherapy (Sanderson 1995, 1998). These documents set standards of care, which if ignored leave the clinician ethically and legally vulnerable. Several states have passed, or are in the process of passing, legislation that gives guidelines the force of law by protecting clinicians who follow guidelines from malpractice litigation (Barlow and Barlow 1995). The implications are clear: failure to provide an empirically validated treatment, when one exists, may constitute malpractice. These guidelines have been adopted by several large behavioral health care organizations (e.g., Merit Behavioral Care) and sent to all providers.

Unfortunately, although empirically supported psychologic treatments exist for depression, clinicians are not necessarily being trained in these approaches (Crits-Christoph et al. 1995; see also Chapters 14 and 15 this volume). This situation has posed a problem for patients and for providers of psychotherapy. Because managed care organizations and federal practice guidelines cannot rely on the delivery of treatments that are not widely available, these treatments are often given secondary status to medication for the treatment of depression, despite their equivalent efficacy (D. H. Barlow 1994; Persons et al. 1996). Thus, although the AHCPR depression guideline's own meta-analysis concludes equivalent efficacy for medication, cognitive-behavioral therapy, and interpersonal therapy, medication receives a stronger endorsement as a first-line treatment.

Recognizing an apparent deficiency in the use and dissemination of empirically supported treatments (ESTs), the American Psychological Association established a task force to identify, promote, and assist in the dissemination of ESTs (Chambless et al. 1998; Woody and Sanderson 1998; up-to-date reports available at www.apa.org/divisions/div12). A major issue for psychotherapy is how to train practitioners in these newer, empirically supported psychotherapies (Chapter 14). At present, this issue pertains to cognitive-behavioral therapy and interpersonal psychotherapy, but as other new empirically supported psychotherapeutic treatments emerge, the issues will remain the same.

A recent survey of clinical psychology internship programs—where clinical psychologists receive the bulk of their supervised clinical experience—revealed that only 59% of programs provided supervision in cognitive therapy for depression and a mere 8% provided supervision in interpersonal psychotherapy (Crits-Christoph et al. 1995). Moreover, having supervision available does not mean that students are required to receive it. For example, only 14% of internship programs required training in cognitive therapy for depression and only 3% required training in interpersonal therapy. Although I am unaware of data from other mental health professionals training programs (e.g., psychiatry and social work), my colleagues from these departments have suggested the data would be no better—and more likely are worse.

If training at the graduate and internship levels is lacking, then one can imagine how difficult it will be to disseminate these treatments for practitioners already in the field. To date, no formal process exists to disseminate and train practitioners in ESTs. With a rapidly changing database, clinicians trained 10 years ago are unlikely to be up to date on the newer, evidence-based psychotherapies. Indeed, most references supporting such therapies have appeared in the past 10 years (Calhoun et al. 1998). How can we motivate clinicians to learn ESTs? Even if they are motivated, how can we disseminate the treatments and provide high-integrity supervision to ensure that clinicians are trained properly? The lack of availability of these treatments, more than the lack of data supporting their efficacy, has diminished the value of psychotherapy for the treatment of depression.

References

Barlow DH: Psychological interventions in the era of managed care. Clinical Psychology: Science and Practice 1:109–122, 1994

Barlow DH, Barlow DG: Guidelines and empirically validated treatments: ships passing in the night? Behavioral Healthcare Tomorrow 4:25–29, 1995

Bennett M: The managed care setting as a framework for clinical practice, in Managed Mental Healthcare: Administrative and Clinical Issues. Edited by Feldman JL, Fitzpatrick RJ. Washington, DC, American Psychiatric Press, 1992, pp 203–218

Calhoun KS, Moras K, Pilkonis PA, et al: Empirically supported treatments: implications for training. J Consult Clin Psychol 66:151–162, 1998

Chambless DL, Baker MJ, Baucom D, et al: Update on empirically validated therapies, II: The Clinical Psychologist 5. 1:3–16, 1998

Crits-Christoph P, Frank E, Chambless DL, et al: Training in empirically validated therapies: what are clinical psychology students learning? Professional Psychology: Research and Practice 26:514–522, 1995

Depression Guideline Panel: Clinical practice guideline number 5, in Depression in Primary Care, Vol 2: Treatment of Major Depression. Rockville, MD, U.S. Department of Health and Human Services, Public Health Service, Agency for Health Care Policy and Research. AHCPR Publication No. 93-0551, 1993

Persons JB, Thase ME, Crits-Christoph P: The role of psychotherapy in the treatment of depression: review of two practice guidelines. Arch Gen Psychiatry 53:301–312, 1996

Sanderson WC: Can psychological interventions meet the new demands of health care? American Journal of Managed Care 1:93–98, 1995

Sanderson WC: The case for evidence-based psychotherapy treatment guidelines. Am J Psychother 52:382–387, 1998

Woody SR, Sanderson WC: Manuals for empirically supported treatments: 1998 update from the task force on psychological interventions. The Clinical Psychologist 51:17–21, 1998

13

Cognitive-Behavioral Therapy of Depression

William C. Sanderson, Ph.D.

Lata K. McGinn, Ph.D.

Cognitive-behavioral therapy (CBT) of depression involves the application of specific, empirically supported strategies focused on depressogenic information processing (e.g., A. T. Beck et al. 1979) and behavior (e.g., Lewinsohn et al. 1986). To alleviate depressive affect, treatment is directed at the following three domains: cognition, behavior, and physiology (see Klosko and Sanderson 1999 for a session-by-session description). In the cognitive domain, patients learn to apply cognitive restructuring techniques so that negatively distorted thoughts underlying depression can be corrected, leading to more logical and adaptive thinking. Within the behavioral domain, techniques such as activity scheduling, social skills training, and assertiveness training are used to remediate behavioral deficits that contribute to and maintain depression (e.g., social withdrawal, loss of social reinforcement). Finally, within the physiologic domain, patients with agitation and anxiety are taught to use imagery, meditation, and relaxation procedures to calm their bodies.

CBT is oriented toward empowering the patient. Within this specific, brief psychotherapeutic treatment modality, the emphasis is on providing patients with skills to offset their depression. One primary goal of CBT is to facilitate the use of treatment techniques outside therapy sessions to create a "positive emotional spiral" wherein patients can implement specific strategies to offset their depressive mood (e.g., cognitive restructuring is used to offset negative thought patterns and the consequent depressive affect; scheduling pleasant activities is used to offset decreased reinforcement secondary to social withdrawal). In the first section of this chapter, we review the major treatment strategies used in CBT for depression, with an emphasis on cognitive therapy, the psychologic intervention with the most empiric support for the treatment of depression (Depression Guideline Panel 1993). In the second part of the chapter, we cover research data attesting to the efficacy of CBT.

Cognitive Therapy

A.T. Beck et al. (1979) developed cognitive therapy as a treatment for depression. Although cognitive therapy incorporates a range of behavioral techniques within its approach, in this chapter we emphasize specific strategies used to change cognition (i.e., cognitive restructuring).

Cognitive restructuring is a therapeutic strategy that focuses directly on the disturbed information processing maintained by depressed patients. Cognitive theories of depression hypothesize that particular negative ways of thinking increase individuals' likelihood of developing and maintaining depression when they experience stressful life events. According to these theories, individuals who possess specific maladaptive cognitive patterns are vulnerable to depression because they tend to engage in negative information processing about themselves and their experiences. Here we present two widely accepted cognitive theories: the cognitive triad and hopelessness theory.

Cognitive Triad

A.T. Beck (1979, 1983) hypothesized that depression-prone individuals possess negative self-schemata (beliefs), which he labeled the *cognitive triad*. Specifically, depressed patients have a negative view of themselves (seeing themselves as worthless, inadequate, unlovable, deficient), their environments (seeing them as overwhelming, filled with obstacles and failure), and their futures (seeing them as hopeless, as though no effort will change the course of their lives). This negative way of thinking

guides their perception, interpretation, and memory of personally relevant experiences, thereby resulting in a negatively biased interpretation
of their personal worlds and, ultimately, in the development of depressive symptoms. For example, a depression-prone individual is more likely to notice and remember situations in which he or she has failed or
does not live up to some personal standard; he or she is also more likely
to discount or ignore successful situations. As a result, the individual
maintains his or her negative sense of self, leading to depression.

Hopelessness Theory

Abramson et al. (1989) proposed a hopelessness theory of depression
formulated from Seligman and colleagues' work on learned helplessness and attribution styles (Seligman 1975; Seligman et al. 1979).
Abramson et al. (1989) hypothesized that when confronted with a negative event, people who exhibit a depressogenic inferential (thinking)
style—defined as the tendency to attribute negative life events to stable
(enduring) and global (widespread) causes—are vulnerable to developing depression because they will infer that 1) negative consequences
will follow from the current negative event, and 2) that the occurrence
of a negative event in their lives means that they are fundamentally
flawed or worthless. For example, consider a woman whose fiancé
breaks off their engagement. She is likely to become hopeless and develop the symptoms of depression if she infers that a consequence of the
break-up is that she will never marry or have children; if she infers that
without a lover she is worthless; or if she attributes the cause of the
break-up to her personality flaws, a stable-global cause that will lead to
many other bad outcomes for her. Thus, according to hopelessness theory, a specific cognitive vulnerability operates to increase the risk for depression through its effects on processing or appraisals of personally
relevant life experiences.

The Process of Cognitive Restructuring

Collaborative empiricism

A.T. Beck (1979) coined the term *collaborative empiricism* to characterize the nature of the therapist–patient relationship in cognitive ther-

apy. The therapist is active and directive and, using the principles of logic and the scientific method, facilitates a rational approach to thinking with regard to the patient's current life circumstances. The patient's thoughts and assumptions are treated as hypotheses that can be tested to verify their accuracy.

To foster a spirit of collaborative empiricism, cognitive-behavioral therapists typically begin treatment by educating patients about their disorder. Helping patients understand the cognitive-behavioral model of depression is particularly important in strengthening the treatment rationale and subsequent patient compliance. When a new technique is introduced, the therapist always begins by presenting the rationale. By educating patients, the therapist builds the therapeutic alliance. When appropriate, relevant research findings are also reviewed (e.g., benefits of CBT versus medication, typical rate of response to treatment). Information covered in session can be bolstered by recommending self-help books and Web sites (e.g., www.cognitivetherapy.com) aimed at educating patients about CBT and depression. The popular self-help book *Feeling Good* (Burns 1980) is of enormous value when applying CBT for depression. It is also valuable for patients to audiotape sessions and review them once or more between sessions.

One of the most important functions of the therapist is to provide structure. First, the therapist and the patient together discuss the goals of therapy. These goals should be specific and concrete (e.g., to decrease depressive symptoms to a score below 10 as measured by the Beck Depression Inventory [BDI] [A. T. Beck et al. 1988], rather than to simply feel better). The therapist continually evaluates with the patient how well therapy is helping the patient progress toward these goals (e.g., whether BDI score is decreasing) and modifies treatment strategies and goals when appropriate.

With regard to overall therapeutic style, the cognitive-behavioral therapist aims to communicate a sense of faith in his or her ability to help the patient. Identifying and responding to negative thoughts about therapy will be important in providing a credible treatment plan for the patient. In fact, the patient should be encouraged to express negative feelings about the therapy so that such factors, which may interfere with treatment, can be dealt with up front. Because patients are unlikely to participate in activities they believe will not ultimately pay off, the more realistic optimism that the therapist can provide, the better. An optimistic, persistent therapeutic style is especially useful in treating depression.

Homework

To maximize rapid treatment response, cognitive-behavioral therapists place great emphasis on the use of homework outside of therapy sessions. By the end of each session, the therapist and the patient should agree on at least one assignment the patient can do to either test beliefs or build skills. The therapist is responsible for facilitating compliance with homework assignments. Although not always the case, patients are often noncompliant with homework because their therapist does not pay enough attention to it; as a result, patients conclude the homework is not important. The therapist can facilitate compliance by providing a rationale that motivates patients, developing homework assignments in collaboration with the patient, following-up with assignments, praising patients when they complete assignments, brainstorming solutions when problems occur rather than labeling the patient as resistant, and pointing out the positive consequences of completing homework assignments.

Guided Discovery

Guided discovery is the technique developed by A.T. Beck (1979) to help patients identify cognitive errors. Guided discovery is essentially based on the Socratic method. Rather than simply pointing out the errors in the patient's thinking (and perhaps seeming to lecture or reprimand patients), the therapist asks specific questions designed to direct (guide) patients to find the errors themselves (discovery). The rationale for this approach is that patients will derive more benefit from discovering their own cognitive distortions than from simply being told what their distortions are. In addition, and perhaps most important, by asking directed questions, the therapist models a process that patients can internalize and learn to use on their own. Merely pointing out patients' distortions is not likely to encourage generalization to other situations and will facilitate dependence on the therapist; in contrast, teaching patients the process of evaluating their thoughts will provide them with a tool they can use in many other situations.

The use of guided discovery highlights a core principle of CBT: As much as possible, the therapist encourages patients to use strategies learned within the context of therapy to generate their own solutions to problems. All strategies used during therapy sessions are ultimately intended to be used by the patient in his or her real world. As is evident from this model, patient noncompliance is a major stumbling block to effective treatment, and this must be dealt with from the outset. Interested readers should see either J. S. Beck (1995) or Klosko and Sanderson (1999) for a thorough discussion of patient noncompliance.

Broad Steps of Cognitive Restructuring

As outlined earlier, cognitive therapy focuses on understanding how patients interpret events in their lives. The therapy is based on the premise that if distorted thoughts and images can be changed, then the accompanying negative emotional states and behaviors will change as well. In this cognitive mediation model of emotion, affect and behavior are seen for the most part as slaves to cognition. If cognition is distorted, then maladaptive affect and dysfunctional behavior will follow. The affect is always in sync with the appraisal. If the patient feels angry, then cognitions associated with threat should be identified; if the patient feels anxious, then cognitions associated with danger should be identified; and so on.

To facilitate cognitive change, patients are encouraged to consider their thoughts and beliefs as hypotheses, to pay attention to all available information, and to revise hypotheses (thoughts) according to incoming information. The following three steps are used to accomplish this goal (see J. S. Beck [1995] for a detailed explanation of cognitive restructuring): 1) monitoring automatic thoughts, 2) analyzing the thoughts, and 3) generating a rational response.

Step 1

Before patients can change the way they think, they must recognize what they are thinking. The thoughts or images on a person's mind are labeled *automatic thoughts*. Thus, the first essential step of cognitive restructuring is to teach people to begin monitoring their automatic thoughts. The best way to begin is to have patients use a change in emotion (e.g., an increase in depression) as a cue to initiate self-monitoring of what was going through their minds. According to cognitive theory, the onset or intensification of emotion is an indication that an automatic thought has occurred. In addition to labeling their thoughts, patients will also label the intensity of their negative affect and note the situation in which the thought occurred. Patients should be encouraged to write down whatever went through their minds. Frequently, patients begin writing their thoughts but then decide to not put them down because they "do not really believe them." Moreover, sometimes the thought is so extreme that when the patient writes it down in, he or she realizes it is an inaccuracy and feels embarrassed to acknowledge it. However, even if thoughts are subsequently discounted, the fact that they occurred, even momentarily, suggests that they most likely had an effect on the person's emotional state at the time. Therefore, therapists must strongly encourage patients to write down any thoughts that pass through their minds and leave the editing for later.

Step 2

After a patient has elucidated his or her thoughts and examined how they influence his or her affect and behavior, the next step is for the therapist and the patient to subject each thought to logical analysis by 1) examining the evidence for the patient's thoughts, 2) determining if any cognitive distortions are present, and 3) attempting to generate alternative hypotheses.

Examining the Evidence Examining evidence is at the heart of a rational approach to life. When the patient's thoughts can be framed in an empiric question, then the patient and the therapist can test the accuracy of these thoughts by examining the evidence. By facilitating this approach, the therapist allows patients to break free of the habitual acceptance of implicit negative thoughts generated by depressogenic schema noted earlier. At this point, cognitions are treated as hypotheses and subjected to logical analysis. Crucial areas to investigate with patients are framed in the following questions:

1. Is there any evidence that supports the thought?
2. Is there any evidence that goes against the thought?

3. If the negative thought is accurate, what can be done to best cope with it?

For example, consider a patient whose depression was exacerbated by the prospect of failing an upcoming examination. The patient's primary negative thought is, "I'm a loser. I'll never pass the test." Because of this expectation, the patient may not study hard and as a result may fail, creating a self-fulfilling prophecy. However, once the negative thought is identified, the therapist and the patient can work together to determine if previous evidence supports the prediction that the patient will fail (e.g., Did the patient fail previous tests? Did he or she pass them? If so, what did the patient do that led to a positive versus a negative outcome?). Once this information is examined in detail, the patient can replace the negative thought with a more accurate thought, such as, "I have passed tests in the past, and although this test is difficult, if I put my effort into it, I can pass this one as well."

An important point to be made here is that the therapist is not trying to get the patient to think in a falsely positive manner (i.e., positive thinking). Rather the goal is to get the patient to see the situation as accurately as possible. If problems exist (e.g., repeatedly failing tests), the therapist can move into a problem-solving mode and help the patient correct behaviors that might be causing the problems (e.g., work on study behavior). This approach will be much more useful and valid than positive thinking in itself.

Identifying Cognitive Distortions   A.T. Beck's (1979) initial work on depression elucidated common errors of logic, or cognitive distortions (Burns 1980), that existed in the information processing styles of depressed patients. The use of cognitive distortions resulted in the patient viewing life events in a way that tended to maintain depression. For example, Beck observed that depressed patients frequently thought in extremes (black-and-white thinking) and, as a result, appraised any less-than-perfect performance as a failure. By identifying cognitive distortions, the therapist can facilitate cognitive restructuring—because it will enable patients to clearly see the errors of logic in their thinking—and the development of more accurate statements (rational responses). Examples of questions that should be applied to the patient's thoughts to uncover cognitive distortions should include the following:

1. Am I looking at things in extremes?
2. Am I taking one instance and seeing it as a pattern?
3. Am I picking out the negative details of a situation, ignoring the rest of the picture?
4. Am I rejecting positive experiences?
5. Am I jumping to a negative conclusion even though I have no facts to support it?
6. Am I magnifying the importance of things or catastrophizing about the consequences of a situation?
7. Am I assuming that something is going to happen because I feel that way?
8. Am I using emotionally charged words that stimulate my negative feelings?
9. Am I seeing myself as responsible for something that I was not in fact responsible for?

For example, after one of her patients dropped out of treatment, a student therapist stated, "I'm a lousy therapist and will have difficulty maintaining patients." On closer examination, she had a total of eight patients, and only one had dropped out. This is an example of the third cognitive distortion: She picked out one negative detail of the situation (the patient dropping out) and ignored the rest of the picture (seven patients currently in treatment). It is also an example of the sixth cognitive distortion: She is magnifying the significance of one event as indicating her total competence ("I'm a lousy therapist"). The second and eighth distortions fit as well: She is taking one event and predicting that it will become a pattern ("I'll have difficulty maintaining patients"), and she is using emotionally charged words ("lousy therapist") rather than something more accurate (e.g., a student therapist is likely to be inexperienced, which may account for the event). Other distortions apply in this situation; the goal is to continue to identify them until all that apply are exhausted.

Generating Alternatives Patients' automatic thoughts represent one interpretation of events. As discussed earlier, a depressed patient's interpretation of events is largely influenced by distorted information processing. Thus, before assuming that any one interpretation is correct, patients are asked to consider all the possibilities by generating alternative hypotheses to their automatic thoughts. This strategy is intended to move patients away from the exclusive use of negatively biased information processing. Continuing with the example of the student therapist, one possibility is that her patient dropped out of treatment because she *was* a lousy therapist. However, there are other alternative hypotheses as well, each of which is equally possible until further information is collected to rule them (or the original hypothesis) out. For example, perhaps the patient dropped out because he felt better, the time of the session was inconvenient, he decided to pursue an alternative treatment (medication), he was financially unable to continue, an unexpected major life event occurred that required his full attention, or perhaps he did not click with the therapist, and so on.

The goal is to generate as many *plausible* alternative explanations as possible. Depressive thinking is rigid in its negativity. When patients step back and generate alternative interpretations of an upsetting event, this process counters and loosens their rigidity. In many instances, none of the alternative hypotheses can be proven, yet each is as plausible as the one that the patient has generated and accepted as true. Thus, increasing patients' awareness of other possibilities gives them a sense of the full picture, demonstrates the frequent subjectivity involved in interpreting events, and highlights their repeated focus on the negative aspects of the situation.

Step 3

After evidence has been reviewed, distortions examined, and alternatives explored, the next step is to generate a rational response (i.e., a more accurate statement about the situation or event). Work done during Step 2 will facilitate the patient's generation of a rational (realistic) response. Thus, the goal in the ongoing example would be to have the student therapist modify the original thought ("I'm a lousy therapist and will have difficulty maintaining patients") to something like, "One patient dropped out and seven patients remain in treatment. I should examine what went wrong in that one instance, but I have to keep in mind that overall, I'm maintaining most of my patients. There are many explanations as to why a patient would drop out of treatment that are as plausible as my negative explanation. Losing one patient does not necessarily predict a problem with keeping patients in general. Also, losing patients is expected to some degree because I am not very experienced. That does not make me a lousy therapist. It's just a function of my current situation that will change over time as I gain more experience and training."

Hypothesis Testing   In many situations, subjectivity does not have to remain. In such instances, hypothesis testing can be conducted. Hypothesis testing involves setting up an experiment to test an interpretation or anticipation of an event to provide more definitive information. In the ongoing example, the student therapist could poll other student therapists and learn about dropout rates in their caseloads. Sometimes this figure can come from the director of the clinic or a supervisor (e.g., on average, 15% of patients drop out). This approach would allow the student therapist to determine the accuracy of her thought (if she has twice as many dropouts as others, perhaps there is a problem, and she should move to a problem-solving mode; if she has the same number or fewer dropouts, her concern is a result of her negative thought pattern). Rather than telling patients how to test the hypothesis, the therapist should ask a series of questions to help the patient uncover the answer on his or her own (guided discovery). Hypothesis testing teaches the patient a process for testing one's thinking pattern, rather than relying on the initial appraisal as fact or as purely subjective.

Problem Solving   More often than not, when depressed patients subject their automatic thoughts to logical principles and empiric testing, they find that their hypotheses are either false or greatly exaggerated. However, sometimes a patient's hypotheses are correct, and the patient is identifying a real problem that requires a solution. Under such circumstances, the therapist should help the patient see his or her task as problem solving. The pessimistic thinking style that accompanies depression interferes with patients' abilities to solve problems—depressed patients tend to view situations as overwhelming and hopeless. By elaborating the problem-solving process, the therapist provides the patient with a strategy to offset this pessimistic thinking style. The following steps are crucial in this process:

1. *Brainstorming solutions.* This involves generating as many solutions as possible, without stopping to evaluate them. Encourage the patient to be creative and thorough.
2. *Looking at the pros and cons of the solutions.* Have the patient list the advantages and disadvantages of each proposed solution.
3. *Choosing the best solution and carrying it out.* Have the patient consider the importance of the various pros and cons and, based on that analysis, choose the solution that seems best and take concrete steps to carry it out.

Continuing with the student therapist example, if her dropout rate was considerably greater than others' in that setting (e.g., her dropout rate was 35% compared with an average of 15%) and no alternative explanations existed (e.g., she tended to take on patients who had a higher likelihood of dropping out, such as adolescents), then the next step would be to move into a problem-solving mode rather than focus on herself as an eternally lousy therapist and give up. The patient and the therapist would brainstorm solutions (e.g., get additional supervision, videotape sessions to get a more precise picture of what is going on, ask for feedback from patients who dropped out), review the pros and cons of each possible solution, and then choose the best one and carry it out to resolve the problem. For example, the chosen solution might be to tape sessions so that the student's supervisor can get a better sense of what may be causing the problem and ultimately work to correct it.

Behavioral Techniques

Lewinsohn (1975) advanced the social learning theory of depression, which posits that depression is a result of changes in reinforcement from environmental interactions. Routes to depression include a loss of positive outcomes (e.g., being complimented by one's employer for a job well done) and an increase in negative outcomes (e.g., being criticized by one's spouse). In depression, a vicious cycle ensues, wherein increased feelings of depression lead to decreased activity, resulting in even less reinforcement, which causes increased depression, and so on (Lewinsohn et al. 1986). This behavioral model posits multiple pathways to depression. First, interactions that have been a source of positive outcomes in the past may no longer be available. For example, the death of a close friend or family member precludes positive interactions from that source, retirement may preclude engagement in a previously satisfying work activity, or an injury may prevent involvement in an enjoyable fitness activity. Second, one may lack the skills needed to achieve positive outcomes in interactions. For example, a lack of assertiveness may result in frequent negative events at work whereby one is continually taken advantage of; a lack of social skills may result in one being alone frequently; or one may set unattainably high standards for performance at work, leading to continuous dissatisfaction. The following sections present a brief overview of the various behavioral strategies used to overcome depression. See Lewinsohn et al. (1986) and Klosko and Sanderson (1999) for more detailed reviews.

Scheduling Pleasant Activities

Whether a cause or a consequence of depression, patients invariably have withdrawn from pleasurable activities. Thus, systematically scheduling and participating in pleasurable events is one way to circumvent the depressive spiral described earlier in this chapter. First, the therapist assists the patient in identifying activities he or she has found pleasant in the past (e.g., going to lunch with a good friend, bicycle riding in the park). Because the patient's recollection is likely to be clouded by depression, a structured assessment of activities (e.g., the Pleasant Events Schedule [Lewinsohn et al. 1986]) is more likely to result in useful information than is merely asking the patient to recall what he or she found enjoyable in the past. It is particularly important to include activities from the following three categories, which have particularly strong connections to mood: positive social interactions (e.g., spending time with a good friend), activities that make one feel useful (e.g., caring for one's child, doing a job well), and activities that are intrinsically pleasant (e.g., a meal at one's favorite restaurant, listening to music) (Lewinsohn et al. 1986). After the events are identified, the therapist and the patient work out a schedule to reintroduce the activities into the patient's life by elaborating specific goals (e.g., goal for the week is to call your good friend and have dinner at one of your favorite restaurants). Because the patient's depressed mood will interfere with his or her ability to anticipate and evaluate positive events, it will be important to focus the patient ahead of time on what was positive about the situation in the past in order to sensitize the patient's information processing. In addition, it is essential to have the patient monitor his or her mood before, during, and after the event to demonstrate the positive effect the event has on the patient's mood, even if the effect is temporary.

Improving Interpersonal Skills

Daily life involves continual social interactions. Depending on the nature of the interactions, it is normal for both positive and negative moods to stem from these interactions. Social learning theory posits that depressed patients may have interpersonal skills deficits that interfere with their ability to gain positive social reinforcement. Two specific areas have received considerable attention in reducing depression: assertiveness training and social skills training (Lewinsohn et al. 1986). Training in these skills allows patients to be more socially effective, ultimately generating feelings of mastery and positive affect, thereby reducing depression. The techniques are quite elaborate and are not described here. Interested readers should consult Klosko and Sanderson (1999) or Lewinsohn et al. (1986) for a detailed overview.

Managing Anxiety and Tension

Patients with depression frequently experience general tension and anxious overarousal. Symptoms such as anxiety, insomnia, and agitation are characteristic of depression and frequently contribute to it. For example, agitation may result in an individual's inability to enjoy a pleasurable event, thus decreasing reinforcement. Insomnia may lead to daytime fatigue and ineffective performance at work. As a result, patients may need to be given physical control strategies to decrease unpleasant overarousal associated with anxiety. Progressive muscle relaxation training is an effective strategy to lower overall arousal levels (Bernstein and Borkovec 1973). Patients who are experiencing anxiety and tension may find that progressive muscle relaxation several times per day reduces overarousal. However, because as many as 50% of patients with depression have a comorbid anxiety disorder (e.g., panic disorder, obsessive-compulsive disorder) (Sanderson et al. 1990), in such cases a specific anxiety disorder–focused intervention may be required to directly address the comorbid syndrome.

Efficacy of Cognitive-Behavioral Therapy for Depression

Since cognitive therapy was formulated by A. T. Beck (1963), numerous studies have demonstrated the efficacy of cognitive therapy for depression. The first landmark study, conducted by Rush et al. (1977), demonstrated that cognitive therapy was more effective than tricyclic antidepressant therapy in patients with clinical depression. In contrast to the findings of previous outcome research that psychotherapies were no more effective than pill placebos and were less effective than antidepressant medications, Rush et al. (1977) were the first to show that a psychosocial treatment was superior to pharmacotherapy in the treatment of depression (Hollon et al. 1991). Furthermore, a follow-up study conducted 12 months after treatment showed that relapse rates were lower among patients who received cognitive therapy (39%) than in those who received antidepressant medication (65%), although this difference did not reach statistical significance (Kovacs et al. 1981).

In the two decades since the initial trial, many controlled trials have been undertaken to replicate these findings. Although many experts now believe that the Rush et al. (1977) study was sufficiently flawed to negate study findings (Hollon et al. 1991), many qualitative and quantitative reviews now conclude that cognitive therapy 1) effectively treats depression, 2) is at least comparable if not superior to medication treatment, and 3) may result in lower rates of relapse in comparison with medication treatments (Dobson 1989; Hollon 1981; Hollon and Beck 1986; Hollon and Najavits 1988; Hollon et al. 1991; Miller and Berman 1983). As a result, cognitive therapy has gained widespread acceptance as a first-line treatment for depression, and CBT is one of only two psychotherapies included in the guidelines for the treatment of depression published by the Agency for Health Care and Policy Research (AHCPR; Depression Guidelines Panel 1993).

However, in the midst of what many have termed a golden age of cognitive therapy, a debate has arisen about the efficacy of cognitive therapy as a treatment for depression. This debate stems in part from the concerns of some researchers regarding the methodologic sufficiency of the studies showing an advantage of cognitive therapy and in large part from the highly visible results of the National Institute of Mental Health Treatment of Depression Collaborative Research Program (TD-CRP) study, which concluded that CBT was not effective in the treatment of severe depression (Elkin et al. 1989). Although the study is flawed in many respects, this single study is threatening to stem the tide in favor of cognitive therapy as a treatment for depression. In the sections that follow, we examine the current state of research on cognitive therapy for depression, present issues of methodologic concern on both sides of the debate, and explore areas of future study. To avoid redundancy with prior reviews of individual studies, our review is focused primarily on meta-analytic studies.

Is Short-Term Cognitive Therapy Effective?

A Review of Meta-Analyses

Several meta-analyses have been conducted to determine the efficacy of CBT in relation to no treatment, pharmacotherapy, and other psychotherapies as well as the relative efficacy of pure cognitive and behavioral components (i.e., cognitive therapy and behavioral therapy). The meta-analyses themselves are not devoid of flaws and vary widely with regard to the number and methodologic stringency of studies reviewed, the size and diagnostic homogeneity of study samples, and the outcome measures and methodology used to conduct the meta-analyses.

In an early meta-analysis using data from Smith et al. (1980), Andrews and Harvey (1981) demonstrated that CBT had comparably larger mean effect sizes ($d = 0.97$) than did placebo controls ($d = 0.55$), other psychotherapies ($d = 0.74$), and counseling ($d = 0.35$). However, the efficacy of CBT is difficult to evaluate, because many available studies on CBT were not included in the original Smith et al. (1980) meta-analysis. Furthermore, the specific efficacy of CBT for depression is difficult to assess because the studies used in the meta-analysis involved patients who had a gamut of neurotic disorders (although most were depressed).

In a meta-analysis of 56 outcome studies, Steinbrueck et al. (1983) found evidence for a superiority of psychotherapy over no treatment and pharmacologic therapies in the treatment of depression but found no differences in efficacy between the different forms of psychotherapy (cognitive, behavioral, marital, and other). Similarly, Nietzel et al. (1987) reported only a nonsignificant trend for the superiority of cognitive treatments over other psychotherapies.

By contrast, a meta-analysis combining 48 studies concluded that CBT was significantly more effective than no treatment, that CBT had somewhat larger treatment effects than did other psychotherapies, and that cognitive therapy and behavioral therapy did not differ with regard to their relative efficacy in treating depression (Miller and Berman 1983). However, results from this meta-analysis must be interpreted with caution because only 10 of the 48 studies involved patients with clinical depression.

A similar flaw is evident in the meta-analysis conducted by Robinson et al. (1990), in which only 35% of the 58 studies involved patients who met formal criteria for a depressive disorder. Results of their analysis found that cognitive-behavioral therapies (CBT, cognitive therapy, or behavioral therapy) were more effective than other psychotherapies (Robinson et al. 1990). Effect sizes for these therapies ranged from 0.85 to 1.02, whereas the effect size for other psychotherapies was approximately 0.49.

Robinson et al. (1990) also found that CBT was more effective than pharmacotherapy and that CBT plus medication was no better than medication or CBT alone. Finally, CBT was found to be slightly more effective than either cognitive therapy or behavioral therapy alone, and cognitive therapy alone was slightly more effective than behavioral therapy alone. However, these findings are tempered by the fact that researcher allegiance was significantly correlated with outcome in the studies used in the meta-analysis. In fact, once researcher allegiance was taken into account, differences in efficacy among the different forms of therapy for depression disappeared.

In one of the better known meta-analyses, Dobson (1989) reviewed 28 studies that included patients with clinical depression only and found that cognitive therapy was clearly more effective than no-treatment or wait-list conditions ($d = -2.15$), other psychotherapies ($d = -0.54$), medication alone ($d = -0.53$), and behavioral therapy alone ($d = -0.46$). Using the BDI as a common measure across studies, Dobson (1989) found that the average cognitive therapy patient did better than 98% of patients in the no-treatment condition, 70% of patients receiving

psychotherapies or medication alone, and 67% of patients receiving behavioral therapy alone.

Dobson's results have been criticized on several accounts. Critics
have commented that Dobson's meta-analyses were drawn from a relatively small number of studies with small sample sizes, that some of the
studies included were not randomized, and that others (e.g., Rush et al.
1977) used less than optimal drug treatments (Glaoguen et al. 1998;
Hollon et al. 1991; Scott 1996). Critics also argued that Dobson's findings of such a clear superiority of cognitive therapy over other treatments may have been influenced by researcher allegiance (which
Dobson did not examine) and may have resulted from his use of the BDI
as the only outcome measure (Robinson et al. 1990). Robinson et al.
(1990) argued that because the BDI was not as widely used then as it is
now, many studies were excluded and, hence, Dobson's study may have
been unrepresentative.

In a reanalysis of the Dobson (1989) data, Gaffan et al. (1995) addressed some of the criticisms leveled against the Dobson study, particularly the issue of researcher allegiance. Using a larger sample (65
studies including Dobson's original 28), study investigators confirmed
the findings of the superiority of cognitive therapy over other treatments
but obtained smaller effect sizes than those found by Dobson. Gaffan
et al. (1995) found that approximately half of the difference observed
between cognitive therapy and other treatments in Dobson's study was
attributable to researcher allegiance. However, when they separately examined the 37 studies published since the Dobson meta-analysis, Gaffan et al. (1995) found that although outcome in these studies was not
correlated with researcher allegiance, the superiority of cognitive therapy over the wait-list control condition, other psychotherapy, and pharmacotherapy was still present, albeit with smaller effect sizes. Their
results also revealed that cognitive therapy plus medication performed
no better than cognitive therapy alone, although allegiance ratings were
much higher for cognitive therapy alone compared with cognitive therapy plus medication.

Two more recent meta-analyses are of particular note because both
included the multisite TDCRP study (Elkin et al. 1989) in their analyses and used more stringent selection criteria than did prior studies. A
meta-analysis conducted by the AHCPR (Depression Guideline Panel

1993) combined data from 22 randomized controlled trials conducted on the treatment of depression. Certain pivotal studies were not included in this meta-analysis because they did not meet the conservative inclusion criteria set by the panel. For example, the only studies used were those in which treatment outcome was reported categorically and intent-to-treat samples could be identified. Using the confidence profile method, the overall efficacy of cognitive therapy alone was found to be 46.6%; for adult outpatients, the efficacy was 46.9%; and for geriatric outpatients, it was 51.3%. cognitive therapy was 30% more effective than the wait-list control condition, 15% more effective than pharmacotherapy, and 9% more effective than pill placebo with clinical management. cognitive therapy alone did not differ in efficacy from other empirically supported psychotherapies as a whole. Individual comparison revealed that cognitive therapy alone (46.6%) did not differ from behavioral therapy alone (55.3%) or interpersonal therapy (IPT) (52.3%) but had higher overall efficacy rates than did brief dynamic therapy (34.8%).

A meta-analysis by Glaoguen et al. (1998) combined 48 controlled trials conducted on depressed outpatients from 1977 to 1996, excluding 30 trials for methodologic reasons. Confirming Dobson's results, Glaoguen et al. (1998) found that cognitive therapy was significantly better than the wait-list control condition, antidepressant medication, and a group of miscellaneous therapies. However, in contrast to Dobson's finding of a clear superiority of cognitive therapy over behavioral therapy, Glaoguen's group found that cognitive therapy was comparable with behavioral therapy alone.

Summary

All meta-analyses found evidence of a clear superiority of cognitive therapy over no-treatment or wait-list control conditions. Six of nine studies found significantly greater treatment effects for cognitive therapy than for other psychotherapies. Of the six studies directly comparing cognitive and behavioral therapies, cognitive therapy outperformed behavioral therapy in three studies and was comparable with behavioral therapy in the other three studies. Finally, cognitive therapy outperformed medication in all five meta-analyses comparing the two treatment modalities.

Taken as a whole, these meta-analyses provide substantial evidence that CBT is an effective treatment for depression, although some findings are tempered when factors such as researcher allegiance are taken into account. As study designs and methodologies become more sophisticated, additional meta-analyses will be necessary to confirm these findings.

Is Cognitive Therapy Effective in Preventing Relapse or Recurrence?

The high degree of relapse (i.e., a continuation of the index episode before recovery) or recurrence (i.e., a new episode after recovery) in depression has made the issue of symptom maintenance a critical one for both psychotherapy and pharmacotherapy researchers. Without additional treatment, the range of relapse appears to vary between 50% and 80% within the first year after recovery from depression (Keller et al. 1982; Lobel and Hirschfeld 1985). Medication studies estimate that symptom relapse or recurrence tends to occur within 6–24 months after treatment is discontinued, findings that have led to a recent development of maintenance treatment strategies for depressed patients with recurrent episodes (Jarrett et al. 1998). Preliminary results show that maintenance-phase treatment with medications such as fluoxetine and imipramine appear to significantly lower the rate of symptom relapse or recurrence in depression (Fava and Kaji 1994; Frank et al. 1990; Kupfer 1992; Montgomery et al. 1988).

CBT has generally been associated with a lower rate of relapse than that found in patients taking medication (see Hollon et al. 1991 for a review). Although methodologies vary significantly between studies, figures suggest that 0%–50% of patients exhibit symptom relapse or recurrence within 1–2 years of discontinuing CBT (Jarrett et al. 1998). Six of the nine meta-analyses reported earlier in this chapter incorporated follow-up data and generally demonstrated that the effects of CBT appear to be maintained over time. Andrews and Harvey (1981) found that the improvement was stable over time for all psychotherapy groups including CBT, with a gradual decline occurring after the first year at an estimated rate of 0.2 effect size units per annum. Similarly, Nietzel et al. (1987) reported that treatment effects were maintained at follow-up (only 70% of studies performed follow-up evaluations). Results from the meta-analysis conducted by Miller and Berman (1983) also demonstrated that effect sizes were stable at follow-up (mean follow-up = 9.5 weeks), leading to the conclusion that the relative efficacy of CBT at posttreatment appeared to predict relative efficacy at follow-up. For the nine studies that conducted follow-up evaluations in the Robinson et al. (1990) meta-analysis, posttreatment and follow-up effect sizes were virtually identical, suggesting that treatment effects were durable over time.

A similar trend was observed in the most recent meta-analyses. In the AHCPR study (Depression Guideline Panel 1993), 7 of the 22 studies incorporated follow-up evaluations and revealed that, compared with pharmacotherapy, cognitive therapy was associated with fewer depressive symptoms and a lower rate of relapse. Three of the seven studies also revealed that patients receiving cognitive therapycognitive therapy had fewer depressive symptoms than did wait-list control subjects at follow-up. Finally, in the Gloaguen et al. (1998) meta-analysis, cognitive therapy was associated with a lower relapse rate as compared with antidepressant treatments.

Despite these findings, the prophylactic effects of CBT have yet to be fully established, due in large part to the difficulty in interpreting results from follow-up studies. Methodologic problems generally observed in such studies include brief follow-up periods; the inclusion of acute nonresponders in follow-up; naturalistic versus controlled follow-up; lack of control subjects; and variabilities in the composition of samples followed, in the timing and nature of assessment, and in defining relapse or recurrence (Depression Guideline Panel 1993; Hollon et al. 1991). The prophylactic value of CBT (and other treatments for depression) has also come into further question following the results of the TDCRP study. In the 18-month naturalistic follow-up of patients receiving treatment in the TDCRP study, all four treatments (CBT, IPT, imipramine, and placebo plus clinical management) were associated with similarly high rates of relapse (Shea et al. 1992). Analyses of the intent-to-treat sample revealed that only 15%–28% of patients did not have major depression or require further treatment at the 18-month follow-up.

Methodologic problems and the results of the TDCRP study notwithstanding, most studies have typically found that CBT provides protection against symptom relapse or recurrence and that it may have a distinct advantage over pharmacotherapy in this respect (Hollon et al. 1991). Nevertheless, relapse or reoccurrence is still a significant issue, and one that has led to a recent focus on developing maintenance strategies for patients who experience recurrent episodes of depression (Jarrett et al. 1998). Two early trials by Blackburn and colleagues examined in treatment responders the preventive effect of a continuation or maintenance phase with cognitive therapy, pharmacotherapy, or a combined treatment. In the first study, Blackburn et al. (1986) demonstrated that acute treatment responders who were provided with maintenance treatment every 6 weeks for an additional 6 months with cognitive therapy or cognitive therapy plus medications had significantly lower rates of relapse (6% and 0%) than did patients who were given maintenance treatment with pharmacotherapy alone (30%). At the 24-month follow-up, patients receiving maintenance cognitive therapy and cognitive therapy plus medication were significantly less likely (23% and 21%, respectively) to have a recurrence than were patients receiving medication alone (78%). In the second study, Blackburn and Moore (1997) examined patients with recurrent depression who received CBT in the short- and long-term phases of treatment, medication in the short- and long-term phases, or medication in the short-term phase and CBT in the long-term phase. Follow-up results conducted at 24 months showed comparable relapse and recurrence rates for all three groups (24%–36%).

Two pilot studies by Jarrett et al. (1998) also shed light on the prophylactic value of cognitive therapy. These investigators evaluated the rates of relapse or recurrence in patients who received an acute trial of cognitive therapy. Treatment responders in the first study were merely given follow-up assessments on a monthly basis, whereas responders in the second study were given cognitive therapy for an additional 10 sessions over a period of 8 months. Relapse rates in the first study were as follows: 40% at 6 months, 45% at 8 months, 50% at 12 months, 67% at 18 months, and 74% at 24 months. By contrast, symptom relapse occurred at a rate of 20% at the 6- and 8-month follow-ups, 27% at 12 months, and 36% at 18 and 24 months. Based on these data, Jarrett et al. (1998) concluded tentatively that extending acute cognitive therapy may be successful in achieving symptom maintenance but they also explored other factors that could have influenced their findings, such as patient gender and therapist competence.

Fava et al. (1998) examined 40 patients who had recurrent depression that had been treated successfully with medications. They randomly assigned the patients to either CBT or clinical management over the next 20 weeks. Antidepressant treatment was slowly tapered and discontinued over this period. Results demonstrated that after drug therapy was discontinued, patients who received CBT were less likely to have residual symptoms than were those receiving clinical management alone. CBT was also associated with significantly lower rates of relapse (25%) as compared with clinical management (80%) at the 2-year follow-up, leading the investigators to conclude that not only is CBT useful in preventing symptom relapse but that an alleviation of residual symptoms via CBT may reduce the risk of relapse in depressed patients.

Summary

Most studies have found that CBT provides protection against symptom relapse or recurrence and may result in lower rates of relapse as compared with pharmacotherapy. Six of the nine meta-analyses presented here incorporated follow-up data and demonstrated that the effects of CBT appear to be stable over time. Among the meta-analyses that compared relapse rates between CBT and medication, CBT appears to have a distinct advantage. However, methodologic problems inherent in follow-up studies make results difficult to interpret. Despite the relatively high maintenance rates, relapse or recurrence is still a significant problem. Recent studies indicate that adding maintenance-phase treatment with CBT may lead to lower rates of symptom relapse or recurrence.

So Why is the Jury Still Out?

Cognitive therapy is more extensively researched than any other psychotherapy for the treatment of unipolar depression, and the breadth of support presented earlier in this chapter appears truly impressive. So why is the jury still out (Jacobson and Hollon 1996a)? Why is there a growing debate about the efficacy of CBT as a first-line treatment for severe depression? These concerns arise in large part from the highly visible results of the TDCRP study, which found that CBT was no more effective than a pill placebo and somewhat less effective than imipramine in the treatment of severe depression (Elkin et al. 1989). As a result, the treatment guidelines prepared by the American Psychiatric

Association and by the AHCPR assert that CBT may be no more effective than a pill placebo in the treatment of severe depression (Depression Guidelines Panel 1993). Although CBT did not differ from other active treatments in treating depression in the full sample of TDCRP study patients, the less-than-impressive performance of CBT in the subsample of patients with severe depression has sparked questions about the role of CBT as an acute treatment for depression per se.

Many investigators now suggest that the TDCRP study was flawed in several important respects. For example, Klein (1996) suggested that the study chose too stringent a level of significance, which led the investigators to understate the superiority of pharmacotherapy over psychotherapy in the subsample of patients with severe depression. Jacobson and Hollon (1996a, 1996b) suggested that the finding within the subsample of patients with severe depression is suspect because it was not robust across the three different sites (CBT was comparable with imipramine at one site, whereas IPT was comparable with imipramine at another site) and because this finding is not consistent with findings from previous studies. Furthermore, Jacobson and Hollon (1996a, 1996b) also point out that there were no differences in the active treatments at the 18-month follow-up, regardless of level of severity. Finally, questions have been raised about allegiance effects and possible differences in the quality of CBT offered at the three different sites, which if confirmed could account for the relatively poor showing of CBT in the study (Jacobson and Hollon 1996a, 1996b).

What is indeed surprising is that a single study, albeit an important one, is shaping current treatment guidelines when none of the multitude of studies comparing drugs with CBT has suggested even a remote advantage of drugs over CBT (see Hollon et al. 1991 for a review). Advocates of CBT suggest that the TDCRP study has gained widespread acceptance because it "corresponds so closely to preconceived notions held by many in the psychiatric community" (Jacobson and Hollon 1996a, p. 74). In contrast, advocates of pharmacotherapy agree that the results of the TDCRP study need to be replicated but argue that its importance is underscored because it is one the few methodologically adequate studies comparing psychotherapy with drugs (Klein 1996).

According to Klein (1996), all previous studies comparing CBT with drugs are methodologically flawed and hence invalid because none included a pill placebo comparison. Unless a pill placebo control is included in studies comparing drugs with psychotherapy, there would be no way of ensuring that pharmacotherapy was adequately implemented and that the study sample was drug responsive (Klein 1996). Jacobson and Hollon (1996a, 1996b) agree that a pill placebo control would strengthen the interpretability of drug–psychotherapy studies, both by increasing the likelihood that treatment differences would be discerned and, in the event that active treatments did not differ, by determining if drugs and psychotherapy were equally effective or ineffective. However, they disagree that the absence of a pill placebo arm nullifies previous findings and assert that studies must independently assess the representativeness of the study sample and the quality of the pharmacotherapy provided. Furthermore, they maintain that it is still important to know the relative efficacy of various treatments for samples regardless of whether they are drug responsive. Other advocates of CBT accuse Klein of circular reasoning by asserting, among other things, that testing for drug responsiveness is a goal of the study (treatment outcome) and not a prestudy requirement (i.e., whether or not the sample is drug responsive) (McNally 1993).

Conclusion Regarding the Empiric Status of Cognitive Therapy

Based on results from the meta-analyses reviewed in this chapter, we suggest that short-term CBT and cognitive therapy alone are effective in the treatment of clinical depression, and in the absence of studies replicating the TDCRP findings of its lesser efficacy among patients with severe depression, we conclude that CBT is still a viable treatment for severe depression. Based on results from the various meta-analyses reviewed here, we also conclude that CBT is more effective than no-treatment and wait-list control conditions and also more effective than other psychotherapies; is at least comparable with antidepressant medications; and has significant evidence attesting to its prophylactic value.

With regard to the question of whether cognitive therapy alone is superior to behavioral therapy or vice versa, findings are muddier. Some meta-analyses find evidence of a clear superiority of cognitive therapy over behavioral therapy, whereas others show no difference between the

two components. Jacobson et al. (1996) found that the comprehensive
CBT treatment combining cognitive and behavioral components did
no better than the cognitive and behavioral components separately.
Furthermore, they showed that the two components were just as effective as the comprehensive treatment in altering negative thinking and
dysfunctional attributional styles, suggesting that both conditions may
arrive at a similar result using different methods.

Future Directions

Although the breadth of support for CBT is impressive, future research
is still necessary to address the concerns raised in this chapter. Additional multicenter studies that compare medications with different forms of
psychotherapy are still needed to confirm the efficacy of short-term
CBT as a treatment for depression. However, for findings to be valid,
active treatments must be administered by clinicians adequately trained
in the various approaches and issues of researcher allegiance and site
differences must be addressed appropriately. Furthermore, whether or
not both sides agree that the absence of a pill placebo control nullifies
prior comparisons between drugs and psychotherapy, it appears that
adding pill placebo controls to future drug–psychotherapy studies is im-
perative, not merely to enhance treatment interpretability but also to address criticisms from pharmacotherapy advocates who will most likely
nullify studies that do not include such controls.

Another control condition that may enhance the interpretation of
treatment outcome data is the placebo plus CBT combination. Findings from the recent multisite study on panic disorder demonstrate that
although combined treatments were more effective than CBT alone in
certain key comparisons, the combined imipramine plus CBT control
condition was no better than the combined placebo plus CBT condition (Barlow 1998). Without such a control, investigators would have
erroneously concluded that CBT plus medication was more effective
than CBT alone for the treatment of panic disorder. Based on these findings, we recommend that future outcome trials on depression include
both a pill placebo alone and a pill placebo plus CBT control condition
to enhance the interpretation of results.

To enhance treatment effects, studies must also examine the relative efficacy of CBT in depressive subtypes that may have characteristics associated with poorer outcome. For example, patients with atypical depression, a new subtype of the mood disorders in DSM-IV (American Psychiatric Association 1994), are less responsive to tricyclic antidepressants than patients with typical depression (Asnis et al. 1995; McGinn et al. 1996). Thus, CBT for atypical depression may need to be modified to address the unique symptoms of this disorder (McGinn et al. 1998). Along the same lines, preliminary evidence indicates that patients with personality disorders may be less responsive to short-term CBT than those without these disorders and that optimal treatment can be accomplished for these patients only if the treatment is modified to address the personality disorders as well (see McGinn et al. 1995 for review). Identifying specific populations who do not respond as well to short-term CBT will lead to the elucidation of factors that must be modified to provide more appropriate treatment.

Finally, future research studies need to evaluate the effectiveness of CBT for depression outside of clinical research centers. The demonstration of treatment efficacy in controlled research environments is only the first step in treatment research. After a positive therapeutic effect has been demonstrated conclusively, generalizability becomes of paramount importance. With regard to CBT for depression, it seems fair to conclude from the data presented in this chapter that CBT is an effective treatment in clinical research settings, but data are not available on the efficacy of CBT for depression when delivered in nonresearch clinical settings to a diverse group of patients. (This situation is not unique to CBT; it applies to other empirically supported treatments such as pharmacologic approaches.) Without data, one must be cautious in generalizing the results from research settings to typical clinical settings because several factors might reduce the efficacy of this treatment (Wolfe 1994). For example, compared with the average clinician, clinicians in research settings are likely to possess greater expertise in the administration of a particular treatment developed in that setting. Thus, because clinician competence may be an important factor for success, one would expect a less favorable outcome in uncontrolled settings where the quality of treatment may not be as good. Although caution may be warranted until data are generated specifically on CBT for depression, it is reassuring to note that data are beginning to appear that support the effectiveness of evidence-based treatments outside of controlled research environments (e.g., Sanderson et al. 1998), and a recent meta-analysis of psychotherapy studies found that the effect sizes of psychotherapy in clinically representative settings are slightly lower (approximately 10%) but comparable with those obtained in clinical research settings (Shadish et al. 1997).

References

Abramson LY, Metalsky GI, Alloy LB: Hopelessness depression: a theory based subtype of depression. Psychol Rev 96:358–372, 1989

American Psychiatric Association: Diagnostic and Statistical Manual of Mental Disorders, 4th Edition. Washington, DC, American Psychiatric Association, 1994

Andrews G, Harvey R: Does psychotherapy benefit neurotic patients? Arch Gen Psychiatry 38:1203–1208, 1981

Asnis GM, McGinn LK, Sanderson WC: Atypical depression: clinical aspects and noradrenergic function. Am J Psychiatry 152:31–36, 1995

Barlow DH (chair): Results from the multi-center clinical trial on the treatment of panic disorder: cognitive behavior treatment versus imipramine versus their combination. Symposium presented at the annual convention of the Association for the Advancement of Behavior Therapy, Washington, DC, November 1998

Beck AT: Thinking and depression: 1. idiosyncratic content and cognitive distortions. Arch Gen Psychiatry 9:324–333, 1963

Beck AT: Cognitive therapy of depression: new perspectives, in Treatment of Depression: Old Controversies and New Approaches. Edited by Clayton PJ, Barrett JE. New York, Raven,1983, pp 265–284

Beck AT, Rush AJ, Shaw B, et al: Cognitive Therapy of Depression. New York, Guilford, 1979

Beck AT, Steer RA, Garbin MG: Psychometric properties of the Beck Depression Inventory: twenty-five years later. Clin Psychol Rev 8:77–100, 1988

Beck JS: Cognitive Therapy: Basics and Beyond. New York, Guilford, 1995

Bernstein DA, Borkovec TD: Progressive Relaxation Training. Champaign, IL, Research Press, 1973

Blackburn IM, Moore RG: Controlled acute and follow-up trial of cognitive therapy and pharmacotherapy in out-patients with recurrent depression. Br J Psychiatry 171:328–334, 1997

Blackburn IM, Eunson KM, Bishop S: A two-year naturalistic follow-up of depressed patients treated with cognitive therapy, pharmacotherapy, and a combination of both. J Affect Disord 10:67–75, 1986

Burns DD: Feeling Good. New York, New American Library, 1980

Depression Guideline Panel: Clinical Practice Guideline, Number 5. Depression in Primary Care, Volume 2: Treatment of Major Depression. Rockville, MD, U.S. Department of Health and Human Services, Public Health Service, Agency for Health Care Policy and Research. AHCPR Publication No. 93-0551, 1993

Dobson K: A meta-analysis of the efficacy of cognitive therapy for depression. J Consult Clin Psychol 57:414–419, 1989

Elkin I, Shea T, Watkins J, et al: National Institute of Mental Health Depression Collaborative Treatment Program. Arch Gen Psychiatry 46:971–982, 1989

Fava M, Kaji J: Continuation and maintenance treatments of major depressive disorder. Psychiatry Ann 24:281–290, 1994

Fava GA, Rafanelli C, Grandi S, et al: Prevention of recurrent depression with cognitive behavior therapy: preliminary findings. Arch Gen Psychiatry 55:816–820, 1998

Frank E, Kupfer DJ, Perel JM, et al: Three year outcomes for maintenance therapies in recurrent depression. Arch Gen Psychiatry 47:1093–1099, 1990

Gaffan EA, Tsaousis I, Kemp-Wheeler SM: Researcher allegiance and meta-analysis: the case of cognitive therapy for depression. J Consult Clin Psychol 63:966–980, 1995

Glaoguen V, Cottraux J, Cucherat M, et al: A meta-analysis of the effects of cognitive therapy in depressed patients. J Affect Disord 49:59–72, 1998

Hollon SD: Comparisons and combinations with alternative approaches, in Behavior Therapy for Depression. Edited by Rehm LP. New York, Academic Press, 1981, pp 33–71

Hollon SD, Beck AT: Cognitive and cognitive-behavioral therapies, in The Handbook of Psychotherapy and Behavior Change: An Empirical Analysis, 2nd Edition. Edited by Garlfield SL, Bergin AE. New York, Wiley, 1986, pp 443–482

Hollon SD, Najavits L: Review of empirical studies on cognitive therapy. American Psychiatric Press Review of Psychiatry, Vol 7. Edited by Frances AJ, Hales RE. Washington, DC, American Psychiatric Press, 1988, pp 643–666

Hollon SD, Shelton RC, Loosen PT: Cognitive therapy and pharmacotherapy for depression. J Consult Clin Psychol 59:88–99, 1991

Jacobson NS, Hollon SD: Cognitive-behavior therapy versus pharmacotherapy: now that the jury's returned its verdict, it's time to present the rest of the evidence. J Consult Clin Psychol 64:74–80, 1996a

Jacobson NS, Hollon, SD: Prospects for future comparisons between drugs and psychotherapy: lessons from the CBT-versus-pharmacotherapy exchange. J Consult Clin Psychol 64:104–108, 1996b

Jacobson NS, Follette WC, Revenstorf D: Psychotherapy outcome research: methods for reporting variability and evaluating clinical significance. Behavior Therapy 15:336–352, 1984

Jacobson NS, Dobson KS, Truax PA: A component analysis of cognitive behavioral treatment for depression. J Consult Clin Psychol 64:295–304, 1996

Jarrett RB, Basco MR, Risser R: Is there a role for continuation phase cognitive therapy for depressed outpatients. J Consult Clin Psychol 66:1036–1040, 1998

Keller MB, Shapiro RW, Lavori P: Relapse in major depressive disorder: analysis with the life table. Arch Gen Psychiatry 39:911–915, 1982

Klein DF: Preventing hung juries about therapy studies. J Consult Clin Psychol 64:81–87, 1996

Klosko JS, Sanderson WC: Depression: Clinical Application of Empirically Supported Psychotherapy. Northvale, NJ, Jason Aronson, 1999

Kovacs M, Rush AJ, Beck AT, et al: Depressed outpatients treated with cognitive therapy or pharmacotherapy. Arch Gen Psychiatry 38:33–39, 1981

Kupfer DJ: Maintenance treatment in recurrent depression. Br J Psychiatry 161:309–316, 1992

Lewinsohn PM: The behavioral study and treatment of depression, in Progress in Behavior Modification. Edited by Hersen M, Eisler RM. New York, Academic Press, 1975, pp 19–64

Lewinsohn PM, Munoz R, Youngren M, et al: Control Your Depression. New York, Fireside, 1986

Lobel B, Hirschfeld RMA: Depression: what we know (DHHS Publ No ADM-85-1318). Rockville, MD, U.S. Department of Health and Human Services, 1985

McGinn LK, Asnis GM, Rubinson E: Clinical and biological validation of atypical depression. Psychiatry Res 60:191–198, 1996

McGinn LK, Young JE, Sanderson WC: When and how to do longer-term therapy...without feeling guilty. Cogn Behav Pract 2:187–212, 1995

McGinn LK, Ortiz C, Sanderson WC, et al: Prevalence and implications of Axis II disorders in patients with atypical depression. Paper presented at the annual convention of the Association for the Advancement of Behavior Therapy, Washington, DC, November 1998

McNally RJ: Methodological controversies in the treatment of panic disorder. J Consult Clin Psychol 64:88–91, 1993

Miller RC, Berman JS: The efficacy of cognitive behavior therapies: a quantitative review of research evidence. Psychol Bull 94:39–53, 1983

Montgomery SA, Dufor H, Brion S, et al: The prophylactic efficacy of fluoxetine in unipolar depression. Br J Psychiatry 153:69–76, 1988

Nietzel MT, Russell RL, Hemmings KA, et al: Clinical significance of psychotherapy for unipolar depression: a meta-analytic approach to social comparison. J Consult Clin Psychol 40:288–294, 1987

Robinson L, Berman J, Neimeyer R: Psychotherapy for the treatment of depression: a comprehensive review of controlled outcome research. Psychol Bull 108:30–49, 1990

Rush A, Beck AT, Kovacs M, et al: Comparative efficacy of cognitive therapy and imipramine in the treatment of depressed patients. Cognitive Therapy Res 1:17–37, 1977

Sanderson WC, Beck AT, Beck J: Syndrome comorbidity in patients with major depression or dysthymia: prevalence and temporal relationships. Am J Psychiatry 147:1025–1028, 1990

Sanderson WC, Raue PJ, Wetzler S: The generalizability of cognitive behavior therapy for panic disorder. Journal of Cognitive Psychotherapy 12:323–331, 1998

Scott J: Cognitive therapy of affective disorders: a review. J Affect Disord 37:1–11, 1996

Seligman MEP: Helplessness: On Depression, Development, and Death. San Francisco, CA, WH Freeman, 1975

Seligman MEP, Abramson LY, Semmel A, et al: Depressive attributional style. J Abnorm Psychol 88:242–247, 1979

Shadish WR, Navarro AM, Crits-Christoph P, et al: Evidence that therapy works in clinically representative conditions. J Consult Clin Psychol 65:355–365, 1997

Shea T, Elkin I, Imber SD, et al: Course of depressive symptoms over follow-up: findings from the NIMH Treatment of Depression Collaborative Research Program. Arch Gen Psychiatry 49:782–787, 1992

Smith ML, Glass GV, Miller TI: The Benefits of Psychotherapy. Baltimore, MD, Johns Hopkins, 1980

Steinbruck SM, Maxwell SE, Howard GS, et al: A meta-analysis of psychotherapy and drug therapy in the treatment of unipolar depression with adults. J Consult Clin Psychol 51:856–863, 1983

Wolfe BE: Adapting psychotherapy outcome research to clinical reality. Journal of Psychotherapy Integration 4:160–166, 1994

CHAPTER 14

Learning the New Psychotherapies

John C. Markowitz, M.D.

Psychotherapy in the United States is changing in response to both scientific developments and economic coercion by managed care. Demand is growing for clinical training in these treatments, both in residency training programs and as continuing medical education. As psychotherapy has changed, training in psychotherapy has changed as well. To some degree, these educational changes reflect the nature of the newer treatment approaches themselves and the science behind them. Psychiatrists and other mental health professionals once used to learn a single psychotherapeutic outlook and intervention: psychodynamic psychotherapy. Indeed, until recently, many psychiatrists understood the term *therapy* as an accepted shorthand for psychodynamic psychotherapy. Such treatment was open ended and typically lengthy. The character or presentation of the patient might determine how supportive or expressive a form of psychodynamic psychotherapy the therapist provided, but the general approach applied regardless of inpatient or outpatient status and regardless of diagnosis.

Open-ended psychotherapy has been abbreviated by the accoun-

Preparation of this chapter was supported in part by grant MH-49635 from the National Institute of Mental Health and from a fund established in The New York Community Trust by DeWitt-Wallace.

tants of managed care. Meanwhile, time-limited psychotherapies, psychodynamic and otherwise, have been developed. A few of the latter have been tested and shown to have efficacy in the treatment of particular psychiatric disorders: cognitive-behavioral therapy (CBT), interpersonal psychotherapy (IPT), and behavioral therapy. To a lesser degree, time-limited psychodynamic psychotherapies have received empirical testing. In this chapter the term *new therapy* refers to focal time-limited psychotherapy in general, but particularly to IPT and to a lesser degree CBT, the preeminent evidence-based focal psychotherapies for depression. This discussion assumes that therapists in the future will develop skills in several psychotherapeutic modalities, choosing among them for particular patients on the basis of empirically derived differential therapeutics (Frances et al. 1984).

The New Therapies

The interpersonal and cognitive-behavioral therapies were developed in the 1960s and 1970s. Hence they are no longer so new, although it has taken time to test their efficacy for major depression, bulimia, and (in the case of CBT) anxiety disorders. Other diagnostically focused research is under way to explore the full range and limits of their acute and longer-term efficacy. Although differing in their theoretical underpinnings, structure, and specific interventions, both IPT and CBT focus on the here and now to help patients improve their coping skills to deal with their current problems. Both treatments are defined in manuals that emphasize certain techniques and proscribe others (Beck et al. 1979; Klerman et al. 1984; Weissman et al. 2000). Both are focal therapies, emphasizing particular patient problems and treatment techniques to solve those problems in order to address specific psychiatric syndromes.

For years, CBT has been disseminated through programs at numerous institutes, especially the Center for Cognitive Therapy in Philadelphia, PA. IPT until recently remained a research intervention, well studied but little practiced outside of research settings. In the past few years, however, increasing demand has encouraged IPT training programs at a few sites in the United States and Canada, in particular at Cornell University in New

York, the University of Pittsburgh, the University of Iowa in Iowa City, and the Clarke Institute in Toronto, Canada.

Cognitive-Behavioral Therapy

Developed by Aaron T. Beck and colleagues, cognitive therapy is based on the principle that automatic, irrational, depressive thoughts (cognitions) accompany and reinforce depressive mood (see Chapter 13). These negative thoughts constitute a cognitive triad of pessimism about the self ("I'm a loser"), the environment ("things are too overwhelming to face"), and the future ("nothing's ever going to get any better"). The automatic thoughts build on long-standing underlying cognitive schemas, or core beliefs, which themselves are negatively charged. Depressed patients believe these mood-congruent thoughts, which not only are painful in themselves but also tend to discourage positive behaviors. The resulting behavioral inhibition leads to further demoralization and a reinforcement of negative thoughts. For example, negative thoughts may lead to social isolation, which confirms the patient's belief that "No one cares about me" and induces further worsening of mood and social withdrawal. In similar fashion, patients with anxiety disorders have threatening cognitions about the dangerousness of their environment (e.g., fear of elevators) or bodily sensations (e.g., palpitations interpreted as an incipient heart attack).

Cognitive therapy helps patients to test the distorted nature of these automatic thoughts rather than take them for granted. If, using a dysfunctional thought record (DTR) grid, the patient can write down, examine, and weigh the evidence for and against these thoughts, he or she may cease to fully believe and act on them. Automatic thoughts can be superseded by more rational responses to situations. This process leads to better functioning and alleviates the depressive episode. Cognitive therapists also frequently combine behavioral interventions with this exploration of cognitions.

Interpersonal Psychotherapy

Developed by the late Gerald L. Klerman along with Myrna M. Weissman and colleagues, IPT defines major depression as a medical illness and helps patients see links between their mood states and life situations. IPT is based on the intuitively reasonable proposition that painful life events disturb mood and vice versa. This proposition is not a causal explanation of major depressive disorder, which is a multidetermined illness, but rather a pragmatic and optimistic treatment strategy. By understanding the relationship between depressed mood and ongoing life problems, the patient can change his or her life role and situation for the better. Improving one's life situation not only is a good thing in itself but also gives the patient a sense of control during a period of perceived helplessness and hopelessness and relieves the depressive episode.

Based on a carefully taken interpersonal history (the *interpersonal inventory*), the therapist offers the patient a formulation (Markowitz and Swartz 1997) linking the onset of the depressive episode to one of four interpersonal problem areas: grief (complicated bereavement), role dispute, role transition, or interpersonal deficits. With the patient's agreement, this formulation then becomes the focus of the remainder of treatment. Sessions focus on the patient's recent mood state, life events, and the relationship between them. When the patient succeeds in an interpersonal encounter, the therapist offers congratulations, reinforcing social skills. If an encounter goes poorly, the therapist and patient link situation to mood and explore alternative interpersonal approaches to handling the problematic situation. For example, if a patient reports a role dispute with her spouse, treatment might review marital arguments or frictions that arise and help the patient to appropriately assert her needs or express anger. Similar to CBT, IPT uses role playing in the office to help the patient prepare for interpersonal encounters and build social skills.

Although IPT and CBT differ and can be distinguished from each other on rating scales (Hill et al. 1992), they also overlap in numerous respects (Table 14–1). The overlap includes not only the so-called common factors of psychotherapy—for example, helping the patient to feel understood and express affect, providing a treatment ritual, offering optimism, and promoting success experiences (J Frank 1971)—but also interventions such as role play. Both approaches are oriented to the patient's present reality (the here and now), seek symptom relief rather than character change (albeit adaptations have been developed to treat personality disorder as well), are defined in manuals, and are circumscribed by time limits. In both approaches, the therapist must fulfill

TABLE **14–1.**   *Characteristics of cognitive-behavioral therapy and interpersonal psychotherapy*

Characteristic	Cognitive-behavioral therapy	Interpersonal psychotherapy
Treatment model	Cognitions affect mood	Medical model of illness; interpersonal situations affect mood
Treatment focus	Distorted cognitions (automatic thoughts)	Interpersonal situations
Techniques	Socratic method; identifying automatic thoughts and schemas	Interpersonal "cheerleading"; exploring options
Role playing	Yes	Yes
Homework	Yes	No
Sessions, *n*	12–20	12–16

similar tasks: to rapidly diagnose the target condition (e.g., major depression), formulate a focus for the time-limited treatment, and maintain that focus for the duration of the treatment.

The New Methods

Manuals

As noted earlier, psychotherapies that have been tested in clinical trials have been defined in manuals (Beck et al. 1979; Klerman et al. 1984; Weissman et al. 1999). These texts provide guidelines for what the therapy is and is not. Reading the manual is a prerequisite to learning the treatment, and the manual subsequently serves as a helpful reference to the therapist. Using a manual as a reference, some gifted therapists need little subsequent supervision. Others, however, can be distracted by the manual, concentrating so hard on technique ("Now what am I supposed to be doing?") or following the written outline of treatment so slavishly that the relationship with the patient may suffer. Supervision of early cases helps to balance the general development of new therapeutic skills with the particular needs of the patient.

Recording of Sessions

The basic training method for psychodynamic psychotherapy has relied on a parallel process of interpersonal distortion. Therapists take notes during or after a treatment session and present the case material to a supervisor. Psychodynamic psychotherapy focuses on the patient's psychodynamic distortions of reality, particularly transferential distortions of the patient's relationship with the therapist. The supervision focuses not only on an understanding of the patient's transferential distortions but also on the therapist's analogous presentation to the supervisor. The supervisor helps the therapist to recognize the patient's behaviors and underlying fantasies as well as to identify related countertransferential issues evoked in the therapist. The realities of the situation are often less important than the alterations of them that patient and therapist make. In this sense, function defines form: The potential inaccuracy of the therapist's report of sessions provides material for discussion. This tradition of secondhand report dates back to the early days of the Berlin Psychoanalytic Institute (Schuster et al. 1972).

This approach has problems. Taking notes during the session is anathema for many therapists and supervisors, because the recording process limits eye contact and potentially distracts both patient and therapist from their own interaction. The notepad may be used as a therapist's defense against affect in the session, dissipating the intensity of the encounter. Alternatively, notes taken after a session often are inaccurate. Although this inaccuracy may be useful as a projective Rorschach test of the therapist, selectively recording the therapist's best or worst moments, such distortion may also omit crucial material from the session. Many therapists have had the sensation of realizing on the way home from the office that the note just written about a patient missed the crux of a session. The new treatments employ new methods. A therapeutic alliance is crucial to the success of any psychotherapy, but treatments such as IPT and CBT are less purely focused on the patient–therapist interaction than is psychodynamic psychotherapy. The actual data—the content of the patient's report elicited by the focal therapy (i.e., in CBT, the patient's automatic thoughts; in IPT, the patient's interpersonal interactions)—are critically important. Thus, treatment records aim not to capture therapist distortions but to retain the true session data.

How is this done? CBT and behavioral therapists rely to a degree on written assessments. In CBT the central (though hardly the sole) such instrument is the DTR, on which the patient records automatic thoughts and the moods and situations in which those cognitions arise. CBT and IPT have tended to rely on videotaping or audiotaping of sessions for two reasons: 1) to allow the assessment of therapist adherence to the treatment approach in research studies and 2) to provide accurate data for supervision.[1] The advantages of taping are apparent: the audio- or videorecorder accurately preserves the data of the session (assuming, of course, that it is left on, that the tape does not run out, and that background noise does not render the record unintelligible). The supervisor and therapist can observe the therapeutic alliance and the raw data the patient reports in addition to how well the therapist has used treatment-specific techniques, avoided extrinsic techniques, and maintained the treatment focus. The supervisor and therapist can hear and (with videotape) see the behavior of the therapist and the patient. Treatment incidents are "caught like a fly in amber" (Chodoff 1972, p. 821), and the tape can be stopped to review key moments in sessions. Videotapes from a treatment library can be used to illustrate exemplary and proscribed interventions.

Taping sessions does have disadvantages. Recording instruments must be set up, which can be a cumbersome task. Therapists must obtain informed written consent from patients and review the requisite confidentiality issues. Many therapists are initially uncomfortable with the idea of taping sessions, particularly with videotaping (Alpert 1996; Friedmann et al. 1978). (We are more voyeurs than exhibitionists.) Early sessions may be distorted by therapist (or less often, patient) discomfort caused by the presence of the camera or tape recorder. Beginning therapists frequently attribute to their patients the reluctance to tape sessions, but patients usually adjust to the taping process more quickly and with less discomfort than do their therapists. Another potential disadvantage is that, even if there is a supervisory hour for each treatment session, stopping the tape and discussing some portions may prevent a review of the entire session. Yet supervision based on treatment notes also may not cover everything. Ideally, diligent therapists should tape

---

[1] Psychodynamic supervision also can work from taped sessions. Indeed, much of the literature on the use of videotape in supervision discusses psychodynamic psychotherapy (e.g., Alpert 1996; Aveline 1992; Friedmann et al. 1978).

sessions, transcribe the tapes, and use the transcription notes as a guide to supervision based on the tape.

Patient Selection

Both IPT and CBT were developed and tested as treatments for particular diagnostic groups, initially for outpatients with major depression. Their success led to adaptations and testing with differing target populations. Finding an appropriate case for a beginning therapist thus should include consideration of diagnostic criteria. For IPT, we recommend that trainees begin with a patient who has major depression, even if their eventual goal is to research a different diagnostic group. For example, dysthymic patients can so discourage a beginning IPT therapist that it is important to start with relatively easy cases of major depression in order to build the therapist's confidence in the treatment. CBT, too, is ideally learned in the context of one of its prime indications, such as major depression or panic disorder.

Serial Assessment

Treatments such as IPT and CBT strive for rapid clinical improvement. In order to monitor the status of the patient and to help the therapist recognize the efficacy of the treatment he or she is learning, the therapist should rate (or have an independent rater rate) symptom measures serially: every 2–4 weeks during treatment. The absolute frequency of the measurements is less important than that they occur regularly, as part of the treatment. Common rating instruments are the Hamilton Depression Rating Scale (Hamilton 1960) and the Beck Depression Inventory (Beck 1978). Ongoing clinical assessment using standardized instruments is good general practice in psychiatric treatment.

Scheduling of Supervision

Supervision is typically scheduled on a weekly basis to keep pace with the rapid developments of time-limited therapy. Supervision may be done individually or with groups of therapists, as time allows. These therapies can be supervised at long distance through the creative combination of audio- or videotaping, overnight mail, and telephone or Internet review.

Goals of Supervision

In open-ended, long-term psychotherapy the goals of supervision may vary and may shift from week to week. The goals of time-limited therapies are based on the particular requirements of these approaches. For treatment studies, supervisory goals are to ensure therapist adherence to the treatment technique and to maximize the potential patient improvement. Supervisors need to help therapists develop particular skills: among others, to rapidly take a history, formulate the case, and develop a focus and then maintain that focus throughout the treatment (Table 14–2).

TABLE **14–2.** *Goals of the new therapies*

Rapid diagnosis of target condition

History taking

Rapid formulation of a focus

Specific interventions in addition to common factors

Maintenance of treatment focus within and across sessions

Adherence: avoiding nonspecific or eclectic approaches

History

In time-limited psychotherapy, time is always at a premium. Yet economy and speed must be balanced with affect: The therapist must avoid the common beginner's mistake of concentrating on data and technique while losing the patient to whom he or she is providing treatment. Psychotherapists used to a longer-term approach may have trouble eliciting a concise history in the early sessions, yet a desultory approach here can be disastrous. An object of the early sessions of a time-limited treatment is to build a treatment alliance while obtaining material that will provide the focus for treatment. Part of this material is a diagnosis (e.g., a major depressive episode) based on DSM-IV symptom criteria (American Psychiatric Association 1994). The rest is a general history that accentuates the material the therapist will use as a focus: characteristic automatic thoughts and thinking patterns for the CBT therapist; object relations or key conflicts for the brief psychodynamic psychotherapist; and patterns of behavior in interpersonal encounters for the IPT therapist. The ability to focus on these issues when taking a history sets a theme for the patient to follow; to some extent, the therapist's focal approach explains the nature and expectations of the therapy even before the full technique has been brought to bear.

Formulation

After obtaining a sufficient history, the therapist produces a formulation for the patient (Markowitz and Swartz 1997). This formulation summarizes the patient's situation, emphasizes its treatability, and provides some explanation of and a framework for the treatment to follow. The IPT therapist asks the patient to explicitly agree to this formulation because it becomes the focus of subsequent treatment—an interpersonal focus on complicated bereavement, a role dispute, role transition, or interpersonal deficits (Klerman et al. 1984; Weissman et al. 1999). Choosing among potential foci is part of the art of therapy. Supervisors can model formulation, but in my experience therapists either grasp the concept quickly or they may never do so. The formulation reflects the therapist's ability to "read" the patient, abstract this reading, and provide succinct feedback. Consider the following example:

> IPT therapist: As we discussed when we did the Hamilton Depression Rating Scale, you are in an episode of major depression. Depression is a medical illness that's not your fault, and it's treatable. From what you've told me, I think your episode has something to do with problems in your marriage: your symptoms developed after things blew up between you and your wife. We call this a role dispute, and it's commonly associated with depression. If you agree with me, we can treat your depression using interpersonal psychotherapy, a treatment that's been shown to effectively treat depression. We'll focus on the relationship between how you feel and how your marriage is going, and we'll see what options you have to change things in your relationship for the better. Although you may have trouble seeing all those options right now because of the depression, there are things you can do to give yourself some control over that situation. If you can resolve your

marital dispute, not only with that be a good thing in itself, but your mood should improve as well. Does that make sense to you?

It takes practice to provide a concise formulation that blends the particulars of the patient's predicament into the therapeutic format.

Some focal psychodynamic psychotherapies focus on a particular relationship pattern (e.g., an Oedipal conflict [Sifneos 1979]) or unconscious dynamic rather than one of the interpersonal areas noted earlier. CBT does not present a single focus as part of its formulation. Although approaches to CBT formulation differ, they tend to present the therapeutic framework of dysfunctional thoughts and attitudes in the course of the first few sessions and to reinforce them thereafter. Therapists may collaborate with the patient to construct a list of problems on which the formulation is based. The formulation may occur at both the overall case level, encompassing the patient's presenting symptoms, and when addressing particular situations that arise in the course of treatment (Persons and Tompkins 1997).

Maintaining Focus

Once the patient agrees to the thematic focus, the therapist must hold the patient to that theme. Different therapies have different methods of maintaining focus. In CBT, the therapist and patient jointly set an agenda for each session, agreeing to address automatic thoughts and distorted cognitions in particular life situations. In IPT, the question that opens each session—"How have things been since we last met?"—in effect sets an agenda in requesting an interval history. The patient can only report a recent event or a mood state; the therapist then links moods to events, helping the patient to see connections and take actions to change his or her life for the better. The elicited recent history leads into a discussion of the focal problem area. Therapists trained in long-term treatment may need supervisory encouragement to actively structure sessions, feeling more comfortable in a more passive and silent role.

Maintaining the focus in IPT seems straightforward in the abstract: emphasizing that depression is an illness, helping the patient to blame the illness rather than himself or herself when warranted, helping the patient to see the connection between the mood disorder and life events, and helping the patient to choose among available options in order to improve his or her life situation and mood. The goal is to focus on here-and-now problems in the patient's current life. In practice, some therapists seemingly get distracted from these basic ideas. Much of supervision involves reviewing taped sessions to point out opportunities, taken and missed, where these points might be made. A good therapist must decide when to let the patient lead the session and when it is appropriate to intervene in order to rouse affect or steer the session back to the agreed-on focus. How much repetition and reinforcement is desirable, and how much is too much? Again, the review of taped sessions can be invaluable to strike the right balance, which may vary from patient to patient and from therapist to therapist.

Difficulties in Learning the New Therapies

Therapist Activity

Silence and the absence of time pressure are among the apparent comforts for therapists providing longer-term therapy. When in doubt, the therapist can simply wait and watch, avoiding the commitment of an intervention until he or she has additional information to confirm the justice of a comment. This is particularly characteristic of psychiatric residents and other trainees: lacking psychotherapeutic experience and confidence and conforming to the pseudo-stereotype of a Freudian model, they often opt for silence. The only psychotherapeutic experience many of these beginners have had is a little long-term psychodynamic psychotherapy, which relies on the free associations of patients and encourages patients to speak at length while therapists listen. When a therapist trained in long-term therapy tries to adjust to time-limited focal therapy, the need for greater therapist activity to intervene and structure treatment can initially be frightening. Some therapists worry that they are violating patient autonomy, putting words or wishes in the patient's mouth—which neither IPT or CBT should do. IPT and CBT therapists learn to take a relaxed, conversational stance, to feel free to speak when warranted. This is not a license for self-indulgence or excessive self-disclosure; the more usual difficulty is in getting the reticent therapist to speak enough to move the therapy forward. A training case or three generally suffices to build therapist confidence in a more interventionist role.

Therapeutic Potency

Psychiatric residents are far more comfortable in encouraging depressed patients about their good prognosis when prescribing medication than when prescribing psychotherapy. Long-term psychotherapy makes no immediate promises to the patient, but a time-limited treatment addresses a particular diagnosis and tells the patient that there is a realistic goal of remission in a matter of weeks. Without a prescription pad, the psychotherapist is putting himself or herself on the line— again, a frightening prospect for a beginning therapist who as yet has no great confidence that he or she can make the therapy work.

Here the track record of these therapies in empirical trials is a great advantage. Unlike earlier therapies, which relied largely on belief in the theories, evidence-based psychotherapies have the support of published randomized clinical outcome studies to prove their efficacy. Indeed, these treatments generally perform comparably to pharmacotherapies for outpatients with major depression. Discussion of the empirical literature in supervision, along with a recognition of the fears of a first-time time-limited therapist, may encourage the novice therapist to proceed. Psychiatric residents who succeed in initial cases often feel greatly empowered by the experience.

Use of Medication

The issue of therapeutic potency is related to the issue of medication use. Many beginning therapists, discouraged by the symptoms of a depressed or otherwise psychiatrically ill patient, may wish to compensate for their lack of therapeutic confidence by suggesting that the patient receive combined treatment with medication and psychotherapy. Although IPT and CBT can each be combined with medication in clinical practice, for teaching purposes it is preferable that the patients receive psychotherapy alone.

Because monotherapy often resolves an episode of major depression (Manning et al. 1992), responding to the therapist's countertransference by prescribing medication may well be counterproductive. The therapist avoids the experience of confronting the patient's painful symptoms and learning not to be overwhelmed by them. Particularly with a relatively simple treatment such as IPT, the therapist who prescribes medication is likely to attribute improvement to the medication rather than to the psychotherapy (and psychotherapist). Hence, supervision of beginning therapists should involve careful case selection (so that pharmacotherapy is not necessary) and attention to therapist fears that evoke the urge to medicate.

Use of the Time Limit

The time pressure induced by the time limit on therapy provides part of the leverage for therapeutic change. This time pressure requires both the patient and the therapist to work hard and fast. Beginning therapists may not like the pressure and accordingly may become vague about the number of sessions that have transpired or are to come. Supervisors need to watch for this and to underscore the importance of setting a firm termination date and of using the time frame to encourage the patient to change.

Mixed Versus Pure Techniques

Some therapists may adopt an eclectic approach and have difficulty sticking to a relatively pure model of the therapy they are learning. Their admixture of techniques may simply reflect a lack of knowledge about the limits and overlaps of different approaches. Or it may reflect an attitude: Why not mix elements of different psychotherapies?

The answer is that specificity, or purity, of technique may matter. E. Frank et al. (1991) found that the purity of IPT—that is, the degree to which therapists kept the treatment thematically in key—was associated with better outcome in the maintenance treatment of recurrent major depression. Indeed, it makes sense that presenting a single model and method to the treatment is one way to maintain a treatment focus. Consistent adherence to a single model teaches the patient a clear method for coping with symptoms and situations. Although the material the patient brings to a particular session may sound cognitive, or interpersonal, or psychodynamic to the therapist, he or she should resist the temptation to switch techniques, and thereby the focus, a maneuver that in the end may succeed only in confusing both patient and therapist. The more rigorous the model, the clearer the message to the patient.

Termination

Once the therapist has gotten the hang of a new treatment and the patient is improving or the depression has remitted, the therapist may decide that this is, after all, a good therapy and that the patient is a good patient. The patient may also express eagerness to continue. At that point the therapist may be sorely tempted to continue treatment indefinitely. The supervisor must reinforce the point that the goals of time-limited therapy are limited: to effect remission of the target syndrome (rather than, for example, to change character) and to provide coping skills in order to forestall its relapse or recurrence. Time may be available in the several-month acute treatment framework to work on more issues than those of the initial focus, but the treatment should not be extended beyond the originally determined time frame. Therapist and patient can learn to address termination—which is played down relative to psychodynamic psychotherapy—as a bittersweet graduation from therapy. The sadness the patient may experience at ending therapy can usefully be distinguished from depressed mood. Even when a patient has had multiple episodes of depression and hence may need continuation and maintenance psychotherapy, the therapeutic dyad should terminate acute treatment and negotiate a new treatment contract.

Data on Learning the New Treatments

Because IPT and CBT were developed in a research context, the process of learning these treatments has received some research attention (e.g., Chevron et al. 1983; Rounsaville et al. 1984, 1986; Weissman et al. 1982). Therapists were trained in IPT in much the manner described above: reading a manual; attending a didactic seminar; and then receiving intensive, hour-for-hour supervision in treating pilot cases.

Weissman et al. (1982) found that of 27 prospective therapists, all of whom had a minimum of 2 years of training in psychodynamic psychotherapy, 23 (85%) were able to complete training cases and receive certification as IPT therapists for research purposes. The trainers found that therapists who were not from medical settings had trouble emphasizing the concept of depression as an illness (admittedly, things may have changed in the many years since this study), some therapists had difficulty focusing on interpersonal problems in the here and now, others followed the manual too rigidly and failed to explore the patient's affect sufficiently, and some had difficulty in using the time limit (Weissman et al. 1982). The same researchers found that whereas interrater reliability of the supervisors' ratings of videotaped sessions was highly significant, no significant relationship existed between the videotape ratings of the psychotherapists and those made on the basis of traditional process note supervision. In other words, the therapist's patient notes drifted far from the reality of the session (Chevron et al. 1983).

Therapist experience played an important role in IPT training. Veteran psychotherapist IPT trainees, who had an average of 14 years of prior psychotherapy experience, were often rated as excellent after having completed a single case. By contrast, therapists with less than 6 years of experience were rated acceptable after one case, and although they improved after a second case, their marks still fell short of excellence (Chevron et al. 1983).

Less experienced psychotherapists, such as psychiatric residents, can be trained to learn the basics of therapies such as IPT (Markowitz 1995) and CBT (Ritchie and White 1992). Residents can compensate for their lack of experience with eagerness and energy, and for the most part they have not yet had the chance to develop treatment styles based on alternative treatment approaches. Residents seem to like these therapies partly because they are practical, emphasizing clinical intervention over theory, and relatively well defined. Even as psychotherapy training declines in psychiatric residency training programs (Altshuler 1990; Rodenhauser 1992), some programs are bolstering their psychotherapy training with CBT and IPT.

We recommend that training programs give residents at least an exposure to treatments such as IPT and CBT no later than the PGY-II training year. This approach gives them frameworks in which to view patients and gives them something to say to depressed inpatients with whom they work. The PGY-III year should include an opportunity to use time-limited, evidence-based focal therapies with outpatients under appropriate supervision. Interested residents may gain further experience in their PGY-IV year.

Training

Training in the new therapies may be obtained in several ways. Numerous cognitive therapy institutes exist, the most famous of which is the Center for Cognitive Therapy in Philadelphia, which offers both intramural and extramural programs. Extramural training involves a few weekend visits over the course of 1 or 2 years of training, with the remainder of the work conducted via long-distance supervision. Therapists tape treatment sessions, send the tapes to their supervisors, and discuss the session by telephone.

Training in IPT has been less widely available, and the paucity of trained therapists makes finding a supervisor more difficult than for other therapies. There are two ways to proceed. In either case, the first step is to read the manual (Klerman et al. 1984; Weissman et al. 2000). The material in the manual may be reinforced by attending courses or workshops, which are increasingly available at professional conferences such as the American Psychiatric Association annual meeting. An IPT workshop was given at the March 1999 American Psychopathological Association meeting. One option is to obtain long-distance individual case supervision with an IPT expert from one of the centers mentioned earlier in this chapter. This is an expensive and labor-intensive approach but is probably the surest way to validate the credentials of a prospective IPT researcher.

An alternative is to convene a group of interested psychotherapists and organize peer supervision. Having read the manual and sometimes having arranged a local workshop, several groups have trained themselves through peer supervision of taped sessions. They have then called in IPT experts to assess their work and have been pronounced accredited. This approach is less costly and develops a cadre of therapists who can collaborate on research. In either case, we recommend that a therapist complete three successful supervised training cases to be considered qualified in IPT.

The variability in current training approaches indicates that this field is still young. Until recently, most IPT therapists were trained solely for research purposes. Experts in CBT, which has far more practitioners, are now trying to establish standards for CBT practice. But neither IPT nor CBT has a formal accreditation board. Nor are there formal guidelines and standards for training. The technology for providing training on a large scale has yet to be developed. The needs for a training bureaucracy and established training standards are issues these therapies must address in order to develop in the future.

References

Alpert MC: Videotaping psychotherapy. J Psychother Pract Res 5:93–105, 1996

Altshuler KZ: Whatever happened to intensive psychotherapy? Am J Psychiatry 147:428–430, 1990

American Psychiatric Association: Diagnostic and Statistical Manual of Mental Disorders, 4th Edition. Washington, DC, American Psychiatric Association, 1994

Aveline M: The use of audio and videotape recordings of therapy sessions in the supervision and practice of dynamic psychotherapy. Br J Psychother 347–358, 1992

Beck AT: Depression Inventory. Philadelphia, PA, Center for Cognitive Therapy, 1978

Beck AT, Rush AJ, Shaw BF, et al: Cognitive Therapy of Depression. New York, Guilford, 1979

Chevron E, Rounsaville B, Rothblum ED, et al: Selecting psychotherapists to participate in psychotherapy outcome studies: relationship between psychotherapist characteristics and assessment of clinical skills. J Nerv Ment Dis 171:348–353,1983

Chodoff P: Supervision of psychotherapy with videotape: pros and cons. Am J Psychiatry 128:819–823, 1972

Frances A, Clarkin JF, Perry S: Differential Therapeutics in Psychiatry: The Art and Science of Treatment Selection. New York, Brunner/Mazel, 1984

Frank E, Kupfer DJ, Wagner EF, et al: Efficacy of interpersonal psychotherapy as a maintenance treatment of recurrent depression. Arch Gen Psychiatry 48:1053–1059, 1991

Frank J: Therapeutic factors in psychotherapy. Am J Psychother 25:350–361, 1971

Friedmann CTH, Yamamoto J, Wolkon GH, et al: Videotape recording of dynamic psychotherapy: supervisory tool or hindrance? Am J Psychiatry 135:388–391, 1978

Hamilton M: A rating scale for depression. J Neurol Neurosurg Psychiatry 25:56–62, 1960

Hill CE, O'Grady KE, Elkin I: Applying the collaborative study psychotherapy rating scale to rate therapist adherence in cognitive-behavior therapy, interpersonal therapy, and clinical management. J Consult Clin Psychol 60:73–79, 1992

Klerman GL, Weissman MM, Rounsaville BJ, et al: Interpersonal Psychotherapy of Depression. New York, Basic Books, 1984

Manning DW, Markowitz JC, Frances AJ: A review of combined psychotherapy and pharmacotherapy in the treatment of depression. J Psychother Pract Res 1:103–116, 1992

Markowitz JC: Teaching interpersonal psychotherapy to psychiatric residents. Academic Psychiatry 19:167–173, 1995

Markowitz JC, Swartz HA: Case formulation in interpersonal psychotherapy of depression, in Handbook of Psychotherapy Case Formulation. Edited by Eels TD. New York, Guilford, 1997, pp 192–222

Persons JB, Tompkins MA: Cognitive-behavioral case formulation, in Handbook of Psychotherapy Case Formulation. Edited by Eels TD. New York, Guilford, 1997, pp 314–339

Ritchie EC, White R: Cognitive therapy training in U.S. psychiatry residency programs. Academic Psychiatry 16:90–95, 1992

Rodenhauser P: Psychiatric residency programs: trends in psychotherapy supervision. Am J Psychother 46:240–249, 1992

Rounsaville BJ, Chevron ES, Weissman MM: Specification of techniques in interpersonal psychotherapy, in Psychotherapy Research: Where Are We and Where Should We Go? Edited by Williams JBW, Spitzer RL. New York, Guilford, 1984

Rounsaville BJ, Chevron ES, Weissman MM, et al: Training therapists to perform interpersonal psychotherapy in clinical trials. Compr Psychiatry 27:364–371, 1986

Schuster DB, Sandt JJ, Thaler OF: The Clinical Supervision of the Psychiatric Resident. New York, Brunner/Mazel, 1972, p 32

Sifneos PE: Short-Term Dynamic Psychotherapy. New York, Plenum, 1979

Weissman MM, Rounsaville BJ, Chevron ES: Training psychotherapists to participate in psychotherapy outcome studies: identifying and dealing with the research requirement. Am J Psychiatry 139:1442–1446, 1982

Weissman MM, Markowitz JC, Klerman GL: Comprehensive Guide to Interpersonal Psychotherapy. New York, Basic Books, 2000

15

The Paradox of Psychotherapy

Too Many, Too Few; Too Much, Too Little

Myrna M. Weissman, Ph.D.

Too Many Psychotherapies

Psychotherapy in the marketplace has been a stunning success (Seligman 1995). More than 200 psychotherapies have been catalogued, treating everything from snake phobias to schizophrenia, and the list is growing. These therapies are administered by a wide range of therapists, from counselors with bachelor degrees to psychoanalytically trained physicians. Some therapies have been specified in manuals; most have not. The therapies often are a hybrid of methods of varying duration for unspecified conditions. There is, however, a problem of credibility.

Too Few Psychotherapies

Only a few psychotherapies have been demonstrated to be efficacious through controlled clinical trials. Many more are probably effective but

Although I take full responsibility for the opinions expressed here, these ideas were enhanced by readings and discussions with many people. Most central are the ideas and writings of my late husband, Gerald L. Klerman, M.D., who died in 1992 but whose thinking was way ahead of his time. Others particularly helpful include Robert Michels, M.D.; Leon Eisenberg, M.D.; Mark Olfson, M.D.; John Markowitz, Ph.D.; Helena Verdeli, Ph.D.; Laura Mufson, Ph.D.; and William Sanderson, Ph.D.

have not been tested. Few therapies meet the efficacy guidelines established by the U.S. Food and Drug Administration (FDA) for psychopharmacologic treatments. If FDA standards existed for psychotherapy today, only two or three psychotherapies would be approved for the treatment of depression (London and Klerman 1982).

Too Much Psychotherapy

Psychotherapy has been overused. How much therapy is enough is a question of popular interest. There is a Woody Allen caricature of the New Yorker: Everyone is in psychotherapy, and half of the population is treating the other half, mostly for minor problems of living. Psychotherapy is described as the cosmetic surgery of the so-called worried well, who receive undefined treatments for ill-defined disorders, for interminable periods of time, at considerable cost, and with no assessment of benefit to patients or their families. Some groups now say that psychotherapy may be toxic and should come with a side-effect warning.

Too Little Psychotherapy

A recent National Health Survey showed that psychotherapy has been decreasing as a treatment for mental disorders. At the same time, pharmacotherapy and alternative treatments have increased (Eisenberg et al. 1998; Ernst et al. 1998). A national study of visits from 1985 to 1995 to physicians specializing in psychiatry showed a significant decrease in the percentage of visits that included psychotherapy and an increase in visits that included psychotropic medication. The mean duration of visits decreased, and the number of visits lasting 10 minutes or less increased. Shortening of visit duration was most evident in patients previously identified as users of psychotherapy—that is, in the young and privately insured (Olfson et al. 1999). Changing financial arrangements, a shift away from psychiatrists as providers of psychotherapy, and new pharmacologic treatments have likely contributed to these changing patterns.

Despite the decrease in psychotherapy, surveys of depressed patients' treatment preferences invariably show that even patients who prefer medication also want psychotherapy. Large populations at risk for depression may refrain from taking drugs, particularly women of child-bearing age, during pregnancy and the lactation period. Moreover, psychotherapy is a recommended treatment for depression in various treatment guidelines. Consumer preference may have led to the overuse of psychotherapy for minor problems of living; however, those so-called minor problems of living are often undiagnosed depression with real morbidity. A host of epidemiologic studies show that most people with major depression have not had their condition diagnosed. Furthermore, in many of those given a diagnosis, the depression remains untreated or undertreated. Fewer depressed patients are receiving psychotherapy than in the past.

Although long-term (1–2 years) and intensive psychotherapy has been the norm in psychiatric residency training programs, the clinical reality is quite different. Under managed care, most depressed patients, if their condition is diagnosed and treated with psychotherapy, receive short-term psychotherapy lasting from one to a maximum of 15 or 20 sessions. The vast majority of Americans receive mental health care through insurance plans that closely monitor the course of treatment, set limits on the length of treatment, and require authorization for further visits or more frequent intervals. The few depressed patients who spend years in psychotherapy now pay the costs themselves. In reality—but not in the public's perception—the Woody Allen caricature of the so-called talking treatment is a relic from the past.

This chapter is based on the following assumptions about psychotherapy:

- Psychotherapy is a useful treatment for depression.
- There is evidence for its efficacy.
- Most depressed patients have psychosocial and interpersonal problems associated with the onset, course, or consequences of their illness that might benefit from psychotherapy.
- Psychotherapy is a useful supplement to medication for many depressed patients.
- Psychotherapy is an important alternative for patients who cannot or will not take medication.

Many controversies surround psychotherapy:

- What is psychotherapy?
- Does psychotherapy work?
- Does psychotherapy work in the real world?
- Does psychotherapy save money?
- Who should receive psychotherapy, for how long, and how often?
- Should psychotherapy be specified?
- Can you read a book and become a therapist?
- Can the research training in psychotherapy be adapted for effectiveness studies?
- What should psychotherapy training include?
- What impact have managed care and guidelines had on clinical care?
- Are new models of psychotherapy needed?

What Is Psychotherapy?

The controversy about psychotherapy is illustrated in a recent exchange between Guze (1998) and Michels (1998) about psychotherapy and managed care. Both agree on the value of psychotherapy, but they disagree on what it is they value. Guze frames psychotherapy as the dialogue and emotional ties that develop between a sick person and his or her caretaker. In his definition, psychotherapy is universal in all medical and psychiatric care. Michels (1998), in contrast, defines psychotherapy as

> a class of therapies provided by some, but not all psychiatrists (and some non physicians as well) to some patients, but not to others. Psychotherapy is based on a theory and has a strategy, it is not simply humanistic and compassionate care by a concerned physician. Psychotherapy may be indicated either for patients with recognizable psychiatric disorders or for persons with problems in living. Some psychiatrists are trained psychotherapists, others are not. Some psychologists and social workers are trained psychotherapists as well. (p. 564)

The differences framed by Guze and Michels are at the heart of the controversies today about indications, reimbursement, and training.

Recommendation

In the research literature, the same differentiation is usually made between psychologic management and specific psychotherapies. Further definition and testing of the efficacy of psychologic management and specific psychotherapies are needed. The National Institute of Mental Health (NIMH) Treatment of Depression Collaborative Research Program included a psychologic management condition in the pharmacotherapy and placebo conditions (Elkin et al. 1989) and showed that placebo plus psychologic management was not as effective as medication or specific psychotherapy (interpersonal psychotherapy [IPT] or cognitive-behavioral therapy [CBT]) for more severely depressed patients. The specification of psychologic management might improve medical and nonmedical care and, if efficacy were demonstrated, might help in reimbursement for health providers' time. Moreover, clear differentiation between the two approaches is needed in any debates about reimbursement for psychotherapy.

Does Psychotherapy Work?

Excellent evidence exists for the efficacy of several time-limited psychotherapies based on controlled clinical trials for the acute treatment of depression and for maintenance treatment (Jorgensen and Bolwig 1998; Thase et al. 1997). The evidence is mostly available for adults. New studies are just being published on adolescents (Brent et al. 1997; Mufson et al. 1999) and geriatric patients (Reynolds et al. 1999; Thase et al. 1997). Because these trials have already been reviewed extensively elsewhere, I will not review them again. The main point is that far more evidence would be useful.

There is no question that far fewer studies have been made of psychotherapy efficacy than of pharmacotherapy efficacy. Efficacy studies in psychotherapy have little or no industry support and no marketing program. A typical drug, before it gets to market, goes through four phases of testing and then undergoes postmarketing surveillance. During these studies, dose feasibility, side effects, drug interactions, and efficacy are tested. Persons who are qualified to conduct Phase 1 studies (i.e., chemists) will not be the same ones conducting the Phase 4 studies (i.e., clinicians). A similar phased model of efficacy is applicable to psychotherapy; however, most psychotherapy trials begin prematurely. Rarely has a series of open trials been conducted. Federal agencies are unlikely to fund open trials. For psychotherapy, dose, specificity, side effects, and indications rarely are tested before an expensive Phase 3 or Phase 4 trial is launched. There is no postmarketing surveillance of psychotherapy.

Recommendation

We need a strategy for Phases 1 through 4 and for postmarketing surveillance studies for psychotherapy. The opportunity for joint ventures with pharmaceutical companies should be accelerated. Several companies have already sponsored the testing of psychotherapy in comparison or combination with pharmacotherapy. For these joint ventures to succeed, psychotherapy has to be an equal partner in them. Interestingly, several of these joint ventures are under way outside of the United States (e.g., in Canada and Australia), where psychotherapy is part of the practice of primary care.

In the mid-1980s, the NIMH initiated a grant program for psychotherapy development. This program is definitely of low profile. Its use and impact should be reviewed. These strategies need to cover the life span. There is only one published efficacy study of individual psychotherapy with depressed adolescents and none with depressed children. The FDA has just required that pharmacotherapy must be tested in children and adolescents if it is to be used. The same requirement should apply to psychotherapy with children and adolescents.

Does Psychotherapy Work in the Real World?

Efficacy trials typically involve randomized clinical assignment whereby investigators exercise considerable control over sample selection, delivery of the intervention, and the conditions under which the intervention occurs. In addition to ruling out competing explanations for patient improvement, these controlled procedures ensure that the intervention is given the best chance of success by reducing variance due to factors associated with heterogenous patients, settings, or therapist styles. The principle is to bias in favor of the effect, so that if the treatment does not work under these ideal conditions, it is unlikely to work under typical clinical practice. In the real world, psychotherapy is given under conditions of varying therapist enthusiasm, training, and skills to patients with multiple psychiatric disorders sometimes complicated by medical problems.

Questions about reimbursement are being raised in the real world. Attention increasingly is being directed toward effectiveness studies. Most effectiveness studies combine clinical outcomes such as symptoms or diagnoses with measures that assess the broader impact of the intervention on various areas of functioning, consumer-based perspectives such as satisfaction with care, use of services, and cost. Psychotherapies generally demonstrate poorer response rates in practice settings than in clinical trials (Woody and Kihlstrom 1997); this is probably true for pharmacotherapy as well.

Although it is important to demonstrate a treatment's efficacy before investigating its effectiveness, there is a pressing public health need to develop strategies for successfully transferring complex mental health treatment technologies, developed under carefully controlled and highly specialized treatment settings, into clinical environments that more broadly represent community care. For psychotherapy with depressed patients, this would include settings in which many depressed patients can be found, for example, in primary care, obstetrics and gynecology, or family practice clinics and for children and adolescents in school-based clinics. Using nonacademic mental health clinics with nonresearch personnel is a challenge. One challenge for psychotherapy effectiveness studies will be to develop feasible, in-service training methods for the therapists in evidence-based treatment.

Recommendation

Effectiveness studies of psychotherapy in depression need to include feasible methods of training, use a range of professionals, and be conducted in settings in which many depressed patients are likely to be found. Outcomes linked to quality of life, such as cost and quality of care, need to be included. These outcomes may be linked to the intervention through a relatively long causal chain. For example, a treatment targets symptom reduction, which may help improve marital relations, which in turn may promote improvements in other areas of functioning such as child care, which may then reduce the use of medical services by the patient or family members. Because effect sizes diminish at each step of the causal pathway, effectiveness studies require large samples.

Does Psychotherapy Save Money?

In an era of constrained public resources, it is critical to know whether a strategy is cost effective. Strategies that achieve equivalent outcomes at lower cost should usually be chosen over more costly alternatives, because they allow more people to receive treatment for any given level of public funding. Few studies have examined the cost effectiveness of mental health treatment for any population (Sturm and Wells 1995). Unmet needs for mental health services may also generate a demand for physical health services. Measuring cost effectiveness for psychotherapy is not straightforward.

The focus in considering cost offset or treatment efficiency has been in the speed of symptom reduction or in decreases in days lost from work, days spent in the hospital, or medical expenditures. Many cost-reduction results have been inferred and not directly assessed (Gabbard et al. 1997). Many outcomes used do not fully reflect the morbidity of illness or the potential target of psychotherapy. It has been well documented that the offspring of depressed parents are at high risk for developing depression and for developing behavioral, school, and health problems (Kramer et al. 1998; McAvay et al. 1999). Cost-offset studies need to have a long-term view, which includes assessment of the impact of the illness on the immediate family and on a range of social functioning. For example, Browne and Steiner (personal communication, 1998) studied 700 primary care patients with dysthymia treated with sertraline, IPT, or both for up to 3 months. The 6-month follow-up results showed the superiority of sertraline, either alone or in combination with IPT, in symptom reduction. However, patients who received IPT, either alone or in combination, had economically important reductions in health and social services expenditures and in expenditures related to social welfare. This study demonstrates the complexity of determining a treatment's cost effectiveness.

Recommendation

Cost-offset assessment of antidepressant treatment should be expanded to include assessment of the nuclear families of depressed patients, particularly offspring and their functioning, as well as health care costs and the cost offset of a range of medical, pediatric, and social services.

Who Should Receive Psychotherapy for Depression, for How Long, and How Often?

Based on controlled clinical trials, candidates for time-limited, evidence-based psychotherapy for acute treatment of depression include nonpsychotic, nonbipolar depressed patients, from adolescents to geriatrics, and particularly patients who cannot take medication. Patients with psychotic delusional depression or bipolar disorder require medication, either alone or in combination with psychotherapy (Depression Guidelines Panel 1993). The concept of time-limited treatment is controversial and unclear and may be misleading. *Time-limited* means that the time is specified in advance, and additional time is renegotiated. It does not necessarily mean restricted coverage. In fact, many depressed patients of all ages and types need treatment over long periods of time, a point stressed in Chapter 11. Major depression fits the model of a chronic illness and often recurs. Although a large number of depressed patients have only one episode, and a small minority have chronic depression, the great majority, about 60%, have recurrences throughout their lifetimes. Treatment, including psychotherapy, should be available when these episodes occur and to prevent future episodes. For patients with multiple episodes, when recurrence is inevitable, prophylaxis treatment may be necessary for long periods of time.

For many patients, having psychotherapy available as needed during periods of stress may be all that is needed. Even in patients with bipolar disorder, a lifelong condition for which psychotropic medications are clearly the major treatment, adjunctive psychotherapy may be helpful in dealing with life events during the acute episodes, in improving medication compliance, or in assisting patients who for any number of reasons may need to discontinue medication (Goodwin and Jamison

1990). Unfortunately, those who control the flow of treatment dollars may not be sufficiently flexible to consider the individual differences among patients as well as the long-term course of the illness.

The relationship of psychotherapy to pharmacotherapy and the need to maintain a flexible attitude in choosing treatment are well illustrated by women of childbearing age who are at high risk for developing depression. Some recent studies indicate that the new psychotropic drugs, when taken during pregnancy, have no long-term effects on offspring. However, many pregnant women refrain from taking these drugs. Psychotherapy can be an alternative to medication if depression occurs during pregnancy. Although a considerable body of evidence supports the efficacy of psychotropic drugs in treating depression, the few studies that included psychotherapy generally found that both medication and time-limited psychotherapy had equal efficacy in reducing depressive symptoms. In general, in the treatment of depression, medication has a faster and more consistent onset of action than psychotherapy; however, Frank et al. (1991) found that psychotherapy alone, delivered once a month over a 36-week period by nonpsychiatrists, prevented recurrence in nearly 70% of patients with severe recurrent depression. If these results can be generalized to depressed pregnant women, psychotherapy could provide an effective alternative to medication during gestation, even in patients who have recurrent depression.

After pregnancy ends, the reintroduction of antidepressants in the postpartum period can pose a problem for women who are nursing. No studies have examined whether antidepressants in breast milk have long-term effects on infants, and little information exists on the short-term effects. In the absence of these data, women who require antidepressants are usually advised to discontinue nursing. In some cases, this medical advice runs counter to strong social and maternal expectations that mothers nurse their babies. The availability of psychotherapy may help woman through the lactation period.

Insurance policies and health care benefits that restrict access to psychotherapy may thus be detrimental to the health of some women who require treatment for depression during pregnancy and the postpartum period and to depressed men and women who do not want to or cannot take medication.

Mental health professionals are under pressure to make therapeutic interventions efficient. Demands for efficiency will focus most heavily on psychotherapy, with most managed care organizations tending to exclude psychotherapy from the benefit package or, if included, limiting the benefit to a few sessions. This exclusion is reflected in the recent Agency for Health Care Policy and Research guidelines that recommend psychotherapy when depression is mild to moderate, nonpsychotic, nonchronic, and not highly recurrent (Depression Guideline Panel 1993). These guidelines would seem to be a great boost for brief time-limited psychotherapies such as IPT or CBT (Beck et al. 1979; Klerman et al. 1984). Unfortunately, most psychiatric illnesses do not fit into the category of being nonchronic or not recurrent. Moreover, primary care practitioners are unlikely to use psychotherapy of any kind.

Recommendation

Treatment decisions should be based on the extensive data on the clinical reality of depression and the populations at high risk and not solely on economic policies or the politics of managed care. Psychotherapy should be reimbursed for acute episodes that may be treated intensively but briefly as well as for recurrent episodes. Some depressed patients may require interventions throughout their lifetime during periods of incipient symptoms. Lifetime caps on coverage need to be reviewed within the clinical context of the condition. The available data suggest that long-term, nonintensive psychotherapy is efficacious for many depressed patients.

Should Psychotherapy Be Specified?

At one time, the diversity of psychotherapists' approaches to patients discouraged research on psychotherapy. Each psychotherapist was considered unique, as was each patient, and there was no way to know what the therapist was doing in the office, with a given patient. Psychotherapy was seen as an art that could not be addressed by science. That outlook has changed.

Treatment manuals constitute a small revolution in psychotherapy research. Manuals follow the tradition of operationalizing criteria, as was done in creating the third edition of the *Diagnostic and Statistical*

Manual of Mental Disorders in the 1980s and in providing guidelines for therapeutic strategies. Manuals provide technical specifications, with scripts for intervention and guidelines on what should be covered and how (Hibbs and Jensen 1996; Luborsky and DuRubeis 1984). Treatment manuals can teach experienced psychotherapists to adapt their styles to a particular approach. Audiotaping or videotaping provides an objective record of how the therapist delivers that treatment and a record that raters can review and score for treatment adherence. A manual can make psychotherapy a relatively uniform, and thus testable, treatment.

Manuals can address the growing demands of third-party payers for accountability; they have become a virtual requirement for psychotherapy studies (Chambless et al. 1998; Sanderson and Woody 1995). Some studies have shown that the therapist's degree of adherence to the manual was significantly associated with patient improvement.

Manuals vary in their depth and clarity. For example, IPT and CBT have been specified in manuals for the treatment of depression in adults (Beck et al. 1979; Klerman et al. 1984; Weissman et al. 1999). These treatments have been adapted for other disorders, sometimes without specific changes. Other adaptations have been defined in great detail (e.g., IPT for dysthymia [Markowitz 1998]; see Klerman and Weissman [1993] for IPT adaptation; CBT for bulimia [Fairburn et al.1993], panic [Barlow and Cerny 1988], anxiety [Barlow and Craske 1994], and social phobia [Turner et al. 1997]). Few manuals have been adapted for children and adolescents (e.g., Lewinsohn et al. 1990; Miller et al. 1997; Mufson et al. 1993; Wilkes et al. 1994).

Recommendation

The development of manuals should be encouraged by academic departments and professional organizations involved in teaching or conducting psychotherapy. Widely used psychotherapies that have not been specified in manuals ought to be. Psychotherapy manuals adapted for the treatment of depression in children and adolescents should be encouraged. Guidelines and standards for the content and procedures of manuals might be developed by professional organizations. Money could be set aside for development of new manuals by professional organizations and by the NIMH (as a prelude to efficacy studies) or by pharmaceutical companies for drug-accompanying studies. An alliance among all three—professional organizations, the NIMH, and pharmaceutical companies—could provide the funds and standards for this undertaking.

Can You Read a Book and Become a Therapist?

We have ample evidence that manuals are not substitutes for psychotherapy training. A manual does not teach psychotherapists how to listen, hear, empathize, and handle one's own feelings and distortions. Manuals teach trained therapists a particular strategy. It is relatively easy for experienced therapists to learn specified therapies. The limitations are usually only ideologic. Although the psychotherapy research literature contains contradictory evidence about the importance of psychotherapist experience, experience effects have been noted consistently. In evaluating 27 potential IPT trainees, on the basis of videotaped samples of their clinical work, we found clinical experience to be the key distinguishing factor. In one research training program, in which trainees had an average of 14 years of experience, we noted a ceiling effect. They reached an average level of "excellent" in learning manual-based therapy with the first supervised case. These therapists grasped and used the techniques simply by reading the manual and attending a didactic seminar. In the course of one to three additional training cases, experienced psychotherapists showed neither significant improvement nor significant deterioration in their excellent performance. In a similar program wherein trainees had less than 6 years of experience, performance in the first training case was rated as "acceptable" on average and significantly improved in the second case (Chevron and Rounsaville 1983).

We concluded that training a skilled therapist in the techniques of a new treatment is not the same as training a novice to do psychotherapy. If psychotherapy training is devalued or eliminated by managed care pressures, therapists will be trained to conduct structured brief therapies without a general background in listening to patients or doing psychotherapy. We found that inexperienced therapists adhered closely to the manual but ended up giving lectures.

Recommendation

Can you read a book and become a psychotherapist? The simple answer is *not well*, if you have little training or experience in psychotherapy. We need better understanding of the quantity and quality of psychotherapy training that is needed to carry out the various specified manual-based treatments. Clearly, more general psychotherapy experience and training results in better adherence and ease of training in IPT. This may not be the case for more structured treatments such as CBT and behavior therapy, although I suspect that more experience and training also are beneficial in these treatments. More structured forms of therapy exist that require less clinical experience. For example, interpersonal counseling was developed for non–mental health professionals (Klerman and Weissman 1993). It relies on clinical judgments as to the professional's verbal skills, warmth and intuitive ability, and interest and comfort in dealing with interpersonal problems. Interpersonal counseling cannot be used to treat serious mental disorders. Standards must be developed for the professional and clinical requirements to carry out different types of psychotherapy. The professional organizations, backed by research, could begin to set standards.

Can the Research Training in Psychotherapy Be Adapted for Effectiveness Studies?

The NIMH Treatment of Depression Collaborative Research Program (comparing CBT, IPT, imipramine, and placebo plus clinical management) set the guidelines for training for psychotherapy efficacy studies (Elkin et al. 1985, 1989; Weissman et al. 1982). These studies have shown the value of video- or audiotapes of actual sessions to improve the accuracy of what the therapist reports during supervision (Chevron and Rounsaville 1983; Rounsaville et al. 1986).

Therapists who meet educational and experiential requirements are taught the basic principles and techniques of the treatment by reading the manual and attending a didactic seminar. They are then required to provide treatment to several patients, video- or audiotape their sessions, and receive supervision based on these tapes. An expert therapist rates a random selection of tapes for adherence to the treatment manual in order to certify the therapists in adherence to the treatment modality, before beginning the trial. These training procedures are not feasible for routine clinical practice or for effectiveness studies. For the latter, many therapists need to be trained in their practice settings (e.g., schools, primary care practices, or mental health settings), and there are budget, time, and physical constraints.

What have these boutique training experiences taught us that can be adapted to the real world or to psychotherapy training programs? First, we learned that there is no substitute for live performance. We found little agreement between the therapist process notes and what was going on in the sessions when viewed on tape. Sometimes therapists rated as highly skilled via process note procedures were rated as far less skilled when tapes were viewed independently (Chevron and Rounsaville 1983). We also found the reverse to be true. Based on this experience we concluded that some documentation of the actual sessions is essential for supervision and for training. Videotapes are more interesting to review than audiotapes; however, audiotapes can substitute and are low tech, low cost, and most feasible.

Training programs in psychotherapy, whether in psychiatry, psychology, social work, or the like, should use the trainees' tapes of actual sessions for teaching, supervision, and quality control. Psychotherapy training programs for efficacy studies usually include funds for monitoring to ensure quality and adherence by random viewing or by listening to tapes of psychotherapy sessions and rating quality (Brook and Lohr 1985).

Training therapists for effectiveness studies is a new challenge. By their very nature, elaborate training as done in efficacy studies is not feasible in these studies. If evidence-based therapies are to be translated into real-world practice, the therapies need to be transportable or they will not be used. Existing personnel need to be able to administer these therapies. If the therapy requires 3 years of training and 1 year of additional training with videotaped supervision, the therapy will remain on the shelf.

Recommendation

New methods of training for effectiveness studies need to incorporate the lessons learned from the efficacy studies and need to approximate in-service training. These new methods could include establishment of minimal criteria of therapist education, experience, and skills; use of audiotapes of actual therapy sessions; supervision in a group format; random checks, using audiotapes for quality control; and established competence criteria.

What Should Psychotherapy Training Include?

You can't give a hair cut or mix a drink for a fee without a license. You don't need a license to give psychotherapy

> *Frances Cournes, paper presented at Rounds,*
> *Columbia University College of Physicians and*
> *Surgeons, Department of Psychiatry, November 1998*

In the United States, approximately 40,000 psychiatrists, 80,000 psychologists, and 120,000 social workers have been licensed to provide psychotherapy. In addition, a large but unknown number of marital, drug, alcohol, group, school, and spiritual counselors; family therapists; clergy; and psychiatric nurses provide various forms of psychotherapy for a fee. Professional disciplines have their own academic and licensing requirements, and insurance companies pay for some but not all therapists. In fact, there is no state regulation or licensing for psychotherapists.

There is considerable reluctance to legislate and license discourse between individuals for the purpose of providing help and support. What are the consequences of not licensing? Do we need a profession of psychotherapy that is independent of academic disciples and requires certification, credentials, regulations, and skills in various approaches? Although professional disciplines have standards for training, psychotherapy will increasingly be carried out by nonmedical professionals or by nonprofessionals with increasingly less training.

Within the professions, a gap exists between clinical training and clinical practice. For example, in 1998 the Resident Review Committee, the oversight body that accredits psychiatric residents, still required long-term psychotherapy experience, which had to include "a sufficient number of patients seen weekly for at least one year under supervision" (Residency Education in Psychiatry 1998). Should resident psychotherapy training be made optional (i.e., selected by psychiatrists interested in careers in psychotherapy) or should it be mandatory? If mandatory, what psychotherapies should be part of training? Kandel (1998) suggests that the mandatory psychotherapy requirement may be responsible for the decrease in psychiatry trainees despite the increased interest in the biology of mental processes:

> We thus are confronting an interesting paradox. While the scientific community...has become interested in the biology of mental processes; the interest of medical students in a psychiatric career is declining...medical students realize that in-so-far as the teaching of psychiatry is often based primarily on doing psychotherapy, a major component of psychiatry as it is now taught does not require a medical education. (p. 467)

Although this decrease has not continued, Kandel makes a good point. Perhaps psychiatric residents could continue to receive as part of their basic education, along with training in diagnosis and psychopharmacology, a core training in listening and hearing patients, dealing with transference and countertransference, and psychologic management (of course, I think all physicians should learn these skills). However, only a few psychiatrists may choose to receive further training in long-term psychotherapy and in the range of time-limited psychotherapies. Psychotherapy could become a subspecialty of psychiatric residency training.

The situation is also paradoxical in mental health professions outside of psychiatry. Although psychotherapy increasingly is being carried out by nonphysicians, training programs in psychology, social work, and counseling do not require training in the evidence-based treatments their trainees will increasingly be called on to administer.

Recommendation

The professions that train psychotherapists should discuss whether a new psychotherapy discipline should be established that cuts across professions. At the very least, psychiatric residency training programs should define the core psychotherapeutic training needed for all residents and then reconsider whether additional training in long-term psychotherapy should be mandatory or optional. Nonmedical training programs (e.g., psychology, social work) that teach psychotherapy should include training in evidence-based psychotherapies. The discordance in psychotherapy practice, research, and training must be addressed. In practice, evidence-based psychotherapies are not widely used. They are a small part of psychology (except for CBT), social work, and psychiatry training programs. Much of the psychotherapy that is reimbursed is short term, yet psychiatric residency programs emphasize training in long-term psychotherapy. Much of the psychotherapy in the future will be carried out by nonphysicians, but they are not required to learn the new psychotherapies. The burden for learning evidence-based psychotherapies falls on the continuing medical education courses, which are variable and unregulated.

What Impact Have Managed Care Guidelines Had on Clinical Care?

The concepts of *consumers* (not patients), *cost containment* (not care), and *providers* (not trained professionals) permeate health care delivery as the 21st century begins (Druss et al. 1998; Eist 1998). The process of care that is managed by health care administrators, with the goal of cutting costs, has affected the treatment of psychiatric disorders perhaps more than other areas of medicine. Cost cutting by managed care companies has so far relied on limiting sessions. To compete, these companies may ultimately have to focus on quality and efficacy (Sanderson 1997; Sanderson and Woody 1995). Psychiatrists are paid primarily to make a diagnosis and prescribe medication, whereas other professionals, at a lower cost, provide psychotherapy, usually for a very limited time (Guze 1998). As a result, psychotherapy is carved out of the psychiatrists' treatment responsibilities. There is debate within the field about what, if anything, should be carved out. Guze (1998) notes that managed care systems generally do not understand the importance of psychotherapy, which he defines as care universal to all medical treatment. He argues that it should not be carved out because this reveals the worst of the Cartesian distinction between mind and body. He argues that psychotherapy should be part of reimbursable physician care for patients with serious mental illnesses and that the bulk of other patients with problems of living (e.g., marital, work, parent–child) be carved out to other professionals. Although one would not argue with Guze's request that psychiatrists be reimbursed for time required for managing severely mentally ill patients, the definition of severe mental illness is unclear. Moreover, psychotherapy without medication is of limited value for the most severely ill patients. Also, many patients with problems of living have chronic or episodic debilitating depressions in which psychotherapy has been shown to be effective.

Michels (1998) argues, and I would agree, that there is no basis for drawing a line between the seriously mentally ill and many others who might benefit from psychotherapy and that the motivation of managed care companies is to limit all psychiatric treatment, not only the amount of time the psychiatrist spends with the seriously mentally ill but also the use of specific psychotherapies. I agree with Michels with one big caveat—his argument is better made with treatments based on evidence of efficacy, from controlled clinical trials. If evidence is not available, guidelines and consensus conferences could have a lesser role in determining standards and reimbursement (Karasu et al. 1993; Persons et al. 1996; Sanderson 1997). This is the standard of care throughout medicine and not just for psychiatric disorders (Ellrodt et al. 1997).

The American Psychological Association assembled a task force in 1993 to define and determine empirically supported treatments (ESTs). The task force set standards for evaluating the efficacy data and for levels of certainty (Chambless et al. 1998; Sanderson 1997). It concluded that training in ESTs needed to be increased and that there was a need to develop and disseminate treatment manuals, to increase training programs with supervised clinical work for continuing education in ESTs, to educate clinicians and third-party payers, and to inform the public about ESTs. The task force called for more manuals of psychodynamic psychotherapy because of its widespread use and for more long-term outcome studies (see Section IV introduction by Sanderson).

Recommendation

To preserve the practice of psychotherapy in the new health care scene, professionals who conduct and test psychotherapy should demonstrate accountability by developing evidence-based practice guidelines, training programs, and methods of dissemination. These guidelines must be more than a review of the field and instead must grapple with criteria for the standard for evidence, much along the lines of the FDA (see Roth and Fonagy 1996). A way must be found to deal with the lag time between evidence from efficacy studies and treatments that are widely used and considered useful by consensus panels but not yet tested. The FDA has allowed a grace period for treatments that were generally regarded as safe and effective but that had not been tested (e.g., digitalis, morphine). This grace period would give the professions time to plan and carry out needed studies.

Are New Models of Psychotherapy Needed?

Psychotherapy typically includes individual face-to-face sessions, sometimes in groups, between therapists and patients. The time and frequency is determined increasingly by the reimbursement patterns of insurance companies. For patients who can afford to pay or who have generous medical insurance, treatment can be open ended and frequent. More economically feasible formats must be developed that consider the patient population, the course of illness, and risk factors. We need to experiment with different formats that meet both patient and economic requirements.

The high rate of major depressive disorder among women of childbearing age, the increased risk in the postpartum period, and the strong relationship between maternal and child depression suggest new opportunities and formats for intervention. I mention here just a few possibilities.

Many depressed women presenting for treatment have small children. Arranging for babysitting, often after a day of work, may not be feasible. To make treatments more accessible we have been offering IPT over the telephone. This approach requires initial assessment of the patient's clinical state and risk of suicide. Many of the women would not have been able to come to psychotherapy, even in the face of a serious depression, because of logistics, inertia, and hopelessness. Because patient satisfaction seems high, Miller and I are currently conducting a clinical trial to test the efficacy of IPT over the telephone. Treatment over the telephone is also being tested with depressed patients seen in family practice (Lynch et al. 1997) and in cancer patients undergoing debilitating chemotherapy (J. Holland, personal communication, 1998). As one patient said to us, "When you are depressed there is an overwhelming need for a realistic approach to time management."

The strong relationship between maternal and childhood depression has been documented in a number of high-risk studies that sampled either the depressed child or the depressed mother. These studies have all focused on the mother's lifetime and not on current depression. Women bringing in their children for treatment of depression might be currently depressed and may be amenable to treatment at that juncture. We surveyed more than 100 mothers who were bringing in their children for treatment of depression at Columbia Presbyterian Medical Center. More than 14% of the mothers were currently experiencing an episode of depression (Ferro et al. 2000). Less than a quarter of these women were in treatment. We are now testing the efficacy of treating the depression in these women to see if treatment has an impact on both the mother and the depressed child.

Posttreatment follow-up and booster sessions need to be available and reimbursable for depressed patients who have had a successful course of treatment but may be undergoing a life stress. The striking results of the Frank et al. (1991) study of monthly IPT as maintenance treatment for severe recurrent depression suggest that infrequent psychotherapy given by nonphysicians can delay relapse or recurrence. Flexibility in the availability of treatment is needed. The notion that regular attendance in prescribed psychotherapy sessions is the norm or even desirable is based on the psychoanalytic psychotherapy of nonpsychotic chronic psychopathology. This practice should not be generalized to all outpatient psychotherapies. After the successful treatment of the acute episode, the schedule for additional treatment is better placed in the patient's hands than in a predetermined protocol. Patient and family education about the signs of relapse and available, accessible treatment are needed to deal with the cost problem in a episodic condition like depression. Perhaps patients could purchase a package of psychotherapy sessions that they could use as needed, after resolution of an acute episode.

For the future, we need:

- Risk-factor research to be translated in order to gain clues about the nature, timing, and sequence of interventions with high-risk individuals in high-risk situations
- More outcome studies related to the presumed mechanisms of action. If CBT is supposed to change cognitions, then cognitive changes should be used as an outcome measure, and they should be proximal to other measures of functioning.
- More efficacy studies of the newer antidepressants in comparison and combination with newer psychotherapies, across the life span and including exploration of dosing and duration of treatment. Comparison studies of drugs and psychotherapy have so far examined the older antidepressants, which had more side effects and were often less well tolerated.
- More effectiveness studies at sites where early intervention might be feasible and appropriate.
- Manuals of psychotherapy for adults adapted to children and adolescents and efficacy and effectiveness studies with these younger and higher-risk populations. Not one controlled clinical trial of individual psychotherapy with prepubertally depressed children has been published.
- To consider that being a patient and talking solo to an adult is not a comfortable role for most people and especially so for adolescents. Group and telephone treatment might be a feasible and more economical treatment for depression in adolescents (Fine 1991).
- Studies that identify the factors that increase treatment adherence as well as studies that determine whether treatment adherence affects outcome.
- To face the fact that the different psychotherapies may not be different in onset, target of action, or side effects. Despite pharmaceutical company claims, this situation is similar to that of pharmacotherapy. Some patients tolerate and respond better to some drugs than to others. The same is most likely true for psychotherapy.

Whether this differential response is related to dose, presumed mechanism of action, context, or side effect is often unclear for drugs and for psychotherapy.

Conclusion

Has anyone not experienced the comfort and therapeutic power of unburdening to a compassionate family member or friend in a safe, nonjudgmental relationship? If psychotherapy is to survive in the marketplace, it must be more than that. In fact, the unclear boundary between human compassion and specific psychotherapy is partly responsible for the current paradoxes. The procedures and boundaries; the necessary training and credentials; the indications and contraindications; the duration, intensity, and possible side effects; and the evidence of efficacy for psychotherapies all need to be specified. Because no industry is supporting this work, as is the case for psychopharmacology, the professional disciplines involved need to give up their guild differences and work together to build an infrastructure of information and planned strategy. Perhaps support from industry will tag along.

The psychiatric professions ought to reconcile their training programs with the reality of health care today. Evidence-based treatment should be taught. If psychiatry is to attract talented residents interested in understanding the biology of mental processes, long-term psychotherapy training may need to be an option, not a mandate. How to accomplish this without giving up the unique psychiatric training in how to talk, listen, and hear patients is a challenge.

The nonmedical disciplines that provide psychotherapy practitioners also need to reconcile their training with the reality of health care today. Their practitioners should develop, test, and learn evidence-based psychotherapy. Because nonmedical practitioners are increasingly the first line of treatment for depression, they need to have more than a passing knowledge of clinical diagnosis, pharmacotherapy, and the high medical comorbidity of most psychiatric disorders. Preoccupation with professional boundaries can lead practitioners to fail to make available effective treatments for depression that can reduce suffering and even save lives.

We need an alliance between psychotherapy researchers and prac-

titioners to replace the current indifference—and more often hostility—on the part of practitioners toward research activities and vice versa.
Some psychotherapy practitioners regard the activities of outcome studies as irrelevant because they feel that psychotherapy is known to be effective and this self-evident truth need not be subjected to experimental
verification. Lurking just below the surface is the fear that research will
prove that psychotherapy is ineffective or less efficacious than drug therapy. The current research direction to move efficacy into effectiveness
studies may help the alliance.

It is held that psychotherapy research violates clinical practice: The
techniques such as standardized interviews, randomization, and fixed
duration are so removed from clinical practice so as to make any generalization from research findings spurious and invalid. It also has been
argued that it is a mistake to apply to psychotherapy a standard derived
from medicine and that psychotherapy is not comparable with medical
modalities such as drugs and surgery; furthermore, the attempt to consider psychotherapy as a treatment modality for specific disorders is partially at the root of the problem in psychotherapy research.

One might imagine that if mental health professionals have no concern about issues of efficacy, then patients, as consumers, might. For the
most part, individual patients and their families trust their therapists and
seldom ask for evidence of efficacy. This situation is changing, partly because of the increased use of psychopharmacologic agents. Patients are
asking for justification of their therapists' prescriptions of psychotherapy, pharmacotherapy, and combinations of the two. An additional challenge is how to require evidence of efficacy without eliminating the
many psychotherapies that are widely used and generally regarded as
safe and effective.

Finally, continuation of psychotherapy as a treatment for depression, available to more than the few who can pay for it out of pocket,
depends largely on evidence for both efficacy and cost offset. The technology for efficacy studies has been well established. The design of cost-
offset studies that take into account both the long-term clinical course
and the imposition on the family structure as potential costs has not
been well established.

My late husband, Gerald L. Klerman, M.D., would have loved participating in these debates and would have had his own ideas on the top-

ic. One idea I know we would share is the patient's right to effective treatment, as he described in his 1990 *American Journal of Psychiatry* article:

> In current psychiatric practice, where there are large areas of ignorance, it behooves individual practitioners and institutions to avoid relying on single treatment approaches or theoretical paradigms.... Treatment programs based only on psychotherapy or only on drugs are subject to criticism. Professionalism required balancing available knowledge, clinical experience and promoting the advancement of scientific knowledge. In the case of psychotherapy such knowledge comes best from controlled trials. (Klerman 1990, p. 417)

References

Barlow DH, Cerny JA: Psychological Treatment of Panic. New York, Guilford, 1988

Barlow DH, Craske MG: Mastery of Your Anxiety and Panic—II. San Antonio, TX, The Psychological Corporation, 1994

Beck AT, Rush A, Shaw B, et al: Cognitive Therapy of Depression. New York, Guilford, 1979

Brent DA, Holder D, Kolko D, et al: A clinical psychotherapy trial for adolescent depression comparing cognitive, family and supportive therapy. Arch Gen Psychiatry. 54:877–885, 1997

Brook RH, Lohr KN. Efficacy, effectiveness, variations, and quality; boundary-crossing research. Med Care 23:710–22, 1985

Chambless DL, Baker MJ, Baucom DH, et al: Update on empirically validated therapies, II. The Clinical Psychologist 5:3–16, 1998

Chevron ES, Rounsaville BJ: Evaluating the clinical skills of psychotherapists; a comparison of techniques. Arch Gen Psychiatry 40:1129–1132, 1983

Depression Guideline Panel: Clinical Practice Guideline, Number 5. Depression in Primary Care, Volume 2: Treatment of Major Depression. Rockville, MD, U.S. Department of Health and Human Services, Public Health Service, Agency for Health Care Policy and Research. AHCPR Publication No. 93-0551, 1993

Druss BG, Allen HM, Bruce ML: Physical health, depressive symptoms and managed care enrollment. Am J Psychiatry 155:878–882, 1998

Eisenberg DM, Davis RB, Ettner SL, et al: Trends in alternative medicine use in the United States, 1990–1997. JAMA 280:1569–1575, 1998

Eist HI: Treatment for major depression in managed care and fee-for-service systems. Am J Psychiatry 155:859–860, 1998

Elkin I, Parloff MB, Hadley SW, et al: National Institute of Mental Health Treatment of Depression Collaborative Research Program: background and research plan. Arch Gen Psychiatry 42:30–36, 1985

Elkin I, Shea T, Watkins JT, et al: National Institute of Mental Health Treatment of Depression Collaborative Research Program: general effectiveness of treatments. Arch Gen Psychiatry 46:971–982, 1989

Ellrodt G, Cook DJ, Lee J, et al: Evidence-based disease management. JAMA 278:1687–1692, 1997

Ernst E, Rand JI, Stevinson C: Complementary therapies for depression. Arch Gen Psychiatry 55:1026–1032, 1998

Fairburn CG, Jones R, Peveler RC, et al: Psychotherapy and bulimia nervosa: Longer-term effects of interpersonal psychotherapy, behavior therapy, and cognitive behavior therapy. Arch Gen Psychiatry 50:419–428, 1993

Ferro T, Verdeli L, Pierre F, et al: Screening for depression in mothers bringing offspring for evaluation or treatment of depression. Am J Psychiatry 157:375–379, 2000

Fine S: Group therapy for adolescent depressive disorder: a comparison of social skills and therapeutic support. J Am Acad Child Adolesc Psychiatry 30:79–85, 1991

Frank E, Kupfer DJ, Wagner EF, et al: Efficacy of interpersonal psychotherapy as maintenance treatment of recurrent depression: contributing factors. Arch Gen Psychiatry. 48:1053–1059, 1991

Gabbard GO, Lazar SG, Hornberger J, et al: The economic impact of psychotherapy: a review. Am J Psychiatry 154:147–155, 1997

Goodwin F, Jamison K: Manic Depressive Illness. New York, Oxford University Press, 1990

Guze SB: Psychotherapy and managed care. Arch Gen Psychiatry 55:561–562, 1998

Hibbs ED, Jensen PS (eds): Psychosocial Treatments for Child and Adolescent Disorders: Empirically Based Strategies for Clinical Practice. Washington DC, American Psychological Association Press, 1996

Jorgensen B, Bolwig DH: The efficacy of psychotherapy in non-bipolar depression: a review. Acta Psychiatr Scand 98:1–13, 1998

Kandel ER: A new intellectual framework for psychiatry. Am J Psychiatry 155:457–469, 1998

Karasu TB, Docherty JP, Gelenberg A, et al: Practice guideline for major depressive disorder in adults. Work group on major depressive disorder. Am J Psychiatry 81–134, 1993

Klerman GL: The psychiatric patient's right to effective treatment: implications. Osheroff V, Chestnut L. Am J Psychiatry 147:409–418, 1990

Klerman GL, Weissman MM (eds): New Applications of Interpersonal Psychotherapy. Washington DC, American Psychiatric Press, 1993

Klerman GL, Weissman MM, Rounsaville BJ, et al: Interpersonal Psychotherapy of Depression. New York, Basic Books, 1984

Klerman GL, Budman S, Berwick D, et al: Efficacy of a brief psychosocial intervention for symptoms of stress and distress among patients in primary care. Med Care 25:1078–1088, 1987

Kramer RA, Warner V, Olfson M, et al: General medical problems among the offspring of depressed parents: a ten year follow-up. J Am Acad Child Adolesc Psychiatry 37:602–611, 1998

Lewinsohn PM, Clarke GN, Hops H: Cognitive-behavioral group treatment of depression in adolescents. Behavior Therapy 21:385–401, 1990

London P, Klerman GL: Evaluating psychotherapy. Am J Psychiatry 139:709–717, 1982

Luborsky L, DeRubeis RJ: The use of psychotherapy treatment manuals: a small revolution in psychotherapy research styles. Clin Psychol Rev 4:5–14, 1984

Lynch D, Tamburrino M, Nagel R: Telephone counseling for patients with minor depression: preliminary findings in a family practice setting. J Fam Pract 44:293–298, 1997

Markowitz JC: Interpersonal Psychotherapy for Dysthymic Disorder. Washington, DC, American Psychiatric Press, 1998

McAvay G, Nunes EV, Zaider TI, et al: Physical health problems in depressed children and nondepressed children and adolescents of parents with opiate dependence. Depression and Anxiety 9:61–69, 1999

Michels R: The role of psychotherapy; psychiatry's resistance to managed care. Arch Gen Psychiatry 55:564, 1998

Miller AL, Rathus JG, Lineham MM, et al: Dialectical behavior therapy adapted for suicidal adolescents. Journal of Practical Psychology and Behavioral Health 3:78–86, 1997

Mufson L, Moreau D, Weissman MM, et al: Interpersonal Psychotherapy for Depressed Adolescents. New York, Guilford, 1993

Mufson L, Weissman MM, Moreau D: The efficacy of interpersonal psychotherapy for depressed adolescents. Arch Gen Psychiatry 56:573–579, 1999

Olfson M, Marcus SC, Pincus HA: Trends in office-based psychiatric practice. Am J Psychiatry 157:451–457, 1999

Persons JB, Thase ME, Crits-Christoph P: The role of psychotherapy in the treatment of depression; review of two practice guidelines. Arch Gen Psychiatry 53:283–290, 1996

Residency Education in Psychiatry. Essential in Residency Training, 1998. Available online at http://www.skisoft.com

Reynolds CF III, Frank E, Perel JM, et al: Nortriptyline and interpersonal psychotherapy as maintenance therapies for recurrent major depression: a randomized controlled trial in patients older than 59 years. JAMA 281:39–45, 1999

Roth A, Fonagy P (eds): What Works for Whom: A Critical Review of Psychotherapy Research. New York, Guilford, 1996

Rounsaville BJ, Chevron ES, Weissman MM, et al: Training therapists to perform interpersonal psychotherapy in clinical trials. Compr Psychiatry 27:364–71, 1986

Sanderson WC: The importance of empirically supported psychological interventions in the new healthcare environment, in Innovation in Clinical Practice: A Source Book, Vol 15. Edited by Vandercreek L, Knapp S, Jackson T. Sarasota, FL, Professional Resource Press, 1997, pp 387–399

Sanderson WC, Woody S: Manuals for Empirically Validated Treatments: A project of the Task Force on Psychological Interventions, Vol 48. Washington, DC, Division of Clinical Psychology, American Psychological Association. The Clinical Psychologist 2:7–11, 1995

Seligman ME: The effectiveness of psychotherapy. The Consumer Reports study. Am Psychol 50:965–974, 1995

Sturm R, Wells KB: How can care for depression become more cost-effective? JAMA 273:51–58, 1995

Thase ME, Greenhouse JB, Frank E, et al: Treatment of major depression with psychotherapy or psychotherapy-pharmacotherapy combinations. Arch Gen Psychiatry. 54:1009–1015, 1997

Turner SM, Beidel DC, Cooley M: Social Effectiveness Therapy: A Program for Overcoming Social Anxiety and Phobia. Toronto, Multi-Health Systems, 1997

Weissman MM, Rounsaville BJ, Chevron E: Training psychotherapists to participate in psychotherapy outcome studies. Am J Psychiatry. 139:1442–1446, 1982

Weissman MM, Markowitz J, Klerman GL: Comprehensive Guide to Interpersonal Psychotherapy. New York, Basic Books, 1999

Wilkes TCR, Belshes G, Rush AV, et al. (eds): Cognitive Therapy for Depressed Adolescents. New York, Guilford, 1994

Woody SR, Kihlstrom LC: Outcomes, quality and cost: integrating psychotherapy and mental health services research. Psychotherapy Research 7:365–381, 1997

Epilogue

Bridge to the 22nd Century

Myrna M. Weissman, Ph.D.

The 189th American Psychopathological Association president, when preparing for the annual meeting in 2099 and bridging the 22nd century, may find this volume charmingly naive and, it is hoped, antiquated. In 2099, the relationship between neurology and psychiatry, courted in 1910 by Adolf Meyer, who held the American Psychopathological Association meeting in conjunction with the meeting of the American Neurological Association, will be scientifically seamless. Understanding of neural circuitry, pathophysiology, genetics, and the plasticity of human behavior in a social context will be more deeply understood. Systematic data on the epidemiology of depression in developing countries and among children of all nations will be available. Monitoring of new epidemics will allow for rapid interventions at primary or secondary levels. By 2099, we will have evolved a health care system that provides appropriate care to everyone, with parity for psychiatric disorders. Understanding of risk factors and early interventions with more targeted drugs will go a long way toward reducing the chronicity, morbidity, and cost of depression.

It was clear even at the end of the 20th century that progress had been made in basic understanding of psychiatric disorders. In 1999 the National Institute of Mental Health sponsored collection of families with early-onset recurrent depression and with bipolar disorder. This information has been used to capitalize on the Human Genome Project and rapidly developing genomic tools coming available in the beginning of the 21st century. Treatment for depression is more targeted, faster, and with fewer side effects and is aimed at the underlying pathophysiology of depression. DSM-III and DSM-IV were a revolution in specifying the symptoms required to make a diagnosis. In the future, DSM-VI may specify the pathophysiology and genetic abnormalities. Thus a crosswalk of DSM-IV with DSM-VI will have many new directions, some forgotten terrain, bridges beyond repair, and roads beyond psychiatry.

On the eve of the 22nd century, there will be numerous new treatments for depression in children and adolescents, and the concentrated effort at the end of the 20th century to develop efficacy data on treatment will have gone a long way in preventing the morbidity in adult life. We will finally understand the role of puberty in the leaping rates of major depression in girls so that prevention is targeted to that age group. We will also have developed better ways for well-trained professionals to provide easy access and early treatment to young people in schools. Congress will continue to see the economic and social benefits of parity in funding of mental health research. Better organizational structures will be formed that allow the efficient yet flexible and creative testing of new treatments. Better ways of determining the effectiveness of treatments in the real world of patient care outside the rarefied laboratories of universities will have been found. Postmarketing surveillance will rapidly detect undue side effects or failures.

Practice guidelines and algorithms that are computerized on the Web and continuously updated will be accepted practice. The economics of treatment delivery will have a clinical face. Although clinical trials may show that all selective serotonin reuptake inhibitors have similar efficacy, individual patients may respond to one and not another. This clinical variability will be widely recognized in formularies and reimbursement in the twenty-second century.

The biologic reductionists will accept new data on the plasticity of human behavior in a social concept and recognize that the environment, whether it is food, abuse, accidents, or family love, can have an early and profound effect on biology. At the same time, psychotherapy advocates will have come to terms with the notion that psychotherapy is not the universal solution for all conditions for indefinite periods. There will be a rapprochement both in science and therapeutics. The 50-minute hour will not be the norm, and great flexibility in the duration, timing, and delivery of psychotherapy will be available. Clinicians will be trained in various psychotherapies, the efficacy of which, like drugs, will have been tested in controlled clinical trials.

The globalization of the pharmaceutical industry, access to the Internet, and the progress in scientific understanding in the 22nd century will ensure that fewer people become depressed and that those who do readily receive effective treatment.

Index

*Page numbers printed in **boldface** type refer to tables or figures.*

Iproniazid, 9, 13–14
Ipsapirone, 68
IPT. *See* Interpersonal
psychotherapy
IRC (Intervention Research
Centers), 209–210
Isoniazid, 10–11

Kielholz, Paul, 9, 15
Klerman, Gerald L., 283,
324–325
Kline, Nathan, 11, 13–14
Knockout genes, 75–76, **77**
Kramer, Peter, 16, 19–20, 26
Kuhn, Roland, 4, 7–9, 11, 14, 19,
20, 25, 26

Largactil. *See* Chlorpromazine
Lasker Prize, 13, 14
Learning the new psychotherapies,
281–298
cognitive-behavioral therapy,
282–283, **285**
data on, 295–297
difficulties in, 292–295
mixed vs. pure techniques,
294–295
termination, 295
therapeutic potency, 293
therapist activity, 292–293
use of medication,
293–294
use of time limit, 294
formulation, 290–291
goals of supervision, 289
history taking, 289–290
interpersonal psychotherapy,
282–284, **285**
maintaining focus, 291–292
manuals, 285, 297, 311–313
patient selection, 288, 309

recording of sessions, 286–288
videotaping or audiotaping,
287–288, 314–316
scheduling of supervision, 288
serial assessment, 288
training, 245–246, 297–298,
313–314
adapting for effectiveness
studies, 314–316
demand for, 281
licensure and requirements
for, 316–318
LEDS (Life Events and Difficulties
Schedule), 115
Licensure, 316
Life Events and Difficulties
Schedule (LEDS), 115
Linkage disequilibrium mapping, 94
Linkage gene maps, 91–92
Listening to Prozac, 16, 19, 25
Lithium, 121, 213
Loomer, Harry, 13, 14
LSD, 20
Lundbeck, 14
Lurie, Max, 10–11, 14

Maintenance treatment
after electroconvulsive therapy,
155–156
depression recurrence and,
130–131
EEG sleep and, 107–111,
110–112
long-term follow-up of
depressed children and
control subjects, 112–113,
114
interpersonal psychotherapy for,
108–109, 130, 142–143, 321
psychobiology and, 105–116
Maintenance Treatment in Late-
Life Depression, 108